Ophthalmic Adverse Events following SARS-CoV-2 Vaccination

Ophthalmic Adverse Events following SARS-CoV-2 Vaccination

Editor

Rohan Bir Singh

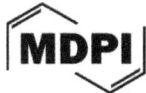

Basel • Beijing • Wuhan • Barcelona • Belgrade • Novi Sad • Cluj • Manchester

Editor
Rohan Bir Singh
Department of
Ophthalmology,
Massachusetts Eye and Ear
Harvard Medical School
Boston
United States

Editorial Office
MDPI
St. Alban-Anlage 66
4052 Basel, Switzerland

This is a reprint of articles from the Special Issue published online in the open access journal *Vaccines* (ISSN 2076-393X) (available at: www.mdpi.com/journal/vaccines/special_issues/QG1CJD5EZP).

For citation purposes, cite each article independently as indicated on the article page online and as indicated below:

Lastname, A.A.; Lastname, B.B. Article Title. *Journal Name* **Year**, *Volume Number*, Page Range.

ISBN 978-3-7258-0154-1 (Hbk)
ISBN 978-3-7258-0153-4 (PDF)
doi.org/10.3390/books978-3-7258-0153-4

© 2024 by the authors. Articles in this book are Open Access and distributed under the Creative Commons Attribution (CC BY) license. The book as a whole is distributed by MDPI under the terms and conditions of the Creative Commons Attribution-NonCommercial-NoDerivs (CC BY-NC-ND) license.

Contents

About the Editor . . . . **vii**

Preface . . . . **ix**

Ho-Man Leung and Sunny Chi-Lik Au
Retinal Vein Occlusion after COVID-19 Vaccination—A Review
Reprinted from: *Vaccines* **2023**, *11*, 1281, doi:10.3390/vaccines11081281 . . . . **1**

Parthopratim Dutta Majumder and Aniruddha Agarwal
Acute Macular Neuroretinopathy and Paracentral Acute Middle Maculopathy during SARS-CoV-2 Infection and Vaccination
Reprinted from: *Vaccines* **2023**, *11*, 474, doi:10.3390/vaccines11020474 . . . . **15**

Lana Kuziez, Taher K. Eleiwa, Muhammad Z. Chauhan, Ahmed B. Sallam, Abdelrahman M. Elhusseiny and Hajirah N. Saeed
Corneal Adverse Events Associated with SARS-CoV-2/COVID-19 Vaccination: A Systematic Review
Reprinted from: *Vaccines* **2023**, *11*, 166, doi:10.3390/vaccines11010166 . . . . **24**

Yasmine Yousra Sadok Cherif, Chakib Djeffal, Hashem Abu Serhan, Ahmed Elnahhas, Hebatallah Yousef, Basant E. Katamesh, et al.
The Characteristics of COVID-19 Vaccine-Associated Uveitis: A Summative Systematic Review
Reprinted from: *Vaccines* **2023**, *11*, 69, doi:10.3390/vaccines11010069 . . . . **45**

Hashem Abu Serhan, Abdelaziz Abdelaal, Mohammad T. Abuawwad, Mohammad J. J. Taha, Sara Irshaidat, Leen Abu Serhan, et al.
Ocular Vascular Events following COVID-19 Vaccines: A Systematic Review
Reprinted from: *Vaccines* **2022**, *10*, 2143, doi:10.3390/vaccines10122143 . . . . **68**

Parul Ichhpujani, Uday Pratap Singh Parmar, Siddharth Duggal and Suresh Kumar
COVID-19 Vaccine-Associated Ocular Adverse Effects: An Overview
Reprinted from: *Vaccines* **2022**, *10*, 1879, doi:10.3390/vaccines10111879 . . . . **82**

Matias Soifer, Nam V. Nguyen, Ryan Leite, Josh Fernandes and Shilpa Kodati
Recurrent Multiple Evanescent White Dot Syndrome (MEWDS) Following First Dose and Booster of the mRNA-1273 COVID-19 Vaccine: Case Report and Review of Literature
Reprinted from: *Vaccines* **2022**, *10*, 1776, doi:10.3390/vaccines10111776 . . . . **103**

Ayman G. Elnahry, Mutaz Y. Al-Nawaflh, Aisha A. Gamal Eldin, Omar Solyman, Ahmed B. Sallam, Paul H. Phillips and Abdelrahman M. Elhusseiny
COVID-19 Vaccine-Associated Optic Neuropathy: A Systematic Review of 45 Patients
Reprinted from: *Vaccines* **2022**, *10*, 1758, doi:10.3390/vaccines10101758 . . . . **111**

Mélanie Hébert, Soumaya Bouhout, Julie Vadboncoeur and Marie-Josée Aubin
Recurrent and De Novo Toxoplasmosis Retinochoroiditis following Coronavirus Disease 2019 Infection or Vaccination
Reprinted from: *Vaccines* **2022**, *10*, 1692, doi:10.3390/vaccines10101692 . . . . **128**

Rohan Bir Singh, Uday Pratap Singh Parmar, Wonkyung Cho and Parul Ichhpujani
Glaucoma Cases Following SARS-CoV-2 Vaccination: A VAERS Database Analysis
Reprinted from: *Vaccines* **2022**, *10*, 1630, doi:10.3390/vaccines10101630 . . . . **136**

Shuntaro Motegi, Takayuki Kanda and Masaru Takeuchi
A Case of Atypical Unilateral Optic Neuritis Following BNT162b2 mRNA COVID-19 Vaccination
Reprinted from: *Vaccines* **2022**, *10*, 1574, doi:10.3390/vaccines10101574 . . . . **148**

About the Editor

Rohan Bir Singh

Dr. Rohan Bir Singh is a fellow at the Laboratory of Corneal Immunology, Transplantation, and Regeneration at the Schepens Eye Research Institute of Massachusetts Eye and Ear, Harvard Medical School, Boston, USA.

His research interests include the immunopathogenesis of dry eye disease, the immunology of corneal graft rejection, and the epidemiology of corneal disorders in the United States. He is a PhD candidate at the Leiden University Medical Center (the Netherlands) with a concentration in ocular immunology. He is also a visiting senior lecturer of ophthalmology and vision sciences at the Adelaide Medical School, University of Adelaide (Australia) and an honorary research associate at the Department of Ophthalmology, Great Ormond Street Institute of Child Health, University College London (United Kingdom).

Dr. Singh has published more than 80 peer-reviewed papers and chapters in leading ophthalmology and immunology journals. He has edited three ophthalmology textbooks and is a member of the editorial boards of several reputed ophthalmology journals.

Preface

In the relentless pursuit of global health and well-being, the scientific community has faced unprecedented challenges, and the advent of the SARS-CoV-2 pandemic has been a defining moment in our collective history. As the world mobilized to develop and deploy vaccines to combat the virus, a remarkable collaboration between researchers, healthcare professionals, and the public unfolded. Vaccination campaigns became a beacon of hope, promising a return to normalcy and a future free from the shackles of the pandemic.

Within this landscape of triumph and hope, it is crucial to delve into the intricacies of the vaccination process and explore the potential consequences. "Ophthalmic Adverse Events Following SARS-CoV-2 Vaccination" emerges as a significant addition to the discourse surrounding the safety and efficacy of the vaccines that have become a cornerstone in our battle against the virus.

The eyes play a pivotal role in our perception of the world. Understanding the ocular effects of the SARS-CoV-2 vaccination is a matter of both scientific curiosity and public health importance. This Special Issue embarks on a journey into the realm of ophthalmic adverse events, providing a comprehensive exploration of the relationship between SARS-CoV-2 vaccination and ocular manifestations.

The genesis of this project lies in the recognition that, while vaccines are essential tools in preventing the spread of infectious diseases, they can occasionally be associated with adverse effects. By focusing specifically on ophthalmic adverse events, we aim to contribute nuanced insights that can inform healthcare professionals, researchers, and the public alike.

The contributors to this volume include ophthalmologists from an array of subspecialties. Their collective expertise lends depth and breadth to the exploration of ophthalmic adverse events, ensuring a multidimensional analysis of the subject matter. Through their contributions, this Reprint aims to bridge the gap between scientific knowledge and public awareness, fostering a dialogue that is both informed and accessible.

In the spirit of scientific inquiry, I acknowledge that our understanding of vaccine-related ocular effects is a dynamic and evolving field. As new data emerge and research advances, it becomes imperative to revisit and refine our perspectives. This Reprint, therefore, represents a snapshot in time—an exploration grounded in the current state of knowledge, with an understanding that future discoveries may further shape our understanding.

In conclusion, this Special Issue is a testament to the resilience of the human spirit and the power of scientific inquiry. As we navigate the complexities of vaccine-related ocular effects, let us embark on this journey with an open mind, a commitment to truth, and an unwavering dedication to the health and well-being of humanity.

Rohan Bir Singh
Editor

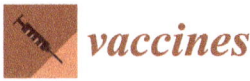

Brief Report

Retinal Vein Occlusion after COVID-19 Vaccination—A Review

Ho-Man Leung [1,*] and Sunny Chi-Lik Au [2]

1. Hospital Authority, Ma Tau Wai 999077, Hong Kong
2. Department of Ophthalmology, Tung Wah Eastern Hospital, So Kon Po 999077, Hong Kong
* Correspondence: hmleung2023@gmail.com

Abstract: *Background* Retinal vein occlusion (RVO) occurring after COVID-19 vaccination has been reported worldwide. Such a sight-threatening condition occurring after COVID-19 vaccination is a menace to ophthalmic health. This article reviews current evidence related to post-COVID-19 vaccination RVO. *Method* A total of 29 relevant articles identified on PubMed in January 2023 were selected for review. *Observation* All cases presented to ophthalmologists with visual loss shortly after COVID-19 vaccination. Mean and median age were both 58. No sex predominance was observed. RVO was diagnosed from findings on dilated fundal examination and ophthalmic imaging. AstraZeneca and BNT vaccines accounted for most cases. Vascular risk factors, e.g., diabetes mellitus and hypertension, were common. Most laboratory tests requested came back unremarkable. Most patients responded well to standard treatment, except those with ophthalmic comorbidities. Visual prognosis was excellent on short-term follow-up. *Discussion* The causality between RVO and COVID-19 vaccination is undeterminable because of the nature of articles, heterogenous reporting styles, contradicting laboratory findings and co-existing vascular risk factors. Vaccine-induced immune thrombotic thrombocytopenia, retinal vasculitis and homocysteinaemia were proposed to explain post-vaccination RVO. Large-scale studies have demonstrated that the incidence of RVO following COVID vaccination is very low. Nevertheless, the effects of boosters on retinal vasculature and ophthalmic health are still unclear. *Conclusions* The benefits of COVID-19 vaccination are believed to outweigh its ophthalmic risks. To ensure safe vaccination, the prior optimisation of comorbidities and post-vaccination monitoring are important. COVID-19 vaccines (including boosters) should be offered with reasonable confidence. Further studies are warranted to elucidate the ophthalmic impact of vaccines.

Keywords: COVID-19; COVID-19 vaccines; retinal artery occlusion; retinal vein occlusion; review

1. Introduction

COVID-19 vaccines have been widely delivered to fight against the COVID-19 pandemic. The health risks of these newly developed vaccines are hot research topics, especially regarding vascular endothelial complications. Several author groups have reported thromboembolic risks of COVID-19 vaccines [1–3], and thus ocular complications such as retinal vein occlusion (RVO) might be possible. With a high global coverage of vaccination [4], it is high time to review the literature regarding COVID-19-vaccine-related RVO.

2. Method

The literature was searched on PubMed on 15 January 2023 using (((vaccine) OR (vaccination) OR (after vaccination) OR (post vaccination)) AND ((COVID-19) OR (COVID) OR (SARS-CoV-2))) AND ((retinal vein occlusion) OR (retinal venous occlusion)). Titles and abstracts were screened.

A total of 37 articles were identified. After screening and review of reference lists of included articles, 29 relevant articles were included.

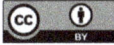

3. Clinical Characteristics of RVO following COVID-19 Vaccination

The age of patients ranged from 13 to 85. The median and mean of patients' ages were both 58. The male to female ratio was around 1:1. These patients presented with visual diminution to ophthalmologists due to visual loss 15 min to 30 days after their last dose of vaccine. About 55% and 39% of cases occurred after the first dose and second dose, respectively. AstraZeneca and BNT vaccine-related RVO comprised most of the cases, while other types of COVID-19 vaccine, for example, Pfizer, Moderna and Covishield, were also reported.

Most patients had their intraocular pressure (IOP) documented. The IOP results, if reported, all fell within the normal range. The anterior segment and fundus were both checked as part of routine ophthalmic examination. No gross abnormalities, except cataracts, were reported on anterior segment examination. Typical fundal abnormalities of RVO on examination led to the diagnosis of RVO in most cases. Optical coherence tomography (OCT) and FA were performed for most of these patients to confirm the diagnosis. Optical coherence tomography angiography was performed in only a minority of cases.

Most centres performed an extensive laboratory work-up for their patients. Examples of abnormalities incidentally detected on work-up were as follows: Mildly reduced platelet count (129×10^9/L) found in one patient with concurrent central retinal artery occlusion (CRAO) and central RVO (CRVO) [5]. One patient had mildly elevated glycated haemoglobin (6.7%) [6]. Raised d-dimer (547 ng/mL) was found in one case [7]. One patient had mildly raised inflammatory markers (erythrocyte sedimentation rate (ESR): 49, C-reactive protein (CRP): 14.6—unit not provided), rheumatoid factors (11, unit not provided) and d-dimer (6077.4 ng/mL) [8]. A mildly elevated homocysteine level was reported in two cases (16.4 and 22.19 micromol/L) [9,10]. Elevated lipid levels (total cholesterol: 227; LDL: 159, unit not provided) and mildly raised ESR (26, unit not provided) were detected from a case of combined CRAO and RVO [11]. Results of laboratory investigations for most other cases were unremarkable. Upon reviewing the past medical history of these cases, it was noted that a number of cases had background vascular risk factors, such as diabetes, hypertension, dyslipidaemia and atrial fibrillation.

The majority of the cases were treated with an intravitreal injection of anti-VEGF (vascular endothelial growth factor), an established treatment of RVO. Two other commonly used alternatives included intravitreal/intravenous corticosteroid and oral aspirin. Most patients reported an improvement in vision and fundal abnormalities resolved at follow-up visits. There were only few non-responders, and this was likely to be related to advanced age, concurrent retinal artery occlusion, which carries poor visual prognosis, and other comorbidities. As all these post-vaccination RVO cases occurred within these last 2 years, no results from long-term follow-up were provided from the case reports.

Summarised clinical information of individual cases can be found in Tables S1 and S2, attached in the Supplementary File. Table 1 presents the essence of clinical information from individual cases.

Table 1. A summary of patients' demographics, comorbidities, presentation, and treatment responses.

Paper	Age/Sex	Vaccine (Dose)	BCVA of the Affected Eye	Interval between Last Dose and Symptom Onset	Comorbidities	Treatment Received	Response to Treatment	Remarks
Ruiz OA et al. [12]	51/F	Moderna (2nd)	8/10	12 days	Hypothyroidism	Not mentioned	VA: 3/10	Concurrent BRAO
Parakh S et al. [9]	31/M	AstraZeneca (1st)	6/9	7 days	Unremarkable	Intravitreal anti-VEGF + folic acid, B6, B12	BCVA 6/6	
Nangia P et al. [13]	13/M	Corbevax	6/7.5	15 days	Unremarkable	Intravenous (IV) pulse methylprednisolone	BCVA 6/6 at 8 months	
Fernández-Vigo JI et al. [14]	69/F	AstraZeneca (1st)	20/100	30 days	Unremarkable	Intravitreal dexamethasone implant	VA: 20/150	Macular atrophy present
Chen Y [7]	72/M	BNT (2nd)	Hand motion	10 days	Unremarkable	Intravitreal aflibercept + intravenous then oral methylprednisolone + pan-retinal photocoagulation	VA: 20/400	Concurrent RAO
Karageorgiou G et al. [15]	60/M	ChAdOx1 (unknown)	20/20	7 days	Obesity	Intravitreal anti-VEGF	Unknown	
Takacs A et al. [10]	35/M	mRNA vaccine (1st)	0.5	14 days	Mild aortic insufficiency, smoker, mild hypertension (139/87 mmHg), lower limb varicosed veins	Aspirin + single dose of intravitreal anti-VEGF	VA: 1.0	
Sodhi PK et al. [10]	43/M	AstraZeneca (1st)	20/630	3 days	Unremarkable	Intravitreal injection of triamcinolone acetonide	VA: 20/200	
Tanaka H et al. [16]	50/F	BNT (1st)	20/25	3 days	Hypertension	Intravitreal ranibizumab	VA: 20/20	
	56/F	BNT (1st)	13/20	3 days	Unremarkable	Intravitreal ranibizumab	VA: 20/20	
Romano D et al. [17]	54/F	AstraZeneca (2nd)	20/400	2 days	Hypertension	Dexamethasone intravitreal implant, laser pan-retinal photocoagulation	VA: 20/200	Ischaemic CRVO
Majumder PD et al. [18]	28/M	AstraZeneca (3rd)	2/60	25 days	Unremarkable	IV pulse and oral steroid	VA: 6/9	

Table 1. Cont.

Paper	Age/Sex	Vaccine (Dose)	BCVA of the Affected Eye	Interval between Last Dose and Symptom Onset	Comorbidities	Treatment Received	Response to Treatment	Remarks
Priluck AZ et al. [19]	57/F	Moderna (2nd)	20/20	3 weeks	Hypertension	Laser, intravitreal anti-VEGF	VA: 20/25	
Sugihara K et al. [20]	38/M	BNT (2nd)	0.9 with myopic correction	2 days	Unremarkable	Intravitreal anti-VEGF	VA: 1.2	
Pur DR et al. [21]	34/M	BNT (1st)	20/20	2 days	Unremarkable	Unknown	VA: 20/20 with residual inferior visual field defect	
Peters MC et al. [22]	71/M	AstraZeneca (1st)	6/60	2 days	Unremarkable	Intravitreal anti-VEGF	Unknown	
Peter MC et al. [22]	58/M	AstraZeneca (1st)	6/18	3 days	Unremarkable	Intravitreal anti-VEGF	Unknown	
	73/F	AstraZeneca (1st)	6/19	3 days	Unremarkable	Intravitreal anti-VEGF	Unknown	
	47/F	Pfizer (1st)	6/9.6	5 days	Hyperthyroidism	Intravitreal anti-VEGF	Unknown	
	36/M	Pfizer (2nd)	6/9	1–3 days	Unremarkable	Intravitreal anti-VEGF	Unknown	
Lee S et al. [11]	34/M	Pfizer (2nd)	Counting finger	10–12 days	Unknown	Intravitreal aflibercept, hyperbaric oxygen, etc.	VA 20/30	Concurrent CRAO
Shah PP et al. [23]	27/F	BNT (2nd)	20/20	26 days	Polycystic ovarian syndrome	Intravitreal anti-VEGF	Significant improvement	
Sonawane NJ et al. [8]	50/M	AstraZeneca (2nd)	6/60	4 days	Diabetes mellitus	Intravitreal anti-VEGF	Unknown	
	43/F	AstraZeneca (2nd)	5/60	3 days	Unremarkable	Close follow-up	Unknown	
Tanaka H et al. [24]	71/F	BNT (2nd)	20/30	1 day	History of BRVO in pre-COVID era, other comorbidities unknown	Intravitreal anti-VEGF	VA: 20/20	
	74/M	BNT (1st)	20/25	1 day	History of BRVO before 1st dose, other comorbidities unknown	Intravitreal anti-VEGF	VA: 20/25	No recurrence detected after 2nd dose

Table 1. *Cont.*

Paper	Age/Sex	Vaccine (Dose)	BCVA of the Affected Eye	Interval between Last Dose and Symptom Onset	Comorbidities	Treatment Received	Response to Treatment	Remarks
Park HS et al. [25]	68/F	AstraZeneca (1st)	Hand motion	1 day	Dyslipidaemia Hypertension	Observe	Unknown	
	76/M	Pfizer (1st)	logMAR 0.8	3 days	Diabetes mellitus, hypertension, old tuberculosis, dementia, end-stage renal disease	Observe	Unknown	
	85/F	Pfizer (2nd)	Counting fingers	1 day		Anti-VEGF	Unknown	
	59/M	AstraZeneca (1st)	logMAR 0.8	2 days	Diabetes mellitus, hypertension	Observe	Unknown	
	61/M	AstraZeneca (1st)	logMAR 0.04	2 days	Unremarkable	Anti-VEGF	Unknown	
	79/M	Pfizer (2nd)	logMAR 0.04	3 days	Diabetes mellitus, early gastric cancer	Anti-VEGF	Unknown	
	77/F	Pfizer (1st)	logMAR 0.8	16 days	Hypertension, chronic hepatitis, colon cancer	Anti-VEGF	Unknown	
	63/M	Pfizer (1st)	logMAR 0.01	13 days	Diabetes mellitus Hypertension	Anti-VEGF	Unknown	
	51/F	AstraZeneca (1st)	logMAR 0.09	21 days	Hypertension	Anti-VEGF	Unknown	
	81/F	Pfizer (1st)	logMAR 0.3	4 days	Hypertension	Observe	Unknown	
	61/M	AstraZeneca (1st)	logMAR 0.9	3 days		Observe	Unknown	
Sacconi E et al. [26]	74/F	Moderna (2nd)	20/40	3 weeks	Atrial fibrillation, breast cancer in remission	Intravitreal anti-VEGF	VA: 20/32	
Ikegami Y et al. [5]	54/F	Moderna (2nd)	No light perception	2 days	Hypothyroidism	Unknown	Unknown	Concurrent CRAO
Endo B et al. [27]	52/M	BNT (1st)	20/20	11 days	Unknown	Intravitreal dexamethasone	Fundal abnormalities improved	
			20/30 [11 days after symptom onset]	N/A	Ditto	Intravitreal anti-VEGF and oral apixaban	VA: 20/20	
Bialasiewicz AA [28]	50/M	BNT (2nd)	0.5	15 min	Atopic dermatitis	low-dose acetylsalicylic acid + monthly intravitreal anti-VEGF injections	VA 1.0	

Table 1. *Cont.*

Paper	Age/Sex	Vaccine (Dose)	BCVA of the Affected Eye	Interval between Last Dose and Symptom Onset	Comorbidities	Treatment Received	Response to Treatment	Remarks
Goyal M et al. [29]	28/M	Sputnik V	6/9	11 days	Unremarkable	Oral prednisolone and apixaban	VA: 6/6	
Da Silva LSC et al. [30]	66/F	AstraZeneca (unknown)	Unknown	16 days	Dyslipidaemia, increased body-mass index, endometrial hypertrophy	Unknown	Unknown	
	51/M	Pfizer (unknown)	Unknown	6 days	Unknown	Unknown	Unknown	
	66/M	AstraZeneca (unknown)	Unknown	4 days	Hypertension	Unknown	Unknown	
	54/F	AstraZeneca (unknown)	Unknown	10 days	Unknown	Unknown	Unknown	
Girbardt C et al. [31]	81/F	Comirnaty (2nd)	0.05	12 days	Hypertension, primary open angle glaucoma	Intravitreal anti-VEGF	Unknown	Concurrent RAO
Choi M et al. [32]	64/M	AstraZeneca (1st)	20/25 (Snellen)	1 day	Unremarkable	Aspirin	Unknown	
	33/F	BNT (2nd)	20/40 (Snellen)	6 days	Unremarkable	Intravitreal anti-VEGF	Unknown	
	48/M	BNT (3rd)	20/125 (Snellen)	6 days	Unremarkable	Intravitreal anti-VEGF	Unknown	
	69/F	AstraZeneca (1st)	20/20 (Snellen)	3 days	Unremarkable	Aspirin	Unknown	
	66/M	AstraZeneca (2nd)	20/20 (Snellen)	7 days	On aspirin for unknown reason, BRVO	Observation	Unknown	
	68/F	AstraZeneca (1st)	Hand motion	1 day	Hypertension, nasal cavity cancer in remission, on aspirin for unknown reason, BRVO	Observation	Unknown	
	74/F	AstraZeneca (2nd)	Hand motion	6 days		Intravitreal anti-VEGF, followed by vitrectomy	Unknown	
	63/F	AstraZeneca (1st)	20/630 (same as pre-vaccination)	3 days	CRVO	Intravitreal anti-VEGF	Unknown	

Table 1. *Cont.*

Paper	Age/Sex	Vaccine (Dose)	BCVA of the Affected Eye	Interval between Last Dose and Symptom Onset	Comorbidities	Treatment Received	Response to Treatment	Remarks
Vujosevic S et al. [33]	69/F	AstraZeneca (1st)	20/32	1 week	Deep vein thrombosis	Laser photocoagulation	VA: 20/20	
	82/F	BNT (2nd)	20/63	2 weeks	Unremarkable	Steroid	VA: 20/40	
	96/F	BNT (2nd)	20/200	1 week	Hypertension, diabetes mellitus	Steroid	VA: 20/200	
	91/F	BNT (2nd)	Counting fingers	1.5 weeks	Unremarkable	Patient refused treatment	VA: Counting fingers	
	78/F	BNT (2nd)	20/25	1 week	Unremarkable	Anti-VEGF	VA: 20/20	
	78/F	BNT (2nd)	20/20	1 week	Unremarkable	None	VA: 20/20	
	70/M	AstraZeneca (1st)	20/20	1 week	Unremarkable	None	VA: 20/20	
	40/M	AstraZeneca (1st)	20/20	2 weeks	Hyperhomocysteinaemia	None	VA: 20/20	
	91/M	BNT (2nd)	20/32	4 weeks	Diabetes mellitus	Steroid	VA: 20/32	
	72/F	BNT (2nd)	20/25	3 weeks	Hypertension, hyperlipidaemia	Steroid	VA: 20/20	
	88/M	BNT (2nd)	20/125	2 weeks	Hypertension, hyperlipidaemia, cardiovascular disease, Alzheimer's disease, "K prostate"	Steroid	VA: 20/125	
	73/F	AstraZeneca (2nd)	Counting fingers	4 weeks	Hypertension, hyperlipidaemia, cardiovascular disease, neuroendocrine tumour	Steroid	VA: Counting fingers	
	65/F	Jcovden (1st)	20/40	1 week	Hypertension, hyperlipidaemia, diabetes mellitus	Steroid	VA: 20/32	
	72/F	AstraZeneca (1st)	20/40	2 weeks	Hypertension, cardiovascular disease	Steroid	VA: 20/50	

Abbreviations: BCVA: best-corrected visual acuity, BNT: BioNTech vaccine, CRAO: central retinal artery occlusion, CRVO: central retinal vein occlusion, F: female, IV: intravenous, M: male, mmHg: millimetre of mercury, RAO: retinal artery occlusion, RVO: retinal vein occlusion, VA: visual acuity and VEGF: vascular endothelial growth factor.

4. Discussion

Latest reviews and studies about post-vaccination RVO.

4.1. Recent Reviews on the Topic

Yeo et al. looked at the literature on post-vaccination retinal vascular occlusion. Their team noted that retinal vascular occlusion took place following the first dose in viral vector vaccines and following the second dose for mRNA vaccines [34]. Apart from RVO, retinal artery occlusion following COVID-vaccination has also been reported around the world [35,36]. Authors found the determination of causality between COVID-19 vaccination and retinal vascular events difficult [34,35,37].

4.2. Recent Relevant Studies Employing Big Data

It has come to our attention that there are two recently published retrospective cohort studies (with propensity score matching) investigating the incidence of retinal vascular occlusion following mRNA COVID-19 vaccination [38,39]. The authors of both studies (Dorney et al., Li et al.) performed statistical analyses on clinical data retrieved from electronic health records from the US.

Dorney et al. stated that the incidence of newly diagnosed retinal vascular occlusion was 3.4 per 100,000 within 21 days of the first dose of mRNA COVID-19 vaccines [39]. No increased risk ratio with statistical significance was observed when compared to the recipients of influenza vaccines and tetanus, diphtheria and pertussis (Tdap) vaccines [39]. Dorney et al. compared the incidence of post-first-dose retinal vascular occlusion to that of post-second-dose, revealing a risk ratio of 2.25 (95% CI: 1.33–3.81) [39].

Li et al. found the hazard ratios of CRVO and branch RVO (BRVO) within 12 weeks of mRNA COVID-19 vaccination (compared to unvaccinated cohort) to be 3.97 (95% CI: 3.02–5.20) and 3.88 (95% CI: 3.02–4.97), respectively [38]. Li et al. also showed an increased risk of retinal vascular occlusion, as well as of all subtypes of retinal vascular occlusion in the vaccinated cohort at 2 years irrespective of sex, age and ethnicity [38].

There are a few points that are worth mentioning. First, the studies focused only on mRNA vaccines. The external validity may be affected, as the results may not be applicable to COVID-19 vaccines of other types [40]. Second, they used different cut-offs for defining vaccine-related retinal vascular occlusion. Li et al. also performed statistical analyses for retinal vascular occlusion that occurred within 2 years of vaccination. The differences in the endpoint selected may have had an influence on the statistical significance of results. On the other hand, whether late-onset RVO is directly related to COVID vaccines is a debatable issue. Thirdly, the populations used for comparison for the two studies were different. Li et al. used unvaccinated subjects for comparison, while Dorney et al. compared recipients of influenza and Tdap vaccines in the pre-COVID era. Lastly, the study by Li et al. placed more emphasis on the relative risks, while Dorney et al. pointed out that the absolute risk was small. The clinical importance of a statistically significant relative risk is equivocal if the absolute risk is very low.

Hashimoto et al. investigated general ocular adverse effects of mRNA vaccines using big data, as well. They obtained data from a database based on a Japanese population [41]. This is one of the few large-scale studies that provide information on the ophthalmic side effects of vaccines in an Asian population. Hashimoto et al. detected a statistically significantly increased risk of retinal vein occlusion following the second dose of mRNA vaccines. Nonetheless, no increased risk of RVO and other ocular events after mRNA COVID vaccination was observed in their self-controlled case series study. The increased risk of RVO following the second dose was thought to be caused by residual confounding [41].

The caveats listed above are not exhaustive. Much caution should be exercised when interpreting studies of these kinds. That said, big data analyses are very promising in ophthalmology and vaccine side effect research. We look forward to studies looking at other types of vaccines and ophthalmic side effect surveillance with the use of big data.

5. Proposed Mechanisms of Suspected Vaccine-Related RVO

The exact mechanisms have yet to be ascertained. On review of the current evidence, three possible mechanisms were raised to explain this phenomenon. Little is known about whether the following mechanisms are independent or synergistic.

5.1. Vaccine-Induced Immune Thrombotic Thrombocytopenia

Chen Y et al. proposed that COVID-19 vaccines may be linked to several post-vaccination new-onset autoimmune conditions, one of which is vaccine-induced immune thrombotic thrombocytopenia (VITT) [42]. The anti-platelet factor 4 (PF4) antibody has been identified to be the culprit of this pathology [43]. The exact pathophysiology of this phenomenon is not certain, but it is believed that it resembles that of heparin-induced thrombocytopenia [44]. A few authors of the articles reviewed here have suggested that VITT may be implicated in vaccine-related RVO.

Nonetheless, the measurement of the anti-PF4 antibody level was only reported in five cases and no positive tests were reported [9,10,32]. That said, no conclusion on the effect of this phenomenon on post-vaccination RVO can be made based on the negative finding in just a few cases. To observe the etiological role of those antibodies in CRVO, it is recommended that the anti-PF4 level should be documented, if possible, in suspected cases of vaccine-related RVO in the future.

5.2. COVID-19 Vaccine as a Trigger in Homocysteinaemia

Parakh S et al. reported a case of RVO after COVID-19 vaccination with mildly elevated homocysteine (22.19 micromol/L) detected on investigation [9]. They attributed the mild homocysteinaemia to recent subclinical COVID-19 infection prior to vaccination (i.e., a very high level of SARS-CoV-2 IgG (>250 U/mL) 15 days after first dose) and suggested that COVID-19 vaccine may trigger venous thromboembolism in background homocysteinaemia ("two-hit hypothesis"). Parakh et al. also cited evidence of the potential effect of vaccines and their adjuvants on endothelial cells and autoimmunity. The theory of ischaemic pre-conditioning was quoted to support their two-hit hypothesis [45].

The validity of this hypothesis is questionable. Homocysteinaemia is known to be associated with arterial thromboembolism; even mild homocysteinaemia carries a risk of arterial thromboembolism [46]. Nonetheless, recent research shows that its association with venous thromboembolic events is unclear and likely quite weak [46], if not absent [47]. On top of this, homocysteine-lowering treatment was not found to reduce the risk of venous thromboembolism [48]. Given the doubtful role of homocysteinaemia, it is difficult to interpret the role of the vaccine in the pathogenesis of RVO together with homocysteinaemia. It may be inappropriate to base the discussion of the role of the vaccine in RVO on a mildly raised homocysteine level.

5.3. Retinal Vasculitis

Another potential new-onset autoimmune condition triggered by COVID-19 vaccines is retinal vasculitis. Ikegami Y et al. and Choi M et al., who noted leaking retinal vessels on patients' FA images, both suggested that an inflammatory state in retinal vasculature induced by COVID-19 vaccines may be the cause of post-vaccination RVO [5,32]. On the other hand, Nangia P et al. suspected that inflammation-induced thromboembolic events may be the reason behind post-vaccination RVO due to a prompt response to systemic anti-inflammatory therapy [13]. Nangia P et al.'s observation corroborates the hypothesis put forth by Ikegami Y et al. However, vessel leakage on FA is not a specific sign for retinal vasculitis.

Other authors proposed that retinal vasculitis may be involved in retinal vein occlusion. Sarpangala S et al. reported a case of CRVO possibly secondary to retinal vasculitis [49]. Vasculitis following immunisation has been observed for other types of vaccines [50,51], although the causal link is unclear [51]. Thromboembolism in vasculitis has been documented, where interleukin (IL)-1 and IL-6 play an important role in vasculitis-related thrombosis [52].

Aside from retinal vasculitis, the current evidence suggests that mRNA vaccines may bring about transient endothelial dysfunction, particularly after the second dose [53]. Endothelial dysfunction itself, whether vasculitis-related or not, can predispose local vasculature to thrombosis [54].

6. How Do We Tell an RVO Is Caused by COVID-19 Vaccination?

Currently, there is no consensus regarding the temporal definition of vaccine-related RVO [55]. Different cut-offs were employed by different authors. From the individual case reports, the interval between symptom onset and vaccination ranged from 15 min to 30 days. In the retrospective case series by Vujosevic S et al., they assumed RVO occurring within 6 weeks to be vaccine-related RVO [33]. Twelve weeks was taken as the cut-off by Hashimoto's team [41]. We noticed that RVO that occurred some time after vaccination was still considered vaccine related. Nevertheless, the effect of vaccination is questionable in cases where the symptom onset was temporally far from the vaccination. In Hashimoto's self-controlled case series, the symptom onset of more than two-thirds of cases occurred more than 3 weeks after vaccination [41]. If the temporal definition vaccine-related RVO was set more strictly, the incidence of genuine vaccine-related RVO would be even lower. On the other hand, Feltgen N et al. suggested that there may be an underestimation of vaccine-related retinal vascular events as the pandemic might restrict patients from seeking medical help [55].

The establishment of causality between RVO and vaccination remains difficult, if not impossible, at this stage. It may be tempting to blame the vaccine in cases where none of the risk factors for RVO were present. A concrete conclusion on causality is difficult to make with the scarcity of cases and defects in the design of studies available. None of the studies available have a study design for the determination of causality. Apart from this, we also noticed that various vascular risk factors were present in quite a number of case reports of post-COVID vaccine RVO. Cardiovascular comorbidities were also common among the cases in a retrospective case series (Vujosevic et al.) [33], case–control studies and case-by-case analysis (Feltgen N et al.) [55], and in a matched cohort and self-controlled case series (Hashimoto Y et al.) [41]. In Hashimoto Y et al.'s analyses, where comorbidities were adjusted, no statistically significant difference in incidence rate ratio was found between the vaccinated and non-vaccinated arms. These vascular risk factors may actually be the genuine reason for post-vaccination RVO, in spite of the role of vaccines being unknown.

7. Ophthalmic Risks with Future Boosters

Very little is known regarding the effect of the third dose and further doses of COVID-19 vaccines on ophthalmic health. To date, only a few case reports of RVO occurring after a third dose have been found, and no conclusion on the causality between vaccination and RVO can be made [24,37,56]. Newer vaccines, such as the bivalent COVID-19 vaccine, have recently been made available in the market and may be used as boosters for populations susceptible to severe COVID-19 [57]. Data regarding the ophthalmic safety of these newer vaccines is still not comprehensive. Continued efforts in surveillance are needed for investigating ophthalmic side effects of further doses and newer types of COVID-19 vaccine.

There are cases where authors have reported the exacerbation and recurrence of past RVO occurring after COVID-19 vaccination. This has resulted in concerns over the safety of the vaccination in this population, including those who suffered from recent post-COVID-19 vaccination RVO [10]. To the best of our knowledge, only two related cases were reported across the world, and one similar case (anti-hepatitis B vaccines) in the 1990s [24,58]. The causality between vaccines and RVO recurrence or exacerbation can still not be confidently established. Caution in patients with a history of RVO should be practised, but it may not be valid to deter patients with such ophthalmic history from receiving vaccinations. To maximise vaccine safety, the optimisation of the general health condition and proper management of underlying medical illnesses prior to vaccination would be of paramount importance.

8. General Discussion

Despite being a sight-threatening condition, post-vaccination RVO, fortunately like other cases of RVO, can be managed effectively with standard treatment. Upon a review of the available evidence, post-vaccination RVO was shown to be a relatively rare ophthalmic adverse event of vaccination. Choi M et al. speculated that COVID-19 vaccines may be the cause of discernibly increased numbers of RVO cases in a short period after vaccination [32]. Such a claim is understandable as there were few cases of RVO that were suspected to be vaccine-related in pre-COVID-19 era. There is, however, insufficient evidence to accuse COVID-19 vaccinations of being one of the potential causes of RVO based on the review of latest evidence. Vaccines may be entirely unrelated to post-vaccination RVO, and the mass vaccination campaigns may have created the illusion of RVO being caused by the vaccines.

In view of the evolution of COVID-19 disease, giving populations further booster doses is gaining popularity worldwide, especially for subjects susceptible to COVID-19. While some studies revealed no statistically significant association between vaccines and venous thromboembolism one month after inoculation with the AstraZeneca vaccine [59,60], there is early evidence showing that the thromboembolic risk of COVID-19 is higher than that of certain vaccines [39,61]. As far as the risk of RVO is concerned, being vaccinated may be safer than being infected.

9. Limitations

This review includes only case reports and studies that were not randomised controlled trials. Causality hence cannot be drawn between RVO and COVID-19 vaccines. The case reports of RVO after COVID-19 vaccination were heterogenous in terms of their reporting style, making direct comparison difficult. Only English articles were included in this review, which may result in bias and an incomplete appraisal of the literature available.

10. Conclusions

COVID-19 vaccination has undoubtedly brought the world immense benefits in terms of public health. Though the long-term ophthalmic risk of COVID-19 vaccines is not known, it is believed that the benefits of vaccination outweigh the potential ophthalmic risk significantly. While we are awaiting the long-term side effect profile of COVID-19 vaccines, COVID-19 vaccination should still be advocated with reasonable reassurance for the benefit of population health. At the same time, the ophthalmic community should stay vigilant for any potential vaccine-related adverse impacts on ophthalmic health.

Supplementary Materials: The following supporting information can be downloaded at: https://www.mdpi.com/article/10.3390/vaccines11081281/s1. Table S1—Patient's demographics, clinical presentation, vaccination record and ophthalmic findings. Table S2—Patient's clinical characteristics, treatment received and response to treatment.

Author Contributions: Concept and design: S.C.-L.A.; Acquisition of data: H.-M.L.; Analysis or interpretation of data: S.C.-L.A. and H.-M.L.; Drafting of the article: H.-M.L. All authors had full access to the data, contributed to the study, approved the final version for publication, and take responsibility for its accuracy and integrity. Contents presented in this manuscript have never been presented or published. All authors have read and agreed to the published version of the manuscript.

Funding: This research received no specific grant from any funding agency in the public, commercial, or not-for-profit sectors.

Institutional Review Board Statement: Not applicable.

Informed Consent Statement: Not applicable.

Data Availability Statement: Not applicable.

Conflicts of Interest: All authors have declared no conflict of interest.

Abbreviation

BNT: BioNTech, BRVO: branch retinal vein occlusion, COVID-19: coronavirus disease 2019; CI: confidence interval, CRAO: central retinal artery occlusion, CRP: C-reactive protein, ESR: erythrocyte sedimentation rate, FA: fluorescein angiogram, IOP: intraocular pressure, OCT: optical coherence tomography, OCTA: optical coherence tomography angiography, RVO: retinal vein occlusion, VITT: vaccine-induced immune thrombocytopenic thrombosis.

References

1. Pottegård, A.; Lund, L.C.; Karlstad, Ø.; Dahl, J.; Andersen, M.; Hallas, J.; Lidegaard, Ø.; Tapia, G.; Gulseth, H.L.; Ruiz, P.L.D.; et al. Arterial events, venous thromboembolism, thrombocytopenia, and bleeding after vaccination with Oxford-AstraZeneca ChAdOx1-S in Denmark and Norway: Population based cohort study. *BMJ* **2021**, *373*, n1114. [CrossRef]
2. Berild, J.D.; Larsen, V.B.; Thiesson, E.M.; Lehtonen, T.; Grøsland, M.; Helgeland, J.; Wolhlfahrt, J.; Hansen, J.V.; Palmu, A.A.; Hviid, A. Analysis of thromboembolic and thrombocytopenic events after the AZD1222, BNT162b2, and MRNA-1273 COVID-19 vaccines in 3 Nordic countries. *JAMA Netw. Open* **2022**, *5*, e2217375. [CrossRef] [PubMed]
3. Schulz, J.B.; Berlit, P.; Diener, H.C.; Gerloff, C.; Greinacher, A.; Klein, C.; Petzold, G.C.; Piccininni, M.; Poli, S.; Röhrig, R.; et al. COVID-19 vaccine-associated cerebral venous thrombosis in Germany. *Ann. Neurol.* **2021**, *90*, 627–639. [CrossRef] [PubMed]
4. World Health Oragnisation. WHO Coronavirus Dashboard. 5 January 2023. Available online: https://covid19.who.int/?mapFilter=vaccinations (accessed on 15 January 2023).
5. Ikegami, Y.; Numaga, J.; Okano, N.; Fukuda, S.; Yamamoto, H.; Terada, Y. Combined central retinal artery and vein occlusion shortly after mRNA-SARS-CoV-2 vaccination. *QJM Int. J. Med.* **2021**, *114*, 884–885. [CrossRef] [PubMed]
6. Sodhi, P.K.; Yadav, A.; Sharma, B.; Sharma, A.; Kumar, P. Central Retinal Vein Occlusion Following the First Dose of COVID Vaccine. *Cureus* **2022**, *14*, e25842. [CrossRef]
7. Chen, Y. Combined central retinal artery occlusion and vein occlusion with exudative retinal detachment following COVID-19 vaccination. *Kaohsiung J. Med. Sci.* **2022**, *38*, 1020–1021. [CrossRef]
8. Sonawane, N.; Yadav, D.; Kota, A.; Singh, H. Central retinal vein occlusion post-COVID-19 vaccination. *Indian J. Ophthalmol.* **2022**, *70*, 308–309. [CrossRef]
9. Parakh, S.; Maheshwari, S.; Das, S.; Vaish, H.; Luthra, G.; Agrawal, R.; Gupta, V.; Luthra, S. Central Retinal Vein Occlusion Post ChAdOx1 nCoV-19 Vaccination–Can It Be Explained by the Two-hit Hypothesis? *J. Ophthalmic Inflamm. Infect.* **2022**, *12*, 34. [CrossRef]
10. Takacs, A.; Ecsedy, M.; Nagy, Z.Z. Possible COVID-19 MRNA Vaccine-Induced Case of Unilateral Central Retinal Vein Occlusion. *Ocul. Immunol. Inflamm.* **2022**, 1–6. [CrossRef]
11. Lee, S.; Sankhala, K.K.; Bose, S.; Gallemore, R.P. Combined central retinal artery and vein occlusion with ischemic optic neuropathy after COVID-19 vaccination. *Int. Med. Case Rep. J.* **2022**, *15*, 7–14. [CrossRef]
12. Ruiz, O.A.G.; González-López, J.J. Simultaneous unilateral central retinal vein occlusion and branch retinal artery occlusion after Coronavirus Disease 2019 (COVID-19) mRNA vaccine. *Arq. Bras. Oftalmol.* **2023**, *87*. [CrossRef] [PubMed]
13. Majumder, P.D.; Nangia, P.; Prakash, V. Retinal venous occlusion in a child following Corbevax COVID-19 vaccination. *Indian J. Ophthalmol.* **2022**, *70*, 3713–3715. [CrossRef] [PubMed]
14. Fernández-Vigo, J.I.; Conde, C.P.; Burgos-Blasco, B.; Fernández-Vigo, J.A. Bilateral retinal vein occlusion after two doses of SARS-CoV-2 adenovirus vector-based vaccine. *J. Français D'ophtalmologie* **2022**, *45*, e397–e399. [CrossRef]
15. Karageorgiou, G.; Chronopoulou, K.; Georgalas, I.; Kandarakis, S.; Tservakis, I.; Petrou, P. Branch retinal vein occlusion following ChAdOx1 nCoV-19 (Oxford-AstraZeneca) vaccine. *Eur. J. Ophthalmol.* **2022**, 11206721221124651. [CrossRef] [PubMed]
16. Tanaka, H.; Nagasato, D.; Nakakura, S.; Nagasawa, T.; Wakuda, H.; Kurusu, A.; Mitamura, Y.; Tabuchi, H. Branch retinal vein occlusion post severe acute respiratory syndrome coronavirus 2 vaccination. *Taiwan J. Ophthalmol.* **2022**, *12*, 202. [PubMed]
17. Romano, D.; Morescalchi, F.; Romano, V.; Semeraro, F. COVID-19 AdenoviralVector Vaccine and Central Retinal Vein Occlusion. *Ocul. Immunol. Inflamm.* **2022**, *30*, 1286–1288. [CrossRef]
18. Majumder, P.D.; Prakash, V. Retinal venous occlusion following COVID-19 vaccination: Report of a case after third dose and review of the literature. *Indian J. Ophthalmol.* **2022**, *70*, 2191–2194. [CrossRef]
19. Priluck, A.Z.; Arevalo, J.F.; Pandit, R.R. Ischemic retinal events after COVID-19 vaccination. *Am. J. Ophthalmol. Case Rep.* **2022**, *26*, 101540. [CrossRef]
20. Sugihara, K.; Kono, M.; Tanito, M. Branch retinal vein occlusion after messenger RNA-Based COVID-19 vaccine. *Case Rep. Ophthalmol.* **2022**, *13*, 28–32. [CrossRef]
21. Pur, D.R.; Bursztyn, L.L.C.D.; Iordanous, Y. Branch retinal vein occlusion in a healthy young man following mRNA COVID-19 vaccination. *Am. J. Ophthalmol. Case Rep.* **2022**, *26*, 101445. [CrossRef]
22. Peters, M.C.; Cheng, S.S.H.; Sharma, A.; Moloney, T.P.; Franzco, S.S.H.C.; Franzco, A.S.; Franzco, T.P.M. Retinal vein occlusion following COVID-19 vaccination. *Clin. Exp. Ophthalmol.* **2022**, *50*, 459–461. [CrossRef]

23. Shah, P.P.; Gelnick, S.; Jonisch, J.; Verma, R. Central retinal vein occlusion following BNT162b2 (Pfizer-BioNTech) COVID-19 messenger RNA vaccine. *Retin. Cases Brief Rep.* **2021**, *17*, 441–444. [CrossRef]
24. Tanaka, H.; Nagasato, D.; Nakakura, S.; Tanabe, H.; Nagasawa, T.; Wakuda, H.; Imada, Y.; Mitamura, Y.; Tabuchi, H. Exacerbation of branch retinal vein occlusion post SARS-CoV2 vaccination: Case reports. *Medicine* **2021**, *100*, e28236. [CrossRef]
25. Park, H.S.; Byun, Y.; Byeon, S.H.; Kim, S.S.; Kim, Y.J.; Lee, C.S. Retinal hemorrhage after SARS-CoV-2 vaccination. *J. Clin. Med.* **2021**, *10*, 5705. [CrossRef]
26. Sacconi, R.; Simona, F.; Forte, P.; Querques, G. Retinal vein occlusion following two doses of mRNA-1237 (moderna) immunization for SARS-CoV-2: A case report. *Ophthalmol. Ther.* **2021**, *11*, 453–458. [CrossRef]
27. Endo, B.; Bahamon, S.; Martínez-Pulgarín, D.F. Central retinal vein occlusion after mRNA SARS-CoV-2 vaccination: A case report. *Indian J. Ophthalmol.* **2021**, *69*, 2865. [CrossRef]
28. Bialasiewicz, A.; Farah-Diab, M.; Mebarki, H. Central retinal vein occlusion occurring immediately after 2nd dose of mRNA SARS-CoV-2 vaccine. *Int. Ophthalmol.* **2021**, *41*, 3889–3892. [CrossRef]
29. Goyal, M.; Murthy, S.; Srinivas, Y. Unilateral retinal vein occlusion in a young, healthy male following Sputnik V vaccination. *Indian J. Ophthalmol.* **2021**, *69*, 3793–3794. [CrossRef] [PubMed]
30. Da Silva, L.S.; Finamor, L.P.; Andrade, G.C.; Lima, L.H.; Zett, C.; Muccioli, C.; Sarraf, E.P.; Marinho, P.M.; Peruchi, J.; Oliveira, R.D.D.L.; et al. Vascular retinal findings after COVID-19 vaccination in 11 cases: A coincidence or consequence? *Arq. Bras. Oftalmol.* **2022**, *85*, 158–165. [CrossRef] [PubMed]
31. Girbardt, C.; Busch, C.; Al-Sheikh, M.; Gunzinger, J.M.; Invernizzi, A.; Xhepa, A.; Unterlauft, J.D.; Rehak, M. Retinal vascular events after mRNA and adenoviral-vectored COVID-19 vaccines—A case series. *Vaccines* **2021**, *9*, 1349. [CrossRef]
32. Choi, M.; Seo, M.-H.; Choi, K.-E.; Lee, S.; Choi, B.; Yun, C.; Kim, S.-W.; Kim, Y.Y. Vision-Threatening Ocular Adverse Events after Vaccination against Coronavirus Disease 2019. *J. Clin. Med.* **2022**, *11*, 3318. [CrossRef]
33. Vujosevic, S.; Limoli, C.; Romano, S.; Vitale, L.; Villani, E.; Nucci, P. Retinal vascular occlusion and SARS-CoV-2 vaccination. *Graefe's Arch. Clin. Exp. Ophthalmol.* **2022**, *260*, 3455–3464. [CrossRef] [PubMed]
34. Yeo, S.; Kim, H.; Lee, J.; Yi, J.; Chung, Y.-R. Retinal vascular occlusions in COVID-19 infection and vaccination: A literature review. *Graefe's Arch. Clin. Exp. Ophthalmol.* **2023**, *261*, 1793–1808. [CrossRef] [PubMed]
35. Su, C.K.Y.; Au, S.C.L. Isolated and combined unilateral central retinal artery and vein occlusions after vaccination. A review of the literature. *J. Stroke Cerebrovasc. Dis.* **2022**, *31*, 106552. [CrossRef]
36. Yeung, M.; Su, C.K.-Y.; Au, S.C.L. Vaccine-related retinal artery occlusion in adults: A review of the current literature. *J. Stroke Cerebrovasc. Dis.* **2022**, 106694. [CrossRef] [PubMed]
37. Sung, S.Y.; Jenny, L.A.; Chang, Y.C.; Wang, N.K.; Liu, P.K. Central Retinal Vein Occlusion in a Young Woman with Diabetes and Hypertension after mRNA-Based COVID-19 Vaccination—A Case Report and Brief Review of the Literature. *Vaccines* **2023**, *11*, 365. [CrossRef]
38. Li, J.-X.; Wang, Y.-H.; Bair, H.; Hsu, S.-B.; Chen, C.; Wei, J.C.-C.; Lin, C.-J. Risk assessment of retinal vascular occlusion after COVID-19 vaccination. *NPJ Vaccines* **2023**, *8*, 64. [CrossRef] [PubMed]
39. Dorney, I.; Shaia, J.; Kaelber, D.C.; Talcott, K.E.; Singh, R.P. Risk of new retinal vascular occlusion after mRNA COVID-19 vaccination within aggregated electronic health record data. *JAMA Ophthalmol.* **2023**, *141*, 441. [CrossRef] [PubMed]
40. Jampol, L.M.; Maguire, M.G. No Red Flags for Risk of Retinal Vascular Occlusion After mRNA COVID-19 Vaccination. *JAMA Ophthalmol.* **2023**, *141*, 447. [CrossRef] [PubMed]
41. Hashimoto, Y.; Yamana, H.; Iwagami, M.; Ono, S.; Takeuchi, Y.; Michihata, N.; Uemura, K.; Yasunaga, H.; Aihara, M.; Kaburaki, T. Ocular Adverse Events after Coronavirus Disease 2019 mRNA Vaccination: Matched Cohort and Self-Controlled Case Series Studies Using a Large Database. *Ophthalmology* **2022**, *130*, 256–264. [CrossRef]
42. Chen, Y.; Xu, Z.; Wang, P.; Li, X.M.; Shuai, Z.W.; Ye, D.Q.; Pan, H.F. New-onset autoimmune phenomena post-COVID-19 vaccination. *Immunology* **2022**, *165*, 386–401. [CrossRef]
43. Scully, M.; Singh, D.; Lown, R.; Poles, A.; Solomon, T.; Levi, M.; Goldblatt, D.; Kotoucek, P.; Thomas, W.; Lester, W. Pathologic antibodies to platelet factor 4 after ChAdOx1 nCoV-19 vaccination. *N. Engl. J. Med.* **2021**, *384*, 2202–2211. [CrossRef] [PubMed]
44. Klok, F.A.; Pai, M.; Huisman, M.V.; Makris, M. Vaccine-induced immune thrombotic thrombocytopenia. *Lancet Haematol.* **2021**, *9*, e73–e80. [CrossRef] [PubMed]
45. Morris, C.F.M.; Tahir, M.; Arshid, S.; Castro, M.S.; Fontes, W. Reconciling the IPC and two-hit models: Dissecting the underlying cellular and molecular mechanisms of two seemingly opposing frameworks. *J. Immunol. Res.* **2015**, *2015*, 697193. [CrossRef]
46. Hirmerová, J. Homocysteine and venous thromboembolism—Is there any link? *Cor et Vasa* **2013**, *55*, e248–e258. [CrossRef]
47. Ospina-Romero, M.; Cannegieter, S.C.; Heijer, M.D.; Doggen, C.J.M.; Rosendaal, F.R.; Lijfering, W.M. Hyperhomocysteinemia and risk of first venous thrombosis: The influence of (unmeasured) confounding factors. *Am. J. Epidemiol.* **2018**, *187*, 1392–1400. [CrossRef] [PubMed]
48. Ray, J.G.; Kearon, C.; Yi, Q.; Sheridan, P.; Lonn, E.; Heart Outcomes Prevention Evaluation 2 (HOPE-2) Investigators. Homocysteine-lowering therapy and risk for venous thromboembolism: A randomized trial. *Ann. Intern. Med.* **2007**, *146*, 761–767. [CrossRef]
49. Kamath, Y.; Sarpangala, S.; George, N.; Kulkarni, C. Central retinal vein occlusion secondary to varicella zoster retinal vasculitis in an immunocompetent individual during the COVID-19 pandemic—A case report. *Indian J. Ophthalmol.* **2021**, *69*, 2532–2535. [CrossRef]

50. Watanabe, T. Vasculitis following influenza vaccination: A review of the literature. *Curr. Rheumatol. Rev.* **2017**, *13*, 188–196. [CrossRef]
51. Bonetto, C.; Trotta, F.; Felicetti, P.; Alarcón, G.S.; Santuccio, C.; Bachtiar, N.S.; Pernus, Y.B.; Chandler, R.; Girolomoni, G.; Hadden, R.D.; et al. Vasculitis as an adverse event following immunization—Systematic literature review. *Vaccine* **2016**, *34*, 6641–6651. [CrossRef]
52. Springer, J.; Villa-Forte, A. Thrombosis in vasculitis. *Curr. Opin. Rheumatol.* **2013**, *25*, 19–25. [CrossRef]
53. Terentes-Printzios, D.; Gardikioti, V.; Solomou, E.; Emmanouil, E.; Gourgouli, I.; Xydis, P.; Christopoulou, G.; Georgakopoulos, C.; Dima, I.; Miliou, A.; et al. The effect of an mRNA vaccine against COVID-19 on endothelial function and arterial stiffness. *Hypertens. Res.* **2022**, *45*, 846–855. [CrossRef]
54. Poredos, P.; Jezovnik, M.K. Endothelial dysfunction and venous thrombosis. *Angiology* **2017**, *69*, 564–567. [CrossRef] [PubMed]
55. Feltgen, N.; Ach, T.; Ziemssen, F.; Quante, C.S.; Gross, O.; Abdin, A.D.; Aisenbrey, S.; Bartram, M.C.; Blum, M.; Brockmann, C.; et al. Retinal Vascular Occlusion after COVID-19 Vaccination: More Coincidence than Causal Relationship? Data from a Retrospective Multicentre Study. *J. Clin. Med.* **2022**, *11*, 5101. [CrossRef] [PubMed]
56. Gironi, M.; D'Aloisio, R.; Verdina, T.; Shkurko, B.; Toto, L.; Mastropasqua, R. Bilateral Branch Retinal Vein Occlusion after mRNA-SARS-CoV-2 Booster Dose Vaccination. *J. Clin. Med.* **2023**, *12*, 1325. [CrossRef] [PubMed]
57. Offit, P.A. Bivalent COVID-19 Vaccines—A Cautionary Tale. *N. Engl. J. Med.* **2023**, *388*, 481–483. [CrossRef]
58. Devin, F.; Roques, G.; Disdier, P.; Rodor, F.; Weiller, P. Occlusion of central retinal vein after hepatitis B vaccination. *Lancet* **1996**, *347*, 1626. [CrossRef]
59. Simpson, C.R.; Shi, T.; Vasileiou, E.; Katikireddi, S.V.; Kerr, S.; Moore, E.; McCowan, C.; Agrawal, U.; Shah, S.A.; Ritchie, L.D.; et al. First-dose ChAdOx1 and BNT162b2 COVID-19 vaccines and thrombocytopenic, thromboembolic and hemorrhagic events in Scotland. *Nat. Med.* **2021**, *27*, 1290–1297. [CrossRef]
60. Simpson, C.R.; Kerr, S.; Katikireddi, S.V.; McCowan, C.; Ritchie, L.D.; Pan, J.; Stock, S.J.; Rudan, I.; Tsang, R.S.M.; de Lusignan, S.; et al. Second-dose ChAdOx1 and BNT162b2 COVID-19 vaccines and thrombocytopenic, thromboembolic and hemorrhagic events in Scotland. *Nat. Commun.* **2022**, *13*, 4800. [CrossRef]
61. Chui, C.S.L.; Fan, M.; Wan, E.Y.F.; Leung, M.T.Y.; Cheung, E.; Yan, V.K.C.; Gao, L.; Ghebremichael-Weldeselassie, Y.; Man, K.K.; Lau, K.K.; et al. Thromboembolic events and hemorrhagic stroke after mRNA (BNT162b2) and inactivated (CoronaVac) COVID-19 vaccination: A self-controlled case series study. *Eclinicalmedicine* **2022**, *50*, 101514. [CrossRef]

Disclaimer/Publisher's Note: The statements, opinions and data contained in all publications are solely those of the individual author(s) and contributor(s) and not of MDPI and/or the editor(s). MDPI and/or the editor(s) disclaim responsibility for any injury to people or property resulting from any ideas, methods, instructions or products referred to in the content.

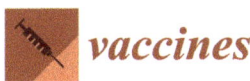

Brief Report

Acute Macular Neuroretinopathy and Paracentral Acute Middle Maculopathy during SARS-CoV-2 Infection and Vaccination

Parthopratim Dutta Majumder [1,*] and Aniruddha Agarwal [2,3,4]

1. Medical Research Foundation, Sankara Nethralaya, 18, College Road, Chennai 600006, India
2. Eye Institute, Cleveland Clinic Abu Dhabi (CCAD), Abu Dhabi P.O. Box 112412, United Arab Emirates
3. Cleveland Clinic Lerner College of Medicine, Case Western Reserve University, Cleveland, OH 44195, USA
4. Department of Ophthalmology, Maastricht University Medical Center, 6211 LK Maastricht, The Netherlands
* Correspondence: drparthopratim@gmail.com; Tel.: +91-44-2827-1616

Abstract: *Purpose*: To review the demographic and clinical profile of patients developing acute macular neuroretinopathy (AMN) or paracentral acute middle maculopathy (PAMM) after receiving coronavirus disease-2019 (COVID-19) vaccination or infection. *Methods*: In this review article, the published literature was searched to determine cases developing either AMN or PAMM after COVID-19 vaccinations or infections. Data, including demographic profile, presenting features, symptoms, diagnosis, and clinical outcomes, were extracted from the selected publications. These parameters were compared between the two groups, i.e., patients developing AMN/PAMM either after vaccination or infection. *Results*: After the literature review, 57 patients developing either AMN ($n = 40$), PAMM ($n = 14$), or both ($n = 3$) after COVID-19 infection ($n = 29$) or vaccination ($n = 28$) were included (mean age: 34.9 ± 14.4 years; $n = 38$; 66.7% females). In 24.6% patients, the diagnosis of COVID-19 infection was preceded by the development of ocular disease. There were no significant differences in the age or gender between the patients developing AMN or PAMM after vaccination or infection ($p > 0.13$). Among the vaccination group, the highest number of patients developing AMN/PAMM were after the Oxford-AstraZeneca ($n = 12$; 42.9%). Patients with vaccination had a significantly early onset of AMN/PAMM compared to those with infection (11.5 ± 17.6 days versus 37.8 ± 43.6 days; $p = 0.001$). *Conclusions*: Both AMN and PAMM are reported to be associated with COVID-19 infections and in persons receiving vaccination against COVID-19. While COVID-19 infections and vaccinations may have a contributory role, other risk factors such as oral contraceptive pills may also play a role in the development of the disease.

Keywords: acute macular neuroretinopathy; paracentral acute middle maculopathy; SARS-CoV-2 infection; COVID-19; vaccination; optical coherence tomography

Citation: Dutta Majumder, P.; Agarwal, A. Acute Macular Neuroretinopathy and Paracentral Acute Middle Maculopathy during SARS-CoV-2 Infection and Vaccination. *Vaccines* **2023**, *11*, 474. https://doi.org/10.3390/vaccines11020474

Academic Editor: Ralph A. Tripp

Received: 21 November 2022
Revised: 9 February 2023
Accepted: 9 February 2023
Published: 17 February 2023

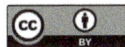

Copyright: © 2023 by the authors. Licensee MDPI, Basel, Switzerland. This article is an open access article distributed under the terms and conditions of the Creative Commons Attribution (CC BY) license (https://creativecommons.org/licenses/by/4.0/).

1. Introduction

Novel SARS-CoV-2 infection is attributed to the result of a hypercoagulable state, which can induce thrombus formation leading to local embolism in the small vessels and micro-vessels of the relevant target organs [1]. Various other pathological events leading to a pro-inflammatory and anti-fibrinolytic state, such as the development of antiphospholipid antibodies and increase in D-dimer levels, were reported to contribute to the hypercoagulable state in patients with COVID-19 [1]. Similarly, several reports of unusual thromboembolic adverse events were reported following the widespread use of anti-SARS-CoV-2 vaccinations. In accordance with the literature, various clinical conditions secondary to thromboembolic and ischemic episodes were reported in the eyes of patients with COVID-19 infection and in patients receiving anti-SARS-CoV-2 vaccinations [2,3].

In a prospective cross-sectional study by Sim et al., one in nine patients with COVID-19 infections had microvascular alterations on ocular imaging, and these signs were observed even in asymptomatic patients with normal vital signs [4]. On the other hand, the exact cause or association between such microvascular changes and COVID-19 vaccination is not clear, but there are several reports that have highlighted the role of vaccine-induced inflammation.

Acute macular neuroretinopathy (AMN) is a rare, outer retinal, microvascular disorder characterized by acute onset wedge-shaped or petaloid perifoveal lesions and ischemia of the deep retinal capillary plexus, involving the external limiting membrane and photoreceptors. Paracentral acute middle maculopathy (PAMM) is also a manifestation of outer retinal ischemia with intermediate/deep retinal capillary plexus involvement but limited to the inner nuclear layer, outer plexiform/nuclear layers. Various systemic risk factors are reported in association with AMN: flu-like illness, fever, oral contraceptive use, systemic shock, antecedent trauma, and dengue fever, among others. A non-specific flu-like illness or fever was reported in almost half of the patients in a review of 101 cases of AMN [5]. PAMM was reported with various other retinal vascular diseases such as retinal vascular occlusions, inflammatory chorioretinopathies, congenital glaucoma, foveal hypoplasia, various intraocular and extraocular surgeries, and systemic vascular diseases, as well as in healthy patients [6]. Recently, there has been an increase in the literature concerning these two entities in patients with SARS-CoV-2 infection and in patients with anti-SARS-CoV-2 vaccinations.

2. Materials and Methods

The study was designed as a review of published AMN and PAMM cases in the literature associated with COVID-19 infections or vaccination. Since the study analyzed published manuscripts, institutional ethics clearance was not required for the study, and there were no informed consent documents. The study adhered to the tenets of the declaration of Helsinki. We conducted a detailed review of the literature on Medline (National Library of Medicine/PUBMED) from December 2020 until 30 September 2022. The search was conducted by two ophthalmologists (retina specialists with fellowship training) using terms such as 'acute macular neuroretinopathy', 'paracentral acute middle maculopathy' AND/OR 'SARS-CoV-2', 'COVID-19', and 'COVID-19 vaccine'. The bibliographies of the retrieved articles were searched thoroughly to find relevant articles.

The manuscripts in the English language were selected for further analysis only. The inclusion criteria were published cases, case series, or original articles of patients with the diagnosis of either AMN, PAMM, or both associated with COVID-19 infection or vaccination. We included studies with either definitive diagnosis of COVID-19 or recipients of COVID vaccination (any approved type of vaccine), including booster doses. Cases without a definitive diagnosis of COVID-19 infection were excluded from this analysis [7]. If a case exhibited pre-existing AMN or PAMM, they were excluded from the analysis. The definition of AMN and PAMM was used based on the published manuscripts, essentially with the help of clinical examination, fundus photography, and multimodal imaging techniques including optical coherence tomography (OCT), fluorescein angiography (FA), and optical coherence tomography angiography (OCTA), whichever were available.

For the purpose of the study, we collected available demographic data from the published cases, including data such as gender, age, ethnicity, and geographic location (if available). The data concerning previous or current COVID-19 infection and vaccination (type, number of doses, and time since last dose) were noted. The medical history of the patients available in the published cases, such as history of drug intake, pre-existing medical conditions, previous surgeries, or ocular findings were noted. The details of the ophthalmic examination and imaging findings were noted for each case. The course of the AMN and PAMM lesions were obtained, and treatments prescribed were also noted. Any additional clinical data such as additional diagnoses, complications, or findings were noted.

The data were collected in a pre-designed data collection sheet by two ophthalmologists. Data analysis was performed using GraphPad Prism® (GraphPad Software Inc., La Jolla, CA, USA) version 6.0. The demographic data were expressed in mean and standard deviation. The parameters between two groups, namely, AMN versus PAMM, and AMN or PAMM after vaccination or after COVID-19 infection were compared using Mann–Whitney U test. Binary data between the groups were analyzed using Chi Square test. The clinical findings, course of the disease, complications and other data were described using descriptive statistics. The total follow-up was also described using mean and standard deviation. The statistical significance was denoted by $p < 0.05$ and 95% confidence interval.

3. Results

A total of 57 cases of AMN and PAMM were obtained after analysis of the published literature. The mean age of all the patients included in the analysis was 34.9 ± 14.4 years. Among them, 29 developed either AMN or PAMM following COVID-19 infections (50.9%) (Table 1), and the other 28 had a history of recent COVID vaccination (49.1%). There were 38 females in the cohort (66.7%). (Tables 1 and 2 describe the demographic features of the patients included in the study). The number of reported cases of AMN ($n = 40$; 70.2%) was higher than PAMM ($n = 14$; 24.6%). PAMM was more commonly seen in patients with COVID-19 infections ($n = 10$) than in patients following vaccinations ($n = 4$). PAMM was associated with central retinal artery occlusion (CRAO) in two patients with COVID-19 infection and in one patient with cilioretinal artery occlusion [8–10]. Turedi and Onal Gunay described the case of a 54-year-old male who developed CRAO two weeks following COVID-19 infection [8]. The laboratory work-up was non-contributory, and ancillary imaging after five days of diagnosis of CRAO revealed a diagnosis of coexisting PAMM [8]. In another case report by Matilde et al., a 41-year-old male presented with an optic neuritis-like picture in the left eye and was treated with pulse corticosteroid therapy. After three days, the patient developed Purtscher-like retinopathy, and a diagnosis of atypical CRAO was considered. OCT of the left eye revealed a PAMM lesion in this patient [9]. Subsequently, the patient tested positive at PCR for COVID-19 infection after he developed flu-like symptoms [9]. Two patients had combined features of AMN and PAMM in patients with the COVID-19 infected group, whereas one such case was reported in a vaccinated patient [11–13].

Table 1. Review of Literature of AMN and PAMM cases in COVID-19 patients.

Author	Age/Sex	Duration (Days)	Laterality	Diagnosis	Presenting Symptoms	Clinical Findings	Outcome
Azar et al. [7]	21/M	NA	Right Eye	AMN	Central Scotoma	NA	Favorable
	28/F	NA	Both Eyes	AMN	Paracentral scotoma	NA	NA
	27/F	NA	Both Eyes	AMN	Paracentral scotoma	NA	NA
	22/F	NA	Right Eye	AMN	Paracentral scotoma	NA	NA
Turedi and Onal Gunay [8]	54/M	14	Right Eye	CRAO + PAMM	Vision loss	Pale, white retina and "cherry-red spot appearance"	
Matilde et al. [9]	41/M	-	Left Eye	atypical CRAO, PAMM	Decreased vision	Initially unremarkable, multiple Purtscher-like CWS, slight retinal whitening around the fovea, and cherry-red spot	Favorable
Ozsaygılı et al. [10]	26/F	14	Left Eye	PAMM	Central Visual Field Defect	Focal area of well-demarcated retinal whitening over the distribution of a CILRA in the superior papillomacular bundle region	Favorable
Gascon et al. [11]	53/M	-	Left Eye	AMN/PAMM	Loss of vision, Negative scotoma, Dyschromatopsia.	Retinal hemorrhages, Roth spots, subtle whitish Parafoveal lesions.	NA
Goyal et al. [12]	32/M	120	Both Eyes	AMN/PAMM	Paracentral and triangular negative scotoma	Triangular deeper retinal greyish-white lesion located superonasal to center of macula in right eye	NA
Preti et al. [14]	70/M	-	Left Eye	AMN	Diaphoresis, Paracentral scotoma, Vision loss	OD: Unremarkable OS: Old scleral buckle	Favorable

Table 1. Cont.

Author	Age/Sex	Duration (Days)	Laterality	Diagnosis	Presenting Symptoms	Clinical Findings	Outcome
Capuano et al. [15]	27/M	-	Left Eye	PAMM	Paracentral scotoma, Dyschromatopsia	Subtle yellowish perifoveal halo	Partial Improvement
	37/F	-	Both Eyes	AMN	Paracentral scotoma	Alternated foveal reflex	Favorable
Naughton et al. [16]	28/M	NA	Both Eyes	PAMM	Decreased vision	CWS, Intraretinal haemorrhages, Retinal pallor in fovea	Favorable
Mace and Pipelet [17]	39/F	2	Both Eyes	AMN	Photopsia, Para-central scotoma	Unremarkable	Persistent
Aidar et al. [18]	71/F	14	Left Eye	AMN	Diminution of vision	Foveal pigment mobilization	No Improvement
Padhy et al. [19]	19/F	14	Both Eyes	PAMM	Scotoma	CWS, subtle white lesions at macula	Favorable
Castro et al. [20]	36/F	63	Both Eyes	PAMM	Blurred vision	Superficial hemorrhages in macula and peripheral retina in left eye	Favorable
Jonathan et al. [21]	47/M	60	Right Eye	PAMM	Paracentral scotoma	Retinal Whitening	Scotoma persisted
Diafas et al. [22]	59/M	14	Both Eyes	AMN	Blurred vision	Unremarkable	Favorable
	24/F	7	Both Eyes	AMN	Paracentral Scotoma.	Perifoveal dark grey patches	No Improvement
Virgo et al. [23]	32/M	16	Right Eye	AMN	Paracentral Scotoma	Unremarkable	NA
	37/F	35	Left Eye	PAMM	Paracentral Scotoma.	Unremarkable	NA
Sonmez et al. [24]	41/F	30	Right Eye	PAMM	Paracentral Scotoma, Decreased Vision	Parafoveal hyper-pigmented round lesion and increased vascular tortuosity	NA
Giacuzzo et al. [25]	23/F	-	Both Eyes	AMN	Photopsias, Paracentral Scotomas	Unremarkable	Favorable
Jalink and Bronkhor [26]	29/F	150	Left Eye	AMN	Paracentral scotoma	Subtle alterations around fovea	Scotoma Unchanged
Zamani et al. [27]	35/F	-	Both Eyes	AMN	Paracentral scotoma, Photopsia	Multiple hemorrhages with white or pale center (Roth's spots)	Died due to pneumonia
David and Fivgas [28]	22/F	-	Both Eyes	AMN	Scotoma	Multiple subtle reddish-brown petaloid lesions radiating from the fovea	NA
Masjedi et al. [29]	29/F	14	Left Eye	AMN	Paracentral scotoma	Unremarkable	Scotoma persisted
Deshmukh et al. [30]	56/F	-	Left Eye	AMN	Paracentral scotoma	Parafoveal retinal whitening	Stable

M = male, F = female, AMN = acute macular neuroretinopathy, PAMM = paracentral acute middle maculopathy, CRAO = central retinal artery occlusion, CWS = cotton wool spot.

In 14 patients (24.6%), the diagnosis or confirmation of COVID-19 infection was preceded by the ocular symptoms and/or signs of AMN/PAMM [11,14,15]. Bilateral involvement was almost similar in both cohorts. The patients who developed AMN and PAMM after COVID-19 vaccinations were relatively younger than the cohort with COVID-19 infection, though it did not reach statistical significance (32.04 ± 13.2 years versus 36.7 ± 14.4 years; $p = 0.13$). Female predilection was more frequently observed in the cohort with COVID vaccination (though not statistically significant) (21 out of 28 patients; 75% versus 18 out of 29 patients; 62%) ($p = 0.29$). Among the female patients, 71% were either on or were using oral contraceptive pills or hormonal devices for birth control.

A total of 21 patients developed AMN and PAMM after the first dose of vaccination, Oxford-AstraZeneca (ChAdOx1-S (recombinant) vaccine) ($n = 12$) was the most common vaccine received by the patients in this group, followed by BNT162b2 (Pfizer Inc./BioNTech SE, Mainz, Germany) (referred to as Pfizer-BioNTech vaccine) and Sinopharm BIBP COVID-19 vaccine (referred to as Sinopharm BIBP vaccine) ($n = 5$ each), mRNA-1273 (Moderna Therapeutics Inc., Cambridge, MA, USA) (referred to as Moderna vaccine) ($n = 4$). One patient developed AMN in both eyes after Ad26.COV2.S (Janssen Pharmaceuticals, Beerse, Belgium) (referred to as Janssen Vaccine). Fourteen patients exhibited bilateral involvement in the vaccinated group, and among them, 12 had AMN and in one patient, both AMN and PAMM were described after COVID-19 vaccination. The details are provided in Table 2.

Table 2. Review of Literature of Cases with AMN and PAMM cases in patients following COVID-19 vaccinations.

Authors	Age/Sex	Duration (Days)	COVID-19 Vaccine (Dose)	Diagnosis	Laterality	Presenting Symptoms	Clinical Features	Outcome
Vinzamuri et al. [13]	35/M	30	Oxford–AstraZeneca (2)	PAMM/AMN	Both Eyes	Blurred vision, Black spots	Unremarkable	Favorable
Diafas et al. [22]	54/M	21	Pfizer–BioNTech (1)	AMN	Left Eye	Photopsia, Small scotoma	Orange–brown oval-shaped lesion superotemporal to the fovea	NA
Jalink and Bronkhorst [26]	42/F	45	Moderna (2)	AMN	Right Eye	Paracentral Scotoma	Faint, brownish circle nasal to the fovea	Favorable
Zaheer et al. [31]	22/F	5	Oxford–AstraZeneca (1)	AMN	Right Eye	Two paracentral scotomas, Flashes	Unremarkable	Stable
Afonso et al [32]	28/F	2	Oxford–AstraZeneca (1)	AMN	Both Eyes	Paracentral Scotoma	Red brown petaloid lesions around the fovea.	Slight improvement
Pichi et al. [33]	NA	5	Sinopharm BIBP (1)	AMN	Left Eye	Vision Loss	NA	Favorable
	NA	NA	Sinopharm BIBP (1)	AMN	NA	NA	NA	
	NA	1 #	Sinopharm BIBP (1)	PAMM	Left Eye	Blurring of vision, Inferior scotoma	A dot hemorrhage superior to the fovea.	NA
Patel and Yonekawa [34]	26/F	2	Janssen (1)	AMN	Both Eyes	Paracentral Scotoma	Unremarkable	NA
Bohler et al. [35]	27/F	2	Oxford–AstraZeneca (1)	AMN	Left Eye	Paracentral Scotoma	Teardrop-shaped macular lesion	NA
Book et al. [36]	21/F	3	Oxford–AstraZeneca (1)	AMN	Both Eyes	Paracentral Scotoma	Circumscribed paracentral dark lesions.	NA
Dehghani et al. [37]	38/M	14	Sinopharm BIBP (1)	PAMM	Right Eye	Flashes of light, Scotoma	Unremarkable	NA
Mambretti et al. [38]	22/F	2	Oxford–AstraZeneca (1)	AMN	Right Eye	Scotoma	Unremarkable	NA
	28/F	2	Oxford–AstraZeneca (1)	AMN	Right Eye	Paracentral scotoma	Unremarkable	NA
Bolletta et al. [39]	24/F	2	Oxford–AstraZeneca (1)	AMN	Both Eyes	Visual field defect	NA	Favorable
Ishibashi et al. [40]	33/F	8	Pfizer–BioNTech (2)	AMN	Left Eye	Field defect	Unremarkable	NA
	62/M	7	Pfizer–BioNTech (2)	PAMM	Left Eye	Visual field defect	Unremarkable	NA
Malerbi et al [41]	50+/F	30	Sinopharm BIBP (1)	PAMM	Both Eyes	Scotoma	Subtle white lesions at the macula in RE and marked lesions in LE	Favorable
Sanjay S et al. [42]	25/F	3	Oxford–AstraZeneca (1)	AMN	Both Eyes	Diminution of Vision, Scotoma	Unremarkable	NA
Drüke D et al. [43]	23/F	1	Oxford–AstraZeneca (1)	AMN	Both Eyes	Paracentral Scotoma	a subtle brownish rimmed lesion parafoveal in the right eye and a bigger blurred lesion nasal to the macula in the left eye	Favorable

Table 2. Cont.

Authors	Age/Sex	Duration (Days)	COVID-19 Vaccine (Dose)	Diagnosis	Laterality	Presenting Symptoms	Clinical Features	Outcome
Valenzuela DA et al. [44]	20/F	2	Pfizer–BioNTech (2)	AMN	Both Eyes	Photopsias, Scotomata	Unremarkable	Favorable
Rennie AT et al. [45]	21/F	3	Moderna (2)	AMN	Both Eyes	Paracentral Scotomas	Perifoveal intraretinal hemorrhage, Reddish-brown perifoveal lesions	Favorable
Bellur S et al. [46]	64/F	3	Moderna (1)	AMN	Both Eyes	Diminution of Vision	Subtle, pigmentary changes in Macula	Mild Improvement
Franchi A et al. [47]	19/F	1	Oxford–AstraZeneca (1)	AMN	Both Eyes	Sudden onset of fortifications	Large, opaque-appearing parafoveal wedge-shaped areas	Favorable
	31/F	2	Oxford–AstraZeneca (1)	AMN	Both Eyes	Sudden onset of fortifications, Paracentral Scotoma	Small opaque-appearing area superior to the fovea	Favorable
	40/F	45	Moderna (2)	AMN	Right Eye	Blurred vision, Photopsia	Pigmentary Changes	Favorable
Gabrielle PH et al. [48]	25/F	1	Oxford–AstraZeneca (1)	AMN	Both Eyes	Paracentral Scotoma, Blackspots	Unremarkable	NA
Chen S and Hodge C [49]	21/F	70	Pfizer–BioNTech (1)	AMN	Left Eye	Paracentral Scotoma	Oval parafoveal lesions	NA

M = male, F = female, AMN = acute macular neuroretinopathy, PAMM = paracentral acute middle maculopathy, # Symptoms started within 20 min of vaccination.

The cohort of patients with COVID-19 vaccination exhibited significantly early onset of AMN and PAMM when compared with the patients with SARS-CoV-2 infection (11.5 ± 17.6 days versus 37.8 ± 43.6 days; p = 0.001). One patient developed ocular symptoms within 20 min of vaccination, along with systemic symptoms such as malignant hypertension [33].

4. Discussion

Since its first description in 1975, one systemic review identified 101 cases of reports of AMN published before December 2014 [5] Our literature review shows a tremendous increase in reports of AMN and PAMM following COVID-19 infection and COVID-19 vaccinations in comparison to the previously published literature on these two clinical entities. The increase in awareness of these clinical entities and the greater use of optical coherence tomography (OCT) and other imaging such as OCT angiography (OCTA) in clinical practice are probably responsible for such an increase in these reports. Furthermore, viral flu-like illness and fever are already known systemic risk factors for AMN. In the published literature, we found a higher proportion of female patients developing AMN and PAMM. This could be attributed to a high percentage (more than 70%) of the female patients using hormone control and OCP that may have contributed to the increased risk of thromboembolic events in patients receiving COVID-19 vaccines. Therefore, due to the presence of confounding factors, our findings do not indicate that females may be more prone to developing retinal ischemic events following COVID-19 infections or vaccinations. This needs further assessment in the future studies.

It may be possible that many cases of AMN and PAMM resulting due to COVID-19 infections or vaccinations may be under-reported. There are other publicly available databases that provide information following adverse events related to vaccination, notably, the Vaccine Adverse Event Reporting System (VAERS), which is co-sponsored by the Centers of Disease Control (CDC) and the United States Food and Drug Administration

(US-FDA). The VAERS is a self-reporting system available to the general population, as well as physicians, who can enter and report adverse events related to their vaccination. Since this is a freely available resource and voluntary in nature, it does not capture all the details regarding the adverse event, and there could be events that are unreported in VAERS database. In our study, we have not performed a VAERS database search. This is because data from VAERS are not peer-reviewed, and therefore, it is inappropriate to combine it with the data obtained from published research for this manuscript. The disease manifestations of AMN and PAMM may also be very subtle in nature. Considering the self-limiting course of these two conditions and possible minimal clinical signs and symptoms, many such cases of AMN/PAMM may have been unnoticed and, hence, were not reported, leading to a reporting bias.

A significant risk of systemic thrombotic complications leading to complement-mediated thrombotic microangiopathy in SARS-CoV-2 infection is now well proven. Our review showed a higher number of PAMM cases in patients with COVID-19 infection. Patients with COVID-19 infection are, thus, at higher risk of developing the acute phase of ischemia of retinal capillary plexuses that may lead to PAMM. To add to it further, PAMM was reported in patients with pulmonary embolism [16] in association with retinal artery occlusions [8,10,12] and raised D-dimer levels [41].

Our study has various limitations including reporting bias, as stated earlier. Other limitations include lack of uniform diagnostic testing and follow-up and lack of treatment guidelines or uniformity. There may be cases where the cause-and-effect association may be weak. It is possible that there could be multiple confounding factors that could exist, leading to the development of AMN and PAMM. Due to the significant interest in the ocular and systemic effects of COVID-19 in the scientific community, it is possible that there could be a publication bias leading to a higher number of reports on AMN and PAMM following either COVID-19 infection or vaccination. The pathophysiological mechanisms of the development of deep retinal ischemia such as AMN or PAMM after vaccination (including vaccines with different mechanisms of action) and COVID-19 infection are still speculative and under investigation. Based on the available reports, it is difficult to conclude which vaccine confers a higher risk of either AMN or PAMM in the recipients.

5. Conclusions and Future Directions

In summary, both COVID-19 infection and vaccination against COVID-19 have been implicated with the development of AMN and PAMM detected using clinical examination and multimodal imaging using OCT and OCTA. The exact strength of this association, or the level of contribution of COVID-19 vaccine/infection in comparison with other risk factors such as OCP, is yet to be ascertained. Patients developing AMN or PAMM after COVID-19 vaccination tend to be younger and develop the disease within a shorter duration of time compared to those developing the disease after COVID-19 infection.

In the future, it is necessary to focus research on the true risk of ischemic events arising from both COVID-19 infections and vaccinations and if there are certain exogenous or endogenous risk factors that contribute to a higher risk of thromboembolic events compared to the general population. With a hope that the future burden of COVID-19 disease will reduce, it will become imperative to understand the real safety and efficacy of the vaccination itself and if there could be improvements in the molecular composition that may reduce adverse events attributed to the vaccine.

Author Contributions: Conceptualization P.D.M. methodology, P.D.M. and A.A.; validation, P.D.M., and A.A.; formal analysis, A.A.; data curation, AA.; writing—original draft preparation, P.D.M.; writing—review and editing, A.A. All authors have read and agreed to the published version of the manuscript.

Funding: This research received no external funding.

Institutional Review Board Statement: Ethical review and approval were waived for this study due to format of the manuscript.

Informed Consent Statement: Not applicable.

Data Availability Statement: Not applicable.

Conflicts of Interest: The authors declare no conflict of interest.

References

1. Kichloo, A.; Dettloff, K.; Aljadah, M.; Albosta, M.; Jamal, S.; Singh, J.; Wani, F.; Kumar, A.; Vallabhaneni, S.; Khan, M.Z. COVID-19 and Hypercoagulability: A Review. *Clin. Appl. Thromb.* **2020**, *26*, 1076029620962853. [CrossRef] [PubMed]
2. Sen, S.; Kannan, N.B.; Kumar, J.; Rajan, R.P.; Kumar, K.; Baliga, G.; Reddy, H.; Upadhyay, A.; Ramasamy, K. Retinal manifestations in patients with SARS-CoV-2 infection and pathogenetic implications: A systematic review. *Int. Ophthalmol.* **2022**, *42*, 323–336. [CrossRef] [PubMed]
3. Dutta Majumder, P.; Prakash, V.J. Retinal venous occlusion following COVID-19 vaccination: Report of a case after third dose and review of the literature. *Indian J. Ophthalmol.* **2022**, *70*, 2191–2194. [CrossRef] [PubMed]
4. Sim, R.; Cheung, G.; Ting, D.; Wong, E.; Wong, T.Y.; Yeo, I.; Wong, C.W. Retinal microvascular signs in COVID-19. *Br. J. Ophthalmol.* **2022**, *106*, 1308–1312. [CrossRef] [PubMed]
5. Bhavsar, K.V.; Lin, S.; Rahimy, E.; Joseph, A.; Freund, K.B.; Sarraf, D.; Cunningham, E.T. Acute macular neuroretinopathy: A comprehensive review of the literature. *Surv. Ophthalmol.* **2016**, *61*, 538–565. [CrossRef]
6. Moura-Coelho, N.; Gaspar, T.; Ferreira, J.T.; Dutra-Medeiros, M.; Cunha, J.P. Paracentral acute middle maculopathy-review of the literature. *Graefes Arch. Clin. Exp. Ophthalmol.* **2020**, *258*, 2583–2596. [CrossRef]
7. Azar, G.; Bonnin, S.; Vasseur, V.; Faure, C.; Salviat, F.; Clermont, C.V.; Titah, C.; Farès, S.; Boulanger, E.; Derrien, S.; et al. Did the COVID-19 Pandemic Increase the Incidence of Acute Macular Neuroretinopathy? *J. Clin. Med.* **2021**, *10*, 5038. [CrossRef]
8. Turedi, N.; Onal Gunay, B. Paracentral acute middle maculopathy in the setting of central retinal artery occlusion following COVID-19 diagnosis. *Eur. J. Ophthalmol.* **2022**, *32*, NP62–NP66. [CrossRef]
9. Matilde, R.; Alberto, P.; Fabio, G.; Leonardo, T.; di Geronimo, N.; Michela, F.; Costantino, S. Multitarget microangiopathy in a young healthy man with COVID-19 disease: A case report. *Indian J. Ophthalmol.* **2022**, *70*, 673–675. [CrossRef]
10. Ozsaygılı, C.; Bayram, N.; Ozdemir, H. Cilioretinal artery occlusion with paracentral acute middle maculopathy associated with COVID-19. *Indian J. Ophthalmol.* **2021**, *69*, 1956–1959. [CrossRef]
11. Gascon, P.; Briantais, A.; Bertrand, E.; Ramtohul, P.; Comet, A.; Beylerian, M.; Sauvan, L.; Swiader, L.; Durand, J.M.; Denis, D. COVID-19-Associated Retinopathy: A Case Report. *Ocul. Immunol. Inflamm.* **2020**, *28*, 1293–1297. [CrossRef]
12. Goyal, M.; Murthy, S.; Annum, S. Retinal Manifestations in Patients Following COVID-19 Infection: A Consecutive Case Series. *Indian J. Ophthalmol.* **2021**, *69*, 1275–1282. Available online: https://pubmed.ncbi.nlm.nih.gov/33913876/ (accessed on 14 September 2022). [CrossRef]
13. Vinzamuri, S.; Pradeep, T.G.; Kotian, R. Bilateral paracentral acute middle maculopathy and acute macular neuroretinopathy following COVID-19 vaccination. *Indian J. Ophthalmol.* **2021**, *69*, 2862–2864. [CrossRef] [PubMed]
14. Preti, R.C.; Zacharias, L.C.; Cunha, L.P.; Monteiro, M.L.R. Acute macular neuroretinopathy as the presenting manifestation of covid-19 infection. *Retin. Cases Brief Rep.* **2022**, *16*, 12–15. [CrossRef] [PubMed]
15. Capuano, V.; Forte, P.; Sacconi, R.; Miere, A.; Mehanna, C.-J.; Barone, C.; Bandello, F.; Souied, E.H.; Querques, G. Acute macular neuroretinopathy as the first stage of SARS-CoV-2 infection. *Eur. J. Ophthalmol.* **2022**. [CrossRef] [PubMed]
16. Naughton, A.; Ong, A.Y.; Gkika, T.; Downes, S. Bilateral paracentral acute middle maculopathy in a SARS-CoV-2-positive patient. *Postgrad. Med. J.* **2021**, *98*, e105–e106. [CrossRef]
17. Macé, T.; Pipelart, V. Acute macular neuroretinopathy and SARS-CoV-2 infection: Case report. *J. Fr. Ophtalmol.* **2021**, *44*, e519–e521. [CrossRef]
18. Aidar, M.N.; Gomes, T.M.; de Almeida, M.Z.H.; de Andrade, E.P.; Serracarbassa, P.D. Low Visual Acuity Due to Acute Macular Neuroretinopathy Associated with COVID-19: A Case Report. *Am. J. Case Rep.* **2021**, *22*, e931169. [CrossRef]
19. Padhy, S.K.; Dcruz, R.P.; Kelgaonkar, A. Paracentral acute middle maculopathy following SARS-CoV-2 infection: The D-dimer hypothesis. *BMJ Case Rep.* **2021**, *14*, e242043. [CrossRef]
20. Castro, C.S.; Ferreira, A.S.; Silva, N.P.; Lume, M.R.; Furtado, M.J. Paracentral Acute Middle Maculopathy After COVID-19 Disease: Multimodal Evaluation. *Retin. Cases Brief Rep.* **2022**, 10–1097. [CrossRef]
21. Jonathan, G.L.; Scott, F.M.; Matthew, K.D. A Case of Post-COVID-19-Associated Paracentral Acute Middle Maculopathy and Giant Cell Arteritis-Like Vasculitis. *J. Neuro-Ophthalmol.* **2021**, *41*, 351–355. [CrossRef]
22. Diafas, A.; Ghadiri, N.; Beare, N.; Madhusudhan, S.; Pearce, I.; Tan, S.Z. Comment on: "Paracentral acute middle maculopathy and acute macular neuroretinopathy following SARS-CoV-2 infection". *Eye* **2022**, *36*, 1507–1509. [CrossRef]
23. Virgo, J.; Mohamed, M. Paracentral acute middle maculopathy and acute macular neuroretinopathy following SARS-CoV-2 infection. *Eye* **2020**, *34*, 2352–2353. [CrossRef]
24. Sonmez, H.K.; Polat, O.A.; Erkan, G. Inner retinal layer ischemia and vision loss after COVID-19 infection: A case report. *Photodiagnosis Photodyn. Ther.* **2021**, *35*, 102406. [CrossRef]
25. Giacuzzo, C.; Eandi, C.M.; Kawasaki, A. Bilateral acute macular neuroretinopathy following COVID-19 infection. *Acta Ophthalmol.* **2022**, *100*, e611–e612. [CrossRef]

26. Jalink, M.B.; Bronkhorst, I.H.G. A Sudden Rise of Patients with Acute Macular Neuroretinopathy during the COVID-19 Pandemic. *Case Rep. Ophthalmol.* **2022**, *13*, 96–103. [CrossRef]
27. Zamani, G.; Ataei Azimi, S.; Aminizadeh, A.; Shams Abadi, E.; Kamandi, M.; Mortazi, H.; Shariat, S.; Abrishami, M. Acute macular neuroretinopathy in a patient with acute myeloid leukemia and deceased by COVID-19: A case report. *J. Ophthalmic Inflamm. Infect.* **2021**, *10*, 39. [CrossRef]
28. David, J.A.; Fivgas, G.D. Acute macular neuroretinopathy associated with COVID-19 infection. *Am. J. Ophthalmol. Case Rep.* **2021**, *24*, 101232. [CrossRef]
29. Masjedi, M.; Pourazizi, M.; Hosseini, N.-S. Acute macular neuroretinopathy as a manifestation of coronavirus disease 2019: A case report. *Clin. Case Rep.* **2021**, *9*, e04976. [CrossRef]
30. Deshmukh, R.; Raharja, A.; Rahman, F.; Petrushkin, H. Optical Coherence Tomography Angiography-Confirmed Paracentral Acute Middle Maculopathy Associated with SARS-COV-2 Infection. *J. Neuro-Ophthalmol. Soc.* **2021**. [CrossRef]
31. Zaheer, N.; Renju, M.P.; Chavan, R. Acute macular neuroretinopathy after COVID-19 vaccination. *Retin. Cases Brief Rep.* **2022**, *16*, 9–11. [CrossRef] [PubMed]
32. Afonso, M.G.; Marques, J.H.; Monteiro, S.; Lume, M.; Abreu, A.C.; Maia, S. Acute macular neuroretinopathy following SARS-CoV-2 vaccination. *Retin. Cases Brief Rep.* **2021**. [CrossRef]
33. Pichi, F.; Aljneibi, S.; Neri, P.; Hay, S.; Dackiw, C.; Ghazi, N.G. Association of Ocular Adverse Events with Inactivated COVID-19 Vaccination in Patients in Abu Dhabi. *JAMA Ophthalmol.* **2021**, *139*, 1131–1135. [CrossRef]
34. Patel, S.N.; Yonekawa, Y. Acute macular neuroretinopathy after SARS-CoV-2 vaccination. *Retin. Cases Brief Rep.* **2022**, *16*, 5–8. [CrossRef] [PubMed]
35. Bøhler, A.D.; Strøm, M.E.; Sandvig, K.U.; Moe, M.C.; Jørstad, Ø.K. Acute macular neuroretinopathy following COVID-19 vaccination. *Eye* **2022**, *36*, 644–645. [CrossRef]
36. Book, B.A.J.; Schmidt, B.; Foerster, A.M.H. Bilateral Acute Macular Neuroretinopathy After Vaccination Against SARS-CoV-2. *JAMA Ophthalmol.* **2021**, *139*, e212471. [CrossRef]
37. Dehghani, A.; Ghanbari, H.; Houshang-Jahromi, M.-H.; Pourazizi, M. Paracentral acute middle maculopathy and COVID-19 vaccination: Causation versus coincidence finding. *Clin. Case Rep.* **2022**, *10*, e05578. [CrossRef]
38. Mambretti, M.; Huemer, J.; Torregrossa, G.; Ullrich, M.; Findl, O.; Casalino, G. Acute Macular Neuroretinopathy following Coronavirus Disease 2019 Vaccination. *Ocul. Immunol. Inflamm.* **2021**, *29*, 730–733. [CrossRef]
39. Bolletta, E.; Iannetta, D.; Mastrofilippo, V.; De Simone, L.; Gozzi, F.; Croci, S.; Bonacini, M.; Belloni, L.; Zerbini, A.; Adani, C.; et al. Uveitis and Other Ocular Complications Following COVID-19 Vaccination. *J. Clin. Med.* **2021**, *10*, 5960. [CrossRef]
40. Ishibashi, K.; Yatsuka, H.; Haruta, M.; Kimoto, K.; Yoshida, S.; Kubota, T. Branch Retinal Artery Occlusions, Paracentral Acute Middle Maculopathy and Acute Macular Neuroretinopathy after COVID-19 Vaccinations. *Clin. Ophthalmol.* **2022**, *16*, 987–992. [CrossRef]
41. Malerbi, F.K.; Schoeps, V.A.; Matos, K.T.F. Paracentral acute middle maculopathy in Susac syndrome after dual exposure to SARS-CoV-2 antigen. *BMJ Case Rep.* **2022**, *10*, e247159. [CrossRef]
42. Sanjay, S.; Kawali, A.; Mahendradas, P. Acute macular neuroretinopathy and COVID-19 vaccination. *Indian J. Ophthalmol.* **2022**, *70*, 345–346. [CrossRef]
43. Drüke, D.; Pleyer, U.; Hoerauf, H.; Feltgen, N.; Bemme, S. Acute macular neuroretinopathy (AMN) following COVID-19 vaccination. *Am. J. Ophthalmol. Case Rep.* **2021**, *24*, 101207. [CrossRef]
44. Valenzuela, D.A.; Groth, S.; Taubenslag, K.J.; Gangaputra, S. Acute macular neuroretinopathy following Pfizer-BioNTech COVID-19 vaccination. *Am. J. Ophthalmol. Case Rep.* **2021**, *24*, 101200. [CrossRef]
45. Rennie, A.T.; DeWeerd, A.J.; Martinez, M.G.; Kay, C.N. Acute Macular Neuroretinopathy Following COVID-19 mRNA Vaccination. *Cureus* **2022**, *14*, e27502. [CrossRef]
46. Bellur, S.; Zeleny, A.; Patronas, M.; Jiramongkolchai, K.; Kodati, S. Bilateral Acute Macular Neuroretinopathy after COVID-19 Vaccination and Infection. *Ocul. Immunol. Inflamm.* **2022**, 1–4. [CrossRef]
47. Franchi, A.; Rauchegger, T.; Palme, C.; Frede, K.; Haas, G.; Blatsios, G.; Kralinger, M.; Zehetner, C. Two Cases of Acute Macular Neuroretinopathy Associated with the Adenovirus-based COVID-19 Vaccine Vaxzevria (Astrazeneca). *Ocul. Immunol. Inflamm.* **2022**, *30*, 1234–1239. [CrossRef]
48. Gabrielle, P.-H.; Baudin, F.; Ben Ghezala, I.; Meillon, C.; Bron, A.M.; Arnould, L.; Creuzot-Garcher, C. Bilateral acute macular neuroretinopathy in a young woman after the first dose of Oxford-AstraZeneca COVID-19 vaccine. *Am. J. Ophthalmol. Case Rep.* **2022**, *25*, 101281. [CrossRef]
49. Chen, S.; Hodge, C. Comment on: "Acute macular neuroretinopathy following COVID-19 vaccination". *Eye* **2022**, *36*, 1513–1514. [CrossRef]

Disclaimer/Publisher's Note: The statements, opinions and data contained in all publications are solely those of the individual author(s) and contributor(s) and not of MDPI and/or the editor(s). MDPI and/or the editor(s) disclaim responsibility for any injury to people or property resulting from any ideas, methods, instructions or products referred to in the content.

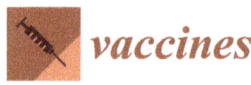

Review

Corneal Adverse Events Associated with SARS-CoV-2/COVID-19 Vaccination: A Systematic Review

Lana Kuziez [1], Taher K. Eleiwa [2], Muhammad Z. Chauhan [3], Ahmed B. Sallam [3], Abdelrahman M. Elhusseiny [3,*] and Hajirah N. Saeed [4,5,6,*]

1. Saint Louis University School of Medicine, St. Louis, MO 63104, USA
2. Department of Ophthalmology, Benha University, Benha 13518, Egypt
3. Department of Ophthalmology, Harvey and Bernice Jones Eye Institute, University of Arkansas for Medical Sciences, Little Rock, AR 72205, USA
4. Department of Ophthalmology, Illinois Eye and Ear Infirmary, University of Illinois at Chicago, Chicago, IL 60661, USA
5. Department of Ophthalmology, Massachusetts Eye and Ear, Harvard Medical School, Boston, MA 02114, USA
6. Department of Ophthalmology, Loyola University Medical Center, Maywood, IL 60611, USA
* Correspondence: amelhusseiny@uams.edu (A.M.E.); hnsaeed@uic.edu (H.N.S.)

Abstract: Vaccines against coronavirus disease 2019 (COVID-19) have played an important global role in reducing morbidity and mortality from COVID-19 infection. While the benefits of vaccination greatly outweigh the risks, adverse events do occur. Non-ocular adverse effects of the vaccines have been well-documented, but descriptions of ophthalmic effects remain limited. This systematic review aims to provide an overview of reported cases of corneal adverse events after receiving vaccination against COVID-19 and to compile existing clinical data to bring attention to these phenomena. Our review discusses corneal graft rejection, including proposed mechanisms, herpetic keratitis, and other reported corneal complications. Ophthalmologists and primary care physicians should be aware of such possible associations.

Keywords: coronavirus; COVID-19 vaccine; corneal complications; corneal graft rejection; keratoplasty; keratitis; viral keratitis; herpes zoster; herpes simplex; vaccination

Citation: Kuziez, L.; Eleiwa, T.K.; Chauhan, M.Z.; Sallam, A.B.; Elhusseiny, A.M.; Saeed, H.N. Corneal Adverse Events Associated with SARS-CoV-2/COVID-19 Vaccination: A Systematic Review. *Vaccines* **2023**, *11*, 166. https://doi.org/10.3390/vaccines11010166

Academic Editor: Rohan Bir Singh

Received: 17 December 2022
Revised: 9 January 2023
Accepted: 10 January 2023
Published: 12 January 2023

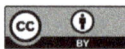

Copyright: © 2023 by the authors. Licensee MDPI, Basel, Switzerland. This article is an open access article distributed under the terms and conditions of the Creative Commons Attribution (CC BY) license (https://creativecommons.org/licenses/by/4.0/).

1. Introduction

Severe acute respiratory syndrome coronavirus 2 (SARS-CoV-2) is a highly transmissible virus that caused the coronavirus disease 2019 (COVID-19) pandemic. COVID-19 is known to have multisystem effects ranging from respiratory failure to coagulopathy [1]. More recently, ophthalmic manifestations of the infection have been identified and include conjunctivitis, scleritis, cranial nerve palsies, orbital inflammatory disease, and various posterior segment diseases [2–4]. The first vaccine against SARS-CoV-2 was made available in late 2020 under emergency authorization by the United States (U.S.) Food and Drug Administration. Since then, various vaccine types have been distributed globally, more than 12 billion doses have been administered, and 67% of the world population has received at least one dose. Despite copious data showing vaccination to be the most effective intervention in mitigating the spread of COVID-19, hesitancy to receive the vaccine continues both in the U.S. and globally, citing low trust in the science and the safety of vaccines [5]. As with almost any intervention, acute adverse effects do occur with SARS-CoV-2 vaccination and have largely been reported to be those common to vaccination in general, though more serious adverse effects may also be associated [6]. Organ-specific adverse events are largely limited to case series and case reports. Case reports and retrospective case series have described possible associations between the administration of the SARS-CoV-2 vaccine and the onset of ophthalmic complications involving the eyelid, orbit, cornea, retina, and other ocular structures [7–15]. There are numerous reports of corneal complications in particular. In this review, we aim to summarize the literature regarding corneal adverse events following SARS-CoV-2 vaccination and address concerns regarding vaccination.

2. Methods

We performed a systematic review of all appropriate literature guided by the Preferred Reporting Items for Systematic Reviews and Meta-Analysis Statement (PRISMA) [16]. We performed a search of all English-language literature on PubMed, searching for publications that matched the search terms "coronavirus", "COVID-19", "SARS-CoV-2", or "severe acute respiratory syndrome", and "cornea" or "corneal", and "vaccine".

The search yielded case reports, case series, systematic reviews, literature reviews, and correspondences. All publications between 1 July 2021 and 1 November 2022 were included. These dates include the first described adverse effects of the SARS-CoV-2 vaccine since its first use in December 2020 to the time of this review. We included all case reports, case series, and correspondences that presented new patient data and reviewed corneal involvement of post-vaccination complications. All systematic reviews, literature reviews, meta-analyses, or replies to the author that did not present new patient data were excluded. One publication was further excluded, as it described the adverse effects of a non-SARS-CoV-2 vaccine. The references of remaining publications were reviewed for inclusion as well. The full texts of all remaining literature were screened and included if any corneal involvement was described. In total, of 93 results meeting search terms and within the desired dates, 32 were excluded based on publication type, one was further excluded due to its description of reactions to a different vaccine, and 15 were excluded due to having no described corneal involvement. In total, 45 publications met the criteria for inclusion (Figure 1). Data collected included age, sex, vaccine type, vaccine dose, the interval from vaccination to symptoms, and treatment. Where appropriate, the manifestations, corneal transplant type, time from transplant to vaccination, and corneal transplant outcomes were recorded. Continuous variables were reported using the mean, standard deviation, and range.

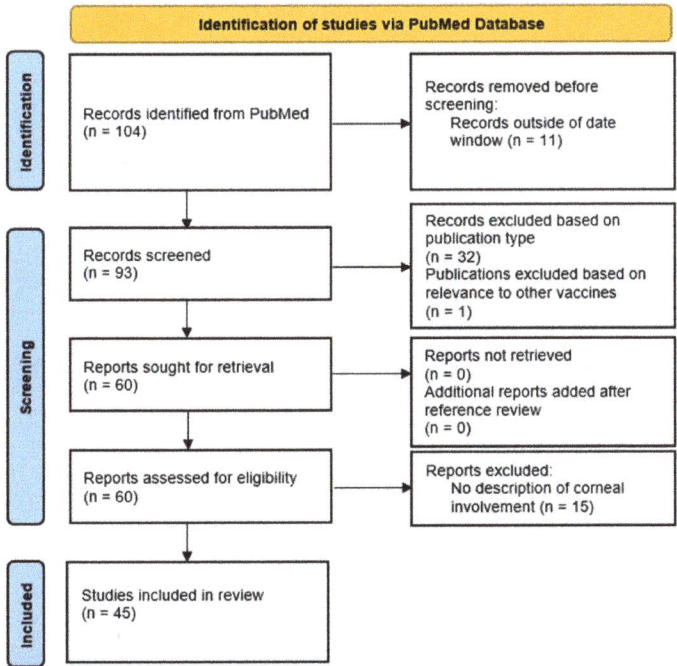

Figure 1. PRISMA flow diagram for this systematic review of the literature.

Cases were categorized based on the described corneal pathology. The quality of studies was evaluated using criteria published by the Task Force for Reporting Adverse Events of the International Society for Pharmacoepidemiology (ISPE) and the International Society of Pharmacovigilance (ISoP) [17]. The criteria include 12 elements: title, demographic, medical history, health status, physical examination, drug identification, dosage, administration/drug reaction interface (representing the interval), concomitant therapies, adverse event, and discussion. Publications were scored 1 point for containing an element and 0 points for the absence of an element. Therefore, publications with all criteria were given 12 points.

3. Results

In review, we identified 45 publications describing corneal complications associated with SARS-CoV-2 vaccination. Twenty publications described corneal graft rejection, 19 described herpetic corneal disease, and 6 case reports described unique corneal pathology. These studies included 90 eyes of 82 patients. In total, we reviewed data for 36 eyes (33 patients) with corneal graft rejection, 46 eyes (43 patients) with herpetic corneal disease, 2 eyes (1 patient) with corneal melting, 2 eyes (1 patient) with corneal edema, 2 eyes (2 patients) with limbal stem cell transplant rejection, 1 eye with peripheral ulcerative keratitis, and 1 eye with marginal keratitis. Information for each case of corneal graft rejection and herpetic keratitis are presented in Tables 1 and 2, respectively. Of note, herpetic disease often refers to herpes simplex or herpes zoster. However, one case, as described later, discusses a case with suspected infection from cytomegalovirus, HSV, or VZV, all part of the herpesvirus family; viral keratitis of another etiology has not been reported in this population. As such, we have referred to all instances of viral keratitis in this review as herpetic keratitis. Furthermore, cases of keratitis associated with herpes simplex are referred to as herpes simplex keratitis (HSK), while cases associated with herpes zoster are referred to as herpes zoster keratitis (HZK); however, HZK with cutaneous V1 dermatomal involvement is referred to as herpes zoster ophthalmicus (HZO).

Table 1. Patient information from reviewed case reports and case series of corneal graft rejection.

Source	Age and Sex	Vaccine and Dose	Vaccine Interval Days *	Transplant Interval *	Type of Transplant	Side	Treatment and Outcome
Abousy et al., 2021 [18]	73 F	BNT162b2 #2	4	8 y	DSAEK	OD	Topical prednisolone and hypertonic ointment; resolution
						OS	
Balidis et al., 2021 [19]	77 F	mRNA-1273 #1	7	12 m	DMEK	OS	Topical, subconjunctival, and IV dexamethasone; improvement on the exam, no further follow-up
	64 F	mRNA-1273 #2	7	3 y	PKP	OD	Topical and intracameral dexamethasone; no improvement and additional interventions NR
	69 M	AZD1222 #1	5	22 m	PKP	OD	Subconjunctival and topical dexamethasone, oral methylprednisolone; resolution
	63 M	AZD1222 #1	10	9 m	DSAEK	OS	Topical dexamethasone; no improvement and additional interventions NR
Crnej et al., 2021 [20]	71 M	BNT162b2 #1	7	5 m	DMEK	OD	Topical dexamethasone and oral valacyclovir; resolution
Eduarda Andrade et al., 2022 [21]	40 M	BNT162b2 #1	6	23 y	PKP	OD	Oral prednisone, topical prednisolone, and subconjunctival dexamethasone; resolution
Forshaw et al., 2022 [22]	94 F	BNT162b2 #1	14	24 m	DMEK	OS	Topical dexamethasone, tobramycin, and hypertonic saline; no improvement, repeat DMEK performed in both eyes
				20 m	DMEK	OD	
Marziali et al., 2022 [23]	15 M	BNT162b2 #1	12	18 m	PKP	OD	Topical dexamethasone; resolution

Table 1. Cont.

Source	Age and Sex	Vaccine and Dose	Vaccine Interval Days *	Transplant Interval *	Type of Transplant	Side	Treatment and Outcome
Mohammadzadeh et al., 2022 [24]	36 F	BBIBP-CorV #1	2	4 y	PKP	OS	Topical betamethasone; improvement on the exam, no further follow-up
	54 F	BBIBP-CorV #1	7	2 y	PKP	OS	Topical betamethasone; resolution
Molero-Senosiain et al., 2022 [25]	72 F	BNT162b2 #1	14	4 y	DSAEK	OD	Topical dexamethasone; resolution
	82 F	BNT162b2 #1	14	4 y	DSAEK	OD	Topical steroid (steroid type NR); resolution
	55 M	AZD1222 #1	7	13 y	PKP	OD	Topical steroid (steroid type NR); resolution
	61 M	AZD1222 #2	30	20 y	PKP	OD	Topical steroid (steroid type NR) and IV methylprednisolone; resolution
	48 F	BNT162b2 #1	30	4 y	PKP	OS	Topical dexamethasone; resolution
Nahata et al., 2022 [26]	28 F	AZD1222 #1	14	11 y	FLEK	OS	Topical prednisolone and homatropine and oral methylprednisolone; resolution
Nioi et al., 2021 [27]	44 F	BNT162b2 #1	13	25 y	PKP	OS	Topical dexamethasone and vitamin D supplementation; resolution
Park et al., 2022 [28]	64 M	AZD1222 #1	2	1 y	DSAEK	OS	Topical and oral steroids (steroid types were NR); resolution
Parmar et al., 2021 [29]	35 M	AZD1222 #1	4	6 m	PKP	OS	Topical prednisolone, topical atropine, and IV methylprednisolone; resolution
Phylactou et al., 2021 [30]	66 F	BNT162b2 #1	7	14 d	DMEK	OD	Topical dexamethasone; resolution
	83 F	BNT162b2 #2	21	6 y	DMEK	OD / OS	Topical dexamethasone; improvement of VA and on the exam, no further follow-up
Rajagopal and Priyanka, 2022 [31]	79 M	AZD1222 #2	42	4 y	PKP	OS	Topical steroids and oral steroids (steroid types were NR); resolution
Rallis et al., 2022 [32]	68 F	BNT162b2 #1	4	4 m	PKP	OS	Topical dexamethasone and oral acyclovir; resolution
Ravichandran and Natarajan, 2021 [33]	62 M	AZD1222 #1	21	2 y	PKP	OD	NR
Shah et al., 2022 [34]	74 M	mRNA-1273 #1	7	3 m	DMEK	NR	Topical prednisolone; improvement of VA and on the exam, no further follow-up
	61 F	mRNA-1273 #2	7	2.5 y	PKP	NR	Topical prednisolone; improvement of VA and on the exam, no further follow-up
	69 F	mRNA-1273 #2	14	6 y	DSAEK	OS	Topical prednisolone and difluprednate; improvement of VA and on the exam, no further follow-up
	77 M	mRNA-1273 #2	7	22 y	PKP	NR	Topical prednisolone; resolution
Simão et al., 2022 [35]	63 F	CoronaVac #1	1	7 y	PKP	OS	Topical dexamethasone, timolol, bimatoprost, and polydimethylsiloxane; no improvement and additional interventions NR
Wasser et al., 2021 [36]	72 M	BNT162b2 #1	13	1 y	PKP	OS	Topical dexamethasone and oral prednisone; resolution
	56 M	BNT162b2 #1	12	25 y	PKP	OD	Topical dexamethasone and oral prednisone; resolution
Yu et al., 2022 [37]	51 M	mRNA-1273 #1	3	3 w	PKP	OD	Topical steroids (steroid type NR); no improvement and additional interventions NR

* Vaccine interval days = days from reported vaccine to presentation or start of symptoms, transplant interval = time from transplant to vaccination, VA = visual acuity, M = male, F = female, NR = not reported, y = year, m = month, w = week, d = day, OD = right eye, OS = left eye, DSAEK = Descemet's membrane and automated endothelial keratoplasty, PKP = penetrating keratoplasty, DMEK = Descemet's membrane endothelial keratoplasty, FLEK = femtosecond laser-assisted endothelial keratoplasty.

Table 2. Overview of reported cases of reactivation or recurrence of viral infections and initial herpetic keratitis.

Source	Age and Sex	Vaccine and Dose	Interval Days *	Eye	Diagnosis (Manifestation)	History of Previous Herpetic Keratitis	Treatment
Al-Dwairi et al., 2022 [38]	50 M	BNT162b2 #1	5	OS	HSK (reduced corneal sensation, dendritic ulcers, ciliary injection, AC cells)	Yes	Topical ACV, moxifloxacin, FML, and oral ACV
Alkhalifa et al., 2021 [39]	42 M	NR #1	4	OD	HSK (conjunctival injection, corneal infiltrate with stromal melting, corneal thinning, descemetocele)	Yes	Oral ACV
	29 F	NR #1	28	OS	HSK (epithelial defect and stromal edema, KP)	Yes	Oral ACV, topical ACV, and FML
Alkwikbi et al., 2022 [40]	18 F	BNT162b2 #2	7	OD	HSK (conjunctival hyperemia, dendritic ulcers, KPs, AC cells)	Yes	topical GCV and lubricant drops
	40 M	BNT162b2 #2	7	OD	HSK (dendritic ulcers)	Yes	topical GCV and oral ACV
	32 M	AZD1222 #2	7	OD	HSK (corneal edema, ciliary congestion, dendritic ulcers)	Yes	oral prednisone and topical cyclopentolate
	29 M	BNT162b2 #2	7	OS	HSK (conjunctival injection, stromal infiltration, dendritic ulcers)	Yes	Topical GCV gel and oral ACV
Bolletta et al., 2021 [41]	83 M	BNT162b2 #2	7	OS	Herpetic keratitis, unspecified (manifestation NR)	Yes	Topical ACV
	79 M	AZD1222 #1	5	OD	Herpetic keratitis, unspecified (manifestation NR)	Yes	Oral VCV, topical dexamethasone
	65 F	BNT162b2 #2	6	OS	Herpetic keratitis, unspecified (manifestation NR)	Yes	Oral VCV, topical dexamethasone
Cohen et al., 2022 [42]	81 F	BNT162b2 #2	3	OD	HZO (Vesicular V1 rash, KPs, conjunctival hyperemia)	Yes	Oral VCV, topical dexamethasone, and cyclopentolate
	74 F	BNT162b2 #3	21	OS	HZO (stromal and epithelial edema, KPs)	Yes	Oral VCV and prednisone, topical dexamethasone, and tropicamide
	63 M	BNT162b2 #3	7	OD	HSK (stromal opacity, Descemet folds, KPs, AC inflammation)	No	Oral ACV, topical dexamethasone, and cyclopentolate

Table 2. Cont.

Source	Age and Sex	Vaccine and Dose	Interval Days *	Eye	Diagnosis (Manifestation)	History of Previous Herpetic Keratitis	Treatment
Fard et al., 2022 [43]	52 M	BNT162b2 #2	1	OD	Herpetic keratitis, unspecified; likely HSK based on the history of recurrent HSK (stromal haze, punctate epithelial erosions)	Yes	Oral ACV, topical trifluridine, and prednisolone
	67 F	mRNA-1273 #1	NR	OS	Herpetic keratitis, unspecified; likely HZK given the history of HZO (epithelial defect without infiltrate)	Yes	Bandage contact lens, oral VCV, and topical FML
Lazzaro et al., 2022 [44]	46 M	BNT162b2 #1	1	OS	HZO (corneal infiltrates, pseudodendrites, vesicular V1 rash)	Yes	Oral VCV and topical GCV
Li et al., 2021 [45]	60 F	CoronaVac #1	2	OD	HSK (dendritic ulcers)	Yes	Topical GCV
	51 M	CoronaVac #2	NR	OS	HZK (corneal edema, Descemet fold, KP, AC inflammation)	No	oral and topical GCV
Mishra et al., 2021 [46]	71 M	NR #1	10	OD	HZK (panuveitis, KP, AC cells and flare, circumcorneal conjunctival congestion)	No	Oral VCV and steroids, topical steroids, intravitreal GCV
Mohammadpour et al., 2022 [47]	30 F	BBIBP-CorV #	14	OS	Herpetic keratitis, unspecified (central corneal opacity and stromal infiltration)	No	Oral VCV, topical betamethasone
Murgova and Balchev, 2022 [48]	56 M	AZD1222 #2	7	OD	Herpetic keratitis, unspecified (paracentral corneal thinning)	Yes	Topical and oral ACV, oral methyl-prednisolone
	89 F	BNT162b2 #2	21	OS	Herpetic keratitis, unspecified (ciliary injection, KPs, AC flare)	Yes	Topical methyl-prednisolone and para-bulbar methylpred-nisolone injections
Pang et al., 2022 [49]	43 F	NR #2	7	OD	Herpetic keratitis, unspecified (manifestations NR)	NR	Topical GCV, tobramycin, and dexamethasone
	55 F	CoronaVac #2	7	OS	Herpetic keratitis, unspecified; likely HSK based on exam findings (dendritic ulcers)	NR	Topical GCV and cyclosporine
	45 F	NR #1	1	OD	Herpetic keratitis, unspecified; likely HZO based on exam findings (conjunctival congestion, corneal ulcer, vesicular V1 rash)	NR	IV GCV, topical GCV, and cyclosporine
	19 M	NR #2	14	OU	Herpetic keratitis, unspecified (manifestations NR)	NR	IV GCV, topical GCV, and cyclosporine

Table 2. Cont.

Source	Age and Sex	Vaccine and Dose	Interval Days *	Eye	Diagnosis (Manifestation)	History of Previous Herpetic Keratitis	Treatment
Rallis et al., 2022 [50]	47 F	AZD1222 #1	4	OS	HSK (anterior uveitis, endotheliitis)	Yes	Oral ACV and topical GCV
	48 M	AZD1222 #1	3	OD	HSK (dendritic ulcers, anterior uveitis)	Yes	Oral ACV and topical GCV
	59 M	AZD1222 #1	4	OU	HSK (OD: dendritic ulcers, OS: geographic ulcer)	No	Oral ACV and topical GCV
	44 M	AZD1222 #1	7	OD	HSK (dendritic ulcers, anterior uveitis)	Yes	Oral ACV and topical GCV
	59 F	AZD1222 #1	5	OD	HZK (pseudodendrites, endotheliitis, anterior uveitis)	Yes	Oral ACV and topical GCV
	65 M	BNT162b2 #1	27	OD	HZO (pseudodendrites, endotheliitis, anterior uveitis, vesicular V1 rash)	No	Oral ACV and topical GCV
	95 M	BNT162b2 #1	25	OS	HZO (pseudodendrites, vesicular V1 rash, anterior uveitis)	No	Oral ACV and topical GCV
	89 M	BNT162b2 #1	13	OS	HZO (pseudodendrites, vesicular V1 rash)	No	Oral ACV and topical GCV
	68 M	BNT162b2 #1	28	OD	HZO (pseudodendrites, vesicular V1 rash)	No	Oral ACV and topical GCV
	87 F	BNT162b2 #1	7	OD	HZO (pseudodendrites, vesicular V1 rash)	No	Oral ACV and topical GCV
Rehman et al., 2022 [51]	35 M	AZD1222 #NR	3	OS	HZO (pinpoint fluorescein-positive lesions, circumcorneal congestion, vesicular V1 rash)	No	Oral VCV, topical ACV, moxifloxacin, and carboxymethylcellulose
	40 M	AZD1222 #NR	28	OS	HZO (conjunctival congestion, vesicular V1 rash)	No	Oral VCV and topical moxifloxacin
Richardson-May et al., 2021 [52]	82 M	AZD1222 #1	1	OS	HSK (reduced corneal sensation, dendritic ulcers)	Yes	Oral ACV and doxycycline, topical GCV, prednisolone, atropine, moxifloxacin
Ryu and Kim, 2022 [53]	87 M	BNT162b2 #2	2	OS	HZK (corneal edema, stromal infiltration, corneal neovascularization, KPs)	Yes	Oral VCV and topical prednisolone
Shan et al., 2022 [54]	19 M	CoronaVac #2	21	OU	Suspected herpetic keratitis (conjunctival hyperemia, rough corneal epithelium, patchy corneal infiltration)	NR	IV GCV and topical GCV, and cyclosporine

Table 2. Cont.

Source	Age and Sex	Vaccine and Dose	Interval Days *	Eye	Diagnosis (Manifestation)	History of Previous Herpetic Keratitis	Treatment
Song et al., 2021 [55]	30 F	BNT162b2 #1	7	OD	HZK (stromal and endothelial infiltration, corneal edema)	Yes	Topical GCV and loteprednol etabonate
You et al., 2022 [56]	74 M	BNT162b2 #2	5	OS	HZK (conjunctival hyperemia, pseudodendrite) and meningitis	No	IV ACV, topical ACV, and levofloxacin

* Interval days = days from reported vaccination to presentation with symptoms, M = male, F = female, OD = right eye, OS = left eye, OU = both eyes, HSK = herpes simplex keratitis, HZO = herpes zoster ophthalmicus, HZK = herpes zoster keratitis, KP = keratic precipitates, AC = anterior chamber, ACV = acyclovir, VCV = valacyclovir, GCV = ganciclovir, FML = fluorometholone, IV = intravenous.

Patients received mRNA, viral vector, or inactivated vaccines, including the CoronaVac (Sinovac Biotech Ltd., Beijing, China), BBIBP-CorV (Sinopharm, Beijing, China), AZD1222 (AstraZeneca, Cambridge, UK), mRNA-1273 (ModernaTX, Inc., Cambridge, MA, USA), and BNT162b2 (BioNTech, Mainz, Germany) vaccines.

The mean quality score of the 45 publications was 11.4 out of 12 possible points. Twenty-five scored 12 points, fourteen scored 11, five scored 10, and one scored 9 (Table 3). Indication of current health status and concomitant therapies were the most commonly missed elements.

Table 3. Quality scores based on criteria per Task Force for Reporting Adverse Events.

Source	Title	Demographic	Current Health Status	Medical History	Physical Examination	Patient Disposition	Drug Identification	Drug Dosage	Drug Reaction Interface	Concomitant Therapies	Adverse Events	Discussion	Total Points
Abousy et al., 2021 [18]	✔	✔	✔	✔	✔	✔	✔	✔	✔		✔	✔	11
Al-Dwairi et al., 2022 [38]	✔	✔	✔	✔	✔	✔	✔	✔	✔	✔	✔	✔	12
Alkhalifa et al., 2021 [39]	✔	✔	✔	✔	✔	✔	✔	✔	✔	✔	✔	✔	12
Alkwikbi et al., 2022 [40]	✔	✔		✔	✔	✔	✔	✔		✔	✔	✔	10
Balidis et al., 2021 [19]	✔	✔	✔	✔	✔	✔	✔	✔	✔	✔	✔	✔	12
Bolletta et al., 2021 [41]	✔	✔	✔	✔	✔	✔	✔	✔	✔	✔	✔	✔	12
Cohen et al., 2022 [42]	✔	✔	✔	✔	✔	✔	✔	✔	✔	✔	✔	✔	12
Crnej et al., 2021 [20]	✔	✔	✔	✔	✔	✔	✔	✔	✔		✔	✔	11
de la Presa et al., 2022 [57]	✔	✔	✔	✔	✔	✔	✔	✔	✔	✔	✔	✔	12
Eduarda Andrade et al., 2022 [21]	✔	✔	✔	✔	✔	✔	✔	✔	✔	✔	✔	✔	12
Fard et al., 2022 [43]	✔	✔	✔	✔	✔	✔	✔	✔	✔	✔	✔	✔	12
Farrell et al., 2022 [58]	✔	✔	✔	✔	✔	✔	✔	✔	✔	✔	✔	✔	12
Forshaw et al., 2022 [22]	✔	✔	✔	✔	✔	✔	✔	✔	✔	✔	✔	✔	12
Gouveau et al., 2022 [59]	✔	✔	✔	✔	✔	✔	✔	✔	✔	✔	✔	✔	12
Khan et al., 2021 [60]	✔	✔	✔	✔	✔	✔	✔	✔	✔	✔	✔	✔	12

Table 3. Cont.

Source	Title	Demographic	Current Health Status	Medical History	Physical Examination	Patient Disposition	Drug Identification	Drug Dosage	Drug Reaction Interface	Concomitant Therapies	Adverse Events	Discussion	Total Points
Lazzaro et al., 2022 [44]	✔	✔		✔	✔	✔	✔	✔	✔		✔	✔	10
Lee and Han, 2022 [61]	✔	✔	✔	✔	✔	✔	✔	✔	✔	✔	✔	✔	12
Li et al., 2021 [45]	✔	✔	✔	✔	✔	✔	✔	✔	✔	✔	✔	✔	12
Marziali et al., 2022 [23]	✔	✔	✔	✔	✔	✔	✔	✔	✔	✔	✔	✔	12
Mishra et al., 2021 [46]	✔	✔	✔	✔	✔	✔	✔	✔	✔		✔	✔	11
Mohammadopur et al., 2022 [47]	✔	✔	✔	✔	✔	✔	✔		✔	✔	✔	✔	11
Mohammadzadeh et al., 2022 [24]	✔	✔	✔	✔	✔	✔	✔	✔	✔	✔	✔	✔	12
Molero-Senosiain et al., 2022 [25]	✔	✔	✔	✔	✔	✔	✔	✔	✔	✔	✔	✔	12
Murgova and Balchev, 2022 [48]	✔	✔		✔	✔	✔	✔	✔	✔		✔	✔	10
Nahata et al., 2022 [26]	✔	✔	✔	✔	✔	✔	✔	✔	✔	✔	✔	✔	12
Nioi et al., 2021 [27]	✔	✔	✔	✔	✔	✔	✔	✔	✔		✔	✔	11
Pang et al., 2022 [49]	✔	✔		✔	✔	✔		✔	✔		✔	✔	9
Park et al., 2022 [28]	✔	✔	✔	✔	✔	✔	✔	✔	✔		✔	✔	11
Parmar et al., 2021 [29]	✔	✔	✔	✔	✔	✔	✔	✔	✔	✔	✔	✔	12
Penbe, 2022 [62]	✔	✔		✔	✔	✔	✔	✔	✔	✔	✔	✔	11
Phylactou et al., 2021 [30]	✔	✔	✔	✔	✔	✔	✔	✔	✔	✔	✔	✔	12
Rajagopal and Priyanka, 2022 [31]	✔	✔	✔	✔	✔	✔	✔	✔	✔		✔	✔	11
Rallis et al., 2021 [32]	✔	✔	✔	✔	✔	✔	✔	✔	✔	✔	✔	✔	12
Rallis et al., 2022 [50]	✔	✔	✔	✔	✔	✔	✔	✔	✔	✔	✔	✔	12
Ravichandran and Natarajan 2021 [33]	✔	✔	✔	✔	✔	✔		✔	✔	✔	✔	✔	11
Rehman et al., 2022 [51]	✔	✔	✔	✔	✔	✔	✔		✔	✔	✔	✔	11
Richardson-May et al., 2021 [52]	✔	✔		✔	✔	✔	✔	✔	✔		✔	✔	10
Ryu and Kim, 2022 [53]	✔	✔	✔	✔	✔	✔	✔	✔	✔		✔	✔	11
Shah et al., 2022 [34]	✔	✔	✔	✔	✔	✔	✔	✔	✔	✔	✔	✔	12
Shan et al., 2022 [54]	✔	✔		✔	✔	✔	✔	✔	✔		✔	✔	10
Simao et al., 2022 [35]	✔	✔	✔	✔	✔	✔	✔	✔	✔	✔	✔	✔	12
Song et al., 2021 [55]	✔	✔	✔	✔	✔	✔	✔	✔	✔		✔	✔	11
Wasser et al., 2021 [36]	✔	✔	✔	✔	✔	✔	✔	✔	✔	✔	✔	✔	12
You et al., 2022 [56]	✔	✔	✔	✔	✔	✔	✔	✔	✔		✔	✔	11
Yu et al., 2022 [37]	✔	✔	✔	✔	✔	✔	✔	✔	✔		✔	✔	11

4. Corneal Graft Rejection

Of the 45 publications we reviewed, 20 described acute corneal graft rejection in 36 eyes of 33 patients. Of the 33 patients, 16 were male, and 17 were female. The mean age was 60.1 ± 16.3 years (median: 63.5; range: 15–94). Acute rejection occurred following the patient's first dose of the vaccine in 26 (72%) eyes and after the patient's second dose in 10 (28%) eyes. There were no reports of rejection after any booster doses. Among all patients, 1 (1 eye, 3%) received the CoronaVac vaccine, 2 (2 eyes, 6%) received the BBIBP-CorV vaccine, 9 (9 eyes, 25%) received the AZD1222 vaccine, 7 (7 eyes, 19%) received the mRNA-1273 vaccine, and 14 (17 eyes, 37%) received the BNT162b2 vaccine. The time from the most recent vaccine to presentation was 11.2 ± 0.4 days (median: 8.5; range: 1–42). Cases were mostly represented by unilateral rejection in the setting of a single graft; however, there were three cases of bilateral corneal graft rejection.

Various keratoplasty techniques were reported, including penetrating keratoplasty (PKP), Descemet's stripping (automated) endothelial keratoplasty (DSAEK), Descemet's membrane endothelial keratoplasty (DMEK), and femtosecond laser-assisted endothelial keratoplasty (FLEK). After reviewing the most recent keratoplasty procedure among the 36 eyes, we found 20 eyes (55.6%) to have undergone a PKP, 1 eye (2.8%) a FLEK, 8 eyes (22.2%) a DMEK, and 7 eyes (19.4%) a DSAEK. The time from the most recent keratoplasty to the reported rejection episode was a mean of 6.2 years and ranged from 14 days to 25 years with a median of 3.5 years. Notably, the standard deviation of the interval time data was greater than the mean, indicating a high variation in the data.

The outcomes of the rejection episodes were mixed. Twenty-two eyes (36%) had resolution, 7 eyes (19%) had improvement, and 6 eyes (17%) had no improvement. The outcome was not reported for 1 eye. Of the 20 eyes that underwent PKP, 14 (70%) had resolution, 2 (10%) had improvement with no further descriptions of the disease course, and 3 (15%) had no improvement (1 outcome was unreported). Of the 8 eyes that underwent DMEK, 2 (25%) had resolution, 4 (50%) had improvement with no further descriptions of disease course, and 2 (25%) had no improvement. Seven eyes underwent DSAEK, and 5 (71%) had resolution; improvement was seen in 1 eye (14%) with no further descriptions of the disease course, and no improvement was seen in 1 eye (14%). Resolution was reported for the one eye that underwent FLEK. Analysis of outcomes by vaccine dose revealed a greater incidence of resolution in patients who had rejection after the first dose versus the second. Among 26 eyes that had rejection after the first vaccine, 18 (69%) had resolution, 3 (12%) had improvement, and 4 (15%) had no improvement; among 10 eyes with rejection after their second dose, 5 (50%) eyes had resolution, 4 (40%) had improvement, and 1 (10%) had no improvement. Comparisons of outcomes by vaccine type demonstrated a similar incidence of resolution in the groups that received the AZD1222 vaccine (7 of 9 eyes, 78%) and the BNT162b2 vaccine (13 of 17 eyes, 76%). The incidence of resolution was lower for the groups that received the BBIBP-CorV (1 of 2 eyes, 50%), mRNA-1273 (1 of 7 eyes, 14%), and the CoronaVac (0 of 1 eye, 0%) vaccines.

Molero-Senosiain et al. reported on five patients who presented symptoms within 1 month of vaccination. One case involved a 72-year-old female with a history of Fuchs endothelial dystrophy (FED) requiring three DSAEKs in her right eye, and three PKPs, and one DSAEK in her left eye, with the most recent surgeries being a DSAEK in the right eye and a PKP in the left, five and eight years prior to presentation, respectively. The authors did not report any underlying risk factors for the multiple graft failures that the patient had [25]. Fourteen days after her first dose of the BNT162b2 vaccine, she presented with blurred vision and a visual acuity (VA) of 20/80 in the right eye. Prior to this episode, she had poor VA in her left eye (counting fingers) due to a failed PKP and a VA of 20/50 in her right eye. Examination revealed graft edema in only the right eye. There were no keratic precipitates (KPs) or anterior chamber reaction. Resolution was achieved by increasing the frequency of her pre-rejection maintenance treatment of topical dexamethasone, and her final VA was 20/60. The second case was an 82-year-old woman with a similar history of FED requiring DSAEK of the right eye four years prior. She presented 14 days following the BNT162b2 vaccine with blurred vision and a reduction in VA from her baseline of 20/40 to 20/100. On exam, she had an edematous graft without KPs and no anterior chamber reaction. Resolution was achieved with topical steroids, and VA improved to 20/60. The remaining three cases in this series involved a 55-year-old male, 61-year-old male, and 48-year-old female, all with a history of keratoconus that was treated with PKP and with pre-rejection VAs of 20/66, 20/100, and 20/45 which worsened to counting fingers, 20/350, and counting fingers, respectively. They all reported blurred vision following the administration of the AZD1222 vaccine. Although all eyes presented with corneal edema, two eyes also had Descemet's membrane folds, one had KPs, and one had an anterior chamber reaction. Treatment for all patients involved topical steroids, although one patient needed intravenous (IV) methylprednisolone after a poor response to topical steroids. All patients achieved reversal of rejection and improvement in vision (20/100 for the female patient and 20/125 for the others).

Similar cases of acute rejection have been reported by Shah et al. in patients receiving the mRNA-1273 vaccine. In their case series, they describe four patients who received the vaccine and developed signs of rejection within two weeks of administration [34]. A 74-year-old male who had a DMEK for pseudophakic bullous keratopathy three months prior and was compliant with once-daily topical fluorometholone reported blurred vision following his first vaccination dose. The exam was significant for a VA of 20/60 from a baseline of 20/25 an endothelial rejection line, KPs, Descemet folds, and corneal edema with a central corneal thickness (CCT) of 743 µm. Within two days of every-2-h prednisolone use, the CCT decreased to 705 µm. He had his second vaccine dose while continuing topical prednisolone and did not experience further complications; after several weeks, his vision improved to 20/40, and CCT further decreased to 655 µm. The authors described another case of a 69-year-old woman with FED requiring bilateral DSAEK 6 years prior and with a pre-rejection VA of 20/25. She presented with a worsening vision in her left eye 14 days after her second dose of the mRNA-1273 vaccine. Slit lamp exam showed conjunctival injection, anterior chamber reaction, and stromal edema (CCT 719 µm) of the left eye; the right eye examination was unremarkable other than the presence of an intact DSAEK graft. Within 3 weeks of topical difluprednate initiation, her VA improved from 20/50 at presentation to 20/30, and there was a resolution of the anterior chamber cell and improvement of stromal edema (CCT 633 µm). The remaining two cases described in this series included a 61-year-old female and a 77-year-old male with a history of a PKP 2.5 and 22 years prior, respectively, and baseline VA of 20/40 and 20/25, respectively. Both patients reported declining vision 1 week after their second dose of the mRNA-1273 vaccine. The exam revealed VA of 20/80 and 20/60 in the affected eyes, respectively, and corneal graft edema, conjunctival inflammation, and KPs in both patients. An endothelial rejection line was also seen in one patient and an anterior chamber reaction in the other. Both patients received topical prednisolone for several weeks with an improvement of VA to 20/60 and 20/40, respectively, and resolution of graft edema, KPs, and conjunctival inflammation. In this series, Shah et al. presented four cases that suggest a temporal association between the mRNA SARS-CoV-2 vaccine and acute corneal graft rejection while recognizing the need for wider population-based and comparative studies to investigate the incidence of graft rejection and any association with SARS-CoV-2 vaccination.

In their case series, Balidis et al. described four cases that responded variably to treatment [19]. They reported on a 77-year-old woman who underwent a DMEK for pseudophakic bullous keratopathy 20 months prior and had three episodes of graft rejection within eight months of transplantation; two episodes were associated with HSK. The third episode required escalation to systemic steroid therapy and coverage for herpetic keratitis; ultimately, the graft failed. After regrafting, the patient continued topical corticosteroids and oral antivirals. At her 12-month appointment post-regraft, her graft was noted to be the clearest since the transplant was performed. Soon after, she received the mRNA-1273 vaccine and noticed blurred vision 7 days later; her exam revealed KPs and corneal edema. Subconjunctival dexamethasone, topical corticosteroids, and hypertonic eye drops did not improve the rejection episode, and she required IV dexamethasone. Improvement was noted at the four-week mark. The authors also reported on a 64-year-old woman with a history of PKP for keratoconus 2 years prior with no complications and a CCT of 470 μm at baseline. One week after the patient's second dose of the mRNA-1273 vaccine, she experienced blurred vision. Anterior chamber reaction and stromal edema (CCT 585 μm) were noted on slit-lamp examination. Topical and intracameral dexamethasone did not achieve resolution, and the edema persisted after four weeks of therapy; the authors did not report any additional interventions. Patient three in this series was a 69-year-old male who underwent PKP of the right eye 22 months prior for post-herpetic corneal scarring. He received the first dose of the AZD1222 vaccine and experienced reduced vision five days later in that eye (VAs not reported). The exam revealed KPs and corneal edema (CCT 757 μm). Treatment involved subconjunctival dexamethasone injections, oral methylprednisolone, and topical dexamethasone. Stromal edema initially did not improve but did so after 8 weeks of treatment (CCT 660 μm). Finally, the authors presented a 63-year-old male with a history of DSAEK of the left eye for FED and repeated DSAEK 9 months prior to presentation due to graft failure. His blurred vision began 10 days after the first dose of the AZD1222 vaccine, with VA reduced to counting fingers at one meter from 20/40 at baseline. Again, corneal edema and KPs were seen. Treatment with topical dexamethasone was begun, but the edema persisted at the 3-week follow-up visit. The authors did not report any further follow-up.

Similar reports of acute graft rejection in patients with various keratoplasty types, variable times since procedure, and repeat graft histories have been made [18,20,26,27,31,33,35–37]. In all cases that reported treatment, patients were treated with topical steroids; in some cases, oral steroids, intracameral dexamethasone, subconjunctival dexamethasone, or IV steroids were used concurrently or subsequently. Despite undergoing prescribed treatment, five total patients reported by Yu et al., Simão et al., Forshaw et al., and Balidis et al. ultimately had graft failure following SARS-CoV-2 vaccination [19,22,35,37]. Yu et al. described a 51-year-old male patient who had acute rejection 3 weeks post-PKP [37]. He was receiving topical steroids but ultimately had graft failure and progression of glaucoma in the setting of increased steroid use. Simão et al. presented a patient who had acute PKP graft rejection after vaccination which improved with topical dexamethasone. After her second dose of the CoronaVac vaccine, she returned with the same clinical presentation; the same treatment was repeated with no recovery, and ultimately had graft failure. Lastly, Forshaw et al. reported on a 94-year-old female with bilateral DMEK rejection 14 days after receiving a SARS-CoV-2 vaccine (unspecified type) [22]. Treatment with topical dexamethasone/tobramycin and hypertonic saline failed to improve her corneal edema. She received a repeat DMEK in both eyes with an overall improved corneal clarity. The remaining two cases were described by Balidis et al. as above.

Discussion

Corneal transplantation is among the most common and successful solid organ transplantations [63]. While rejection is understood to be rare following vaccination in general, the phenomenon is likely underreported [45,64]. A survey of cornea specialists in 2021 revealed at least 34 anecdotal keratoplasty rejection episodes related to vaccines, but that same study also noted that only four articles describing a total of 12 cases of an association between recent vaccination and corneal transplant rejection had been published over 30 years [65]. High-quality studies on the association between vaccines and corneal graft rejection have not been done, and the evidence is thus far inconclusive. While no formal pathophysiologic link has been made between the two, a review of post-vaccination corneal graft rejection revealed associations between rejection and influenza, tetanus, hepatitis B, yellow fever, recombinant zoster, and SARS-CoV-2 vaccines [64].

Our literature review revealed 33 cases (36 eyes) of corneal graft rejection after SARS-CoV-2 vaccination, more reported cases than with any other vaccine. There are many biases that may account for this difference, but it is a difference that has not been prospectively explored and one that needs further study. On the other hand, Busin et al. examined 77 diagnosed cases of rejection among 2062 patients that received corneal transplants between January 2018 and December 2021 [66]. They found no notable increase in the number of eyes with graft rejection in 2021 when vaccination was widely implemented. In further analysis, the authors compared the incidence of graft rejection in the "risk period" (the first 60 days after vaccination) versus the incidence outside of the risk period. They found no significant increase in the incidence of rejection within the risk period. Additionally, they analyzed rejection data for patients who received a cornea transplant before receiving their SARS-CoV-2 vaccine and those who received a transplant after the vaccine and again found no significant differences. Similarly, a multi-country study by Roberts et al. found no increase in the number of corneal graft rejection cases diagnosed per month after vaccination programs were widely implemented versus in the periods prior to lockdowns and during lockdowns [67]. The data presented by both Busin et al. and Roberts et al. do not support an association between SARS-CoV-2 vaccination and corneal graft rejection. However, all published data together provide insight into the need for analysis on a greater scale to establish vaccine safety in patients with corneal grafts.

Based on the limited dataset in this review, it appears that rejection was less likely to fully resolve after DMEK as compared to PKP or DSAEK. This is an association that warrants further study, but may be due to the often lower dosage and potency of topical steroid regimen post-DMEK as compared to other forms of corneal transplantation. Clinicians should be aware of a possible association between SARS-CoV-2 vaccination and corneal graft rejection, report associations when found and take this into consideration in clinical management. It is important to note the high degree of reversibility of corneal graft rejection with appropriate management and re-emphasize the benefit of SARS-CoV-2 vaccination for individuals and communities. Clinicians may consider increasing topical steroid use in the peri-vaccination period as a relatively low-risk potentially prophylactic measure to mitigate graft rejection.

The cornea is among the few tissues in the body that have immune privilege. The unique avascular anatomy as well as the absence of lymphatic tissue within the cornea prevent access by the immune system. Additionally, the corneal layers express low amounts of major histocompatibility complexes (MHC) I and II, limiting the immune response against antigens. Regulatory T cells (Tregs) have an important role in downregulation of immune responses in the cornea. Expression of surface molecules on these cells, including cytotoxic T lymphocyte antigen-4, programmed cell death ligand-1, and forkhead box protein 3 (Foxp3), as well as secretion of interleukin-10 and transforming growth factor-β work to suppress immune activation by inhibiting activities of antigen presenting cells and CD4+ T cells and inhibiting interferon gamma production [63,68,69]. While dendritic cells exist in the central and peripheral cornea, they are suppressed by interleukin-1 receptor antagonist expressed in the cornea, further reinforcing the cornea's exclusion from immune surveillance [68]. These mechanisms and others promote survival of corneal allografts. It has been hypothesized that the immune system activation and dysregulation occurring after vaccination may threaten these barriers and expose the corneal graft and foreign antigens to the immune system, mediating rejection [70].

Cross-reactivity between the SARS-CoV-2 antigen and MHC-antigen complexes has been proposed as a mechanism for acute rejection following SARS-CoV-2 vaccination. The BNT162b2 and the mRNA-1723 vaccines are lipid-encapsulated mRNA molecules encoding the spike protein, which is the target antigen for the humoral immune response. After vaccination, anti-spike protein titers are elevated. At this time, antibodies that are cross-reactive with corneal graft donor molecules may produce an immune response, thereby mediating rejection [30]. Another proposed mechanism is based on observed corneal responses during states of inflammatory stress. In response to stress, MHC class II and co-stimulatory molecule expression is induced in corneal epithelial cells and dendritic cells. Such inflammatory stress may be induced after vaccination and lead to allosensitization by presentation of donor antigens [68]. Similarly, inflammation within the host bed has been demonstrated to decrease the expression of Foxp3 in Tregs and disrupt differentiation of Tregs, potentially weakening the multiple mechanisms for immune modulation by Tregs [71]. Furthermore, SARS-CoV-2 vaccines elicit strong humoral and cellular immune responses, as seen with other vaccines, including a Th1-biased CD4+ response. CD4+ Th1 cells are mediators of corneal graft rejection and may play a role here [32,72].

Another possible mechanism may include an immune reaction to vaccination adjuvants, which are used to enhance the body's immune response and lower the frequency and amount of vaccine needed to obtain adequate preventive immunity [49].

5. Herpetic Keratitis

Of the literature included in this review, 19 publications described the occurrence of herpetic keratitis after SARS-CoV-2 vaccination in 46 eyes of 43 patients. Twenty-six patients (60.4%) were male. Mean age was 55.7 ± 21.3 years (median: 55; range: 18–95). One patient (1 eye, 2%) received the mRNA1273 vaccine, 1 patient (1 eye, 2%) received the BBIBP-CorV vaccine, 22 patients (22 eyes, 48%) received the BNT162b2 vaccine, 4 patients (5 eyes, 11%) received the CoronaVac vaccine, and 12 patients (13 eyes, 28%) received the AZD1222 vaccine. Vaccine type was not recorded for 3 patients (4 eyes, 9%). Symptoms began an average of 9.5 ± 8.4 days (median 7; range 1–28) after vaccination in the 41 patients for which this interval was reported. Vaccination to symptom interval was not reported for 2 patients (2 eyes). Twenty-one patients (22 eyes, 49%) reported symptoms after their first vaccine, 17 patients (19 eyes, 33%) had symptoms exclusively after their second vaccine, and 2 patients (2 eyes, 5%) had symptoms after their third vaccination/booster. Three patients (4 eyes, 9%) had symptom recurrence after receiving a subsequent vaccine dose. Vaccine dose number was unreported for 3 patients. Fourteen patients (15 eyes, 33%) were diagnosed with herpes simplex keratitis (HSK) while 16 patients (16 eyes, 35%) were diagnosed with herpes zoster keratitis (HZK/HZO). Six studies involving 15 eyes of 13 patients did not specify which type of herpes virus infection was diagnosed, although based on history and exam it is likely that two of these eyes were HSK and two were HZK. Additionally, 25 patients (25 eyes, 54%) had a known history of herpetic keratitis prior to presentation for acute reactivation or recurrence of disease following vaccination.

All cases of herpetic keratitis (HK) with reported outcomes had improvement or resolution. Of the 41 eyes with reported outcomes, 24 (59%) had resolution and 17 (41%) had improvement. Of the 13 eyes with HSK and reported outcomes, 7 (54%) had resolution and 6 (46%) had improvement. Among 16 eyes diagnosed with HZK/HZO, 9 eyes (56%) had resolution and 7 (44%) had improvement. In the group diagnosed with HK after the first vaccine dose (22 eyes), 15 (68%) had resolution and 7 (32%) had improvement. In the group with HK after the second vaccine dose (14 eyes), 9 eyes (64%) had improvement and 5 eyes (36%) had resolution. Resolution was seen in the 2 eyes with HK after the third vaccine dose (100%). Among the 22 eyes with HK after receiving the BNT162b2 vaccine, 11 (52%) had resolution and 10 (48%) had improvement (outcome was unreported for 1 eye). Of the 13 eyes that had HK after receiving the AZD1222 vaccine, 8 (67%) had resolution and 4 (33%) had improvement (outcome was unreported for 1 eye). Five eyes had HK after receiving the CoronaVac vaccine and 2 (40%) had resolution while 3 (60%) had improvement. One eye with HK after receiving the BBIBP-CorV vaccine had resolution after treatment.

Al-Dwairi et al. described a case of a 50-year-old man with a history of PKP of the left eye for corneal opacity from a previous episode of herpetic keratitis years prior [38]. He received pre- and post-operative subconjunctival anti-vascular endothelial growth factor injections and had been on oral acyclovir and topical prednisolone for over a year until 7 months before his presentation. He presented almost two years post-operatively with redness, tearing, and pain in his left eye following vaccination one week prior with the BNT162b2 vaccine. The examination was significant for multiple dendritic ulcers in the graft with ciliary injection and anterior chamber cells consistent with recurrence of HSK. He ultimately had resolution of the ulcers after topical acyclovir and moxifloxacin as well as lubricant eye drops for 2 weeks. Li et al. presented a similar case of a 60-year-old woman with a history of PKP for corneal scarring due to HSK [45]. She had no episodes of acute rejection or keratitis until two days after receiving the inactivated CoronaVac vaccine. Characteristic dendritic ulcers were seen on slit lamp examination. Treatment with topical ganciclovir and discontinuation of topical steroids resolved the recurrent HSK in two weeks. The patient went on to receive her second dose of the vaccine while using topical ganciclovir without any issues.

Several cases of HZK after SARS-CoV-2 vaccination have also been reported. You et al. presented a unique case of VZV reactivation and meningitis in a 74-year-old male who initially presented with headache, forehead pain, left eyelid swelling, and photophobia [56]. He had had the second dose of the BNT162b2 vaccine 5 days prior. On exam, skin lesions involved the ophthalmic distribution of the trigeminal nerve. Ocular exam revealed pseudodendrites of the cornea, conjunctival chemosis, and hyperemia. Further investigation of the headache involved cerebrospinal fluid studies which were indicative of meningitis due to VZV. He received IV acyclovir, topical acyclovir, and topical levofloxacin. He had improvement within 3 days. Twenty days after discharge, he returned with a central epithelial defect of the same eye. Treatment was initiated with a bandage contact lens and a topical solution of ofloxacin and recombinant human epithelial growth factor. Over two months, the epithelium healed and at 6 months, exam findings were stable with some stromal haze.

Shan et al. presented a case of a 19-year-old man with no ophthalmic history who developed a suspected herpetic keratitis after both the second and third dose of the CoronaVac vaccine [54]. He initially presented three weeks after his second dose with blurred vision in both eyes and was treated with topical ganciclovir and levofloxacin but had no relief. He was later admitted for worsening symptoms and exam findings of conjunctival hyperemia, irregular corneal epithelium, and patchy corneal infiltrates. He received IV ganciclovir, topical ganciclovir, and topical cyclosporine. Within 1 week, his symptoms resolved, and exam findings and vision were improved. He received the third dose of the CoronaVac vaccine 18 months later with a recurrence of the same symptoms; exam findings were consistent with those of the previous episode. He again received topical ganciclovir and topical cyclosporine. He also received oral acyclovir and ganciclovir. At the follow-up one week later, his exam had improved, symptoms resolved, and VA returned to 20/20. Unique to this case is the recurrence of corneal disease with repeat vaccination suggesting an association between the vaccine and viral reactivation in the cornea.

Of the 14 patients with HSV reactivation, 12 had a previous history of HSK. Of the two cases with no previous HSK history, one developed into recurrent HSK after its manifestation after both the first and second doses of the vaccine. In their case series, Rallis et al. included the case of a 59-year old-male with no history of herpetic ocular disease who developed bilateral keratitis 4 days after receiving the AZD1222 vaccine [50]. Exam revealed right sided corneal dendrites and a geographic ulcer of the left eye. He received topical ganciclovir and topical corticosteroids, and oral acyclovir. Complete resolution was noted after two weeks. After his second dose of the AZD1222 vaccine, he had recurrence of herpetic keratitis. No further treatment or follow-up was reported. In contrast, of the 16 patients with HZK, only 6 had a previous history of HZK or HZO. Patients with no history of herpetic keratitis had a mean age of 56 ± 22.8 years (median 57; range 19–95); 28% were female, and 72% were male. Among patients with recurrent herpetic keratitis, the mean age was 55.6 ± 20.6 years (median 53; range 18–89); 48% were female and 52% were male. Other cases of reactivation and recurrence of HSV and VZV as described in Table 2, involved typical presentations of such infections. Treatment for herpetic keratitis included topical antivirals, oral antivirals, or a combination of both with or without additional agents.

Interestingly, a recent study using the Centers for Disease Control and Prevention Vaccine Adverse Events Reporting System demonstrated a temporal association between vaccine-associated uveitis (VAU) and SARS-CoV-2 vaccination. Among 491 patients diagnosed with VAU, 249 (20.76%) had herpes ophthalmicus (unspecified) [9]. They also noted that the benefits of vaccination outweigh the risks of VAU but that physicians should be aware of this association.

Discussion

The reported adverse effects of the SARS-CoV-2 vaccines have included the reactivation of viral diseases, particularly herpes simplex and herpes zoster. In addition to other cutaneous reactions, McMahon et al. described 4 cases of herpes simplex flares and 10 cases of herpes zoster from among 414 reported cutaneous effects of the SARS-CoV-2 vaccine within an international database [73]. Ozdemir et al. similarly reported herpes zoster in two healthy young patients following vaccination [74]. Additional literature presents similar cases of reactivation of latent herpetic infection after vaccination [75]. In their review of the Vaccine Adverse Events Reporting System, Gringeri et al. identified 5934 cases of herpes zoster and 273 of herpes simplex infection after receiving the BNT162b2 vaccine [76]. These cases included 60 (1.01%) cases of "ophthalmic herpes zoster" and 6 (2.20%) cases of "ophthalmic herpes simplex". They found a reporting odds ratio of 1.49 for herpes zoster and 1.51 for herpes simplex. Barda et al. found a similar risk ratio for herpes zoster of 1.43, but an unremarkable risk ratio for herpes simplex infection for the same vaccine [77]. However, Shasha et al. found a risk ratio for herpes zoster that was inconclusive for the same vaccine [78]. Conflicting evidence in the literature regarding the SARS-CoV-2 vaccines and their potential effects on latent viral disease reveals the need for further research.

In herpetic infections of the trigeminal distribution in general, the virus resides in the trigeminal ganglion after primary infection. Reactivation along the ophthalmic branch can cause corneal disease. Little is known about the potential pathogenesis of herpetic reactivation after SARS-CoV-2 vaccines, and it is unclear what role the vaccines may have on recurrent versus new-onset herpetic keratitis. Known triggers of herpes virus reactivation are induced in severe COVID-19 infections, including fever and physical stress and may be implicated in the case of vaccination [79]. It has been hypothesized that lymphopenia and lymphocyte exhaustion during the course of a severe COVID-19 infection may also contribute to reactivation [80,81]. Additionally, in the post-vaccination state, stimulation of the immune system is induced, involving increases in T-helper type 1 CD4+ and CD8+ cells. This stimulation in cellular immunity may cause a shift of naïve CD8+ cells, overwhelming the ability of virus-specific CD8+ cells to control the latent virus [82]. An additional hypothesis describes the response of toll-like receptor (TLR) signaling to vaccination against COVID-19. TLRs are known to be involved in the reactivation process of herpes viruses and serve to maintain the latency of the virus in the host. Vaccination also stimulates the release of inflammatory cytokines, which induce T and B cell immune responses but disturb antigen expression, lowering the threshold for reactivation [80,83].

6. Others

A single case of corneal melt after SARS-CoV-2 vaccination was reported in the literature by Khan et al. [60]. They presented the case of a 48-year-old man with a two-week history of blurred vision, photophobia, pain, and watering in both eyes. He had received the first dose of the AZD1222 vaccine 3 weeks before the start of his symptoms. On exam, he had conjunctival and ciliary congestion, with corneal melt, uveal tissue prolapse, and bilateral massive choroidal detachments found on B-scan ultrasonography. Workup for underlying autoimmune or infectious etiologies was negative. Ultimately, the patient required PKP in both eyes.

A case of bilateral corneal edema was reported by Lee and Han [61]. A 55-year-old female with a history of uneventful cataract surgery two months prior presented with sudden visual disturbance and ocular pain six days after receiving the AZD1222 vaccine. Her vision at presentation had worsened from 20/20 at baseline to 20/30 bilaterally. Slit-lamp examination revealed mild bilateral corneal edema with a CCT of the right and left eyes of 580 µm and 594 µm, respectively. Endothelial cell density was 2849/mm^2 in the right eye and 2778/mm^2 in the left eye. After two weeks of topical prednisolone use, her vision improved to 20/25 bilaterally, and the corneal edema had resolved in the right eye with minimal residual edema of the left eye; CCTs improved to 553 µm and 579 µm of the right and left eyes, respectively.

Marginal keratitis as an adverse effect was reported in one case by Farrell et al. [58]. A 66-year-old female presented with worsening right eye pain and redness 2.5 weeks after receiving the first dose of the mRNA-1273 vaccine. She self-medicated with antibiotic eye drops from symptom onset with no improvement. On exam, the right eye had a significant conjunctival injection, infiltrates of the cornea, and peripheral corneal vascularization. There were no epithelial defects, anterior chamber abnormalities, or discharge. The left eye was unremarkable. She was diagnosed with marginal keratitis of the right eye and started topical antibiotics and corticosteroids and had improvement within several days.

Gouveau et al. and de la Presa et al. have reported on patients experiencing rejection of limbal allografts following SARS-CoV-2 vaccination. The first by Gouveau et al. described a 72-year-old male with a history of chemical injury and subsequent keratolimbal allograft of the right eye (KLAL) 6.5 years prior; he had an uneventful post-operative course and later had a PKP and cataract extraction/intraocular lens implantation 15 months and 3.5 years after the KLAL, respectively [59]. He tolerated his medication regimen of oral tacrolimus, topical prednisolone, dorzolamide-timolol, and cyclosporine well His tacrolimus dosage was eventually decreased, and his subsequent lab work showed subtherapeutic tacrolimus levels. On routine follow-up 1 month after receiving the second dose of the BNT162b2 vaccine, he was noted to have chemosis as well as perilimbal engorgement and tortuous vessels. However, there was no corneal edema, KPs, anterior chamber reaction, or epithelial rejection line. The patient declined oral steroids and was started on topical difluprednate and tacrolimus, and his oral tacrolimus dosage was increased. Within 4 months, the KLAL segments showed improvement. In their similar case study, de la Presa et al. presented a 27-year-old with a history of limbal-stem cell deficiency secondary to contact lens use and subsequent living-related conjunctival limbal allograft (LR-CLAL) of her right eye approximately 4.5 years prior [57]. She was maintained on mycophenolate mofetil (MMF) and topical prednisolone for years with no noted complications at her regular follow-up appointments. However, 15 days after receiving the first dose of the mRNA-1273 vaccine, she presented with redness and irritation in her right eye. Exam revealed conjunctival hyperemia sparing the LR-CLAL graft and an epithelial rejection line along the limbus with no corneal infiltrates or edema. She was started on topical difluprednate, and oral prednisone, and her MMF was increased. Her symptoms improved over several days, and by two weeks, improvements were seen on the exam (fading epithelial rejection line and resolution of hyperemia). She received the second dose of the vaccine while still on increased topical and systemic immunosuppression with no complications.

Lastly, Penbe described a single case of peripheral ulcerative keratitis in a 76-year-old man with a history of PKP of the left eye 10 years prior who presented with right eye pain and blurred vision two weeks after receiving the CoronaVac vaccine [62]. On presentation, he had peripheral stromal infiltration spanning 180 degrees, corneal necrosis from the temporal limbus to the visual axis, and nodular scleritis of the right eye. The left eye had no acute changes but was opaque from the previous pathology. Work-up for autoimmune etiology was negative. He was empirically treated with IV methylprednisolone and topical moxifloxacin, dexamethasone, cyclosporine, cyclopentolate, flurbiprofen, and autologous serum drops. He was later transitioned to oral prednisone, azathioprine, and doxycycline. He received several amniotic membrane grafts over 5 weeks, and the corneal defect resolved. However, his VA had improved minimally from finger counting at 10 cm at presentation to finger counting at one meter. In the setting of an opaque left corneal graft, the decision to pursue PKP was ultimately made to restore vision to 20/100. In the postoperative follow-up 4 weeks later, the right eye corneal graft was clear.

7. Conclusions

Since efforts directed toward vaccinating the global population against COVID-19 began in 2021, cases of ophthalmologic adverse events occurring in the post-vaccination period have been reported. In this review, we presented cases of corneal complications following SARS-CoV-2 vaccination and discussed mechanisms theorized to be involved in acute corneal graft rejection and herpetic keratitis post-vaccination. Despite the 66 cases reviewed here, a causal relationship between the two events cannot be definitively established; more data are needed to better understand the potential interactions of the vaccine with the cornea and its effect on immune response. More data are also needed to make any correlations between ocular outcomes after COVID-19-associated corneal graft rejection and herpetic keratitis, and the variables described by the ISPE and the ISoP, including medical and medication history. Regardless, the benefits of vaccination appear to outweigh the risks and in the absence of new evidence suggesting otherwise, ophthalmologists should continue to recommend vaccination against COVID-19 for patients. At the same time, patients who have a history of corneal transplantation or herpetic keratitis should be closely monitored after vaccination and should be counseled on the signs and symptoms of graft rejection and herpetic reactivation, respectively.

Author Contributions: Conceptualization, A.M.E.; methodology, A.M.E.; formal analysis, L.K., T.K.E. and M.Z.C.; investigation, L.K.; resources, A.M.E. and L.K.; data curation, L.K.; writing—original draft preparation, L.K., A.M.E. and H.N.S.; writing—review and editing, H.N.S., A.B.S. and A.M.E.; visualization, L.K. All authors have read and agreed to the published version of the manuscript.

Funding: This research received no external funding.

Institutional Review Board Statement: Not applicable.

Informed Consent Statement: Not applicable.

Data Availability Statement: Not applicable.

Conflicts of Interest: The authors declare no conflict of interest.

References

1. Roberts, C.M.; Levi, M.; McKee, M.; Schilling, R.; Lim, W.S.; Grocott, M.P.W. COVID-19: A complex multisystem disorder. *Br. J. Anaesth.* **2020**, *125*, 238–242. [CrossRef] [PubMed]
2. Hu, K.; Patel, J.; Swiston, C.; Patel, B.C. Ophthalmic Manifestations Of Coronavirus (COVID-19). In *StatPearls*; StatPearls Publishing: Treasure Island, FL, USA, 2022.
3. Eleiwa, T.; Abdelrahman, S.N.; ElSheikh, R.H.; Elhusseiny, A.M. Orbital inflammatory disease associated with COVID-19 infection. *J. AAPOS* **2021**, *25*, 232–234. [CrossRef]
4. Eleiwa, T.K.; Elmaghrabi, A.; Helal, H.G.; Abdelrahman, S.N.; ElSheikh, R.H.; Elhusseiny, A.M. Phlyctenular Keratoconjunctivitis in a Patient With COVID-19 Infection. *Cornea* **2021**, *40*, 1502–1504. [CrossRef]
5. Lazarus, J.V.; Wyka, K.; White, T.M.; Picchio, C.A.; Rabin, K.; Ratzan, S.C.; Parsons Leigh, J.; Hu, J.; El-Mohandes, A. Revisiting COVID-19 vaccine hesitancy around the world using data from 23 countries in 2021. *Nat. Commun.* **2022**, *13*, 3801. [CrossRef] [PubMed]
6. Demasi, M. FDA urged to publish follow-up studies on COVID-19 vaccine safety signals. *BMJ* **2022**, *379*, o2527. [CrossRef] [PubMed]
7. Haseeb, A.A.; Solyman, O.; Abushanab, M.M.; Abo Obaia, A.S.; Elhusseiny, A.M. Ocular Complications Following Vaccination for COVID-19: A One-Year Retrospective. *Vaccines* **2022**, *10*, 342. [CrossRef]
8. Eleiwa, T.K.; Gaier, E.D.; Haseeb, A.; ElSheikh, R.H.; Sallam, A.B.; Elhusseiny, A.M. Adverse Ocular Events following COVID-19 Vaccination. *Inflamm. Res.* **2021**, *70*, 1005–1009. [CrossRef]
9. Singh, R.B.; Singh Parmar, U.P.; Kahale, F.; Agarwal, A.; Tsui, E. Vaccine-associated uveitis following SARS-CoV-2 vaccination: A CDC-VAERS database analysis. *Ophthalmology* **2022**. [CrossRef]
10. Ng, X.L.; Betzler, B.K.; Testi, I.; Ho, S.L.; Tien, M.; Ngo, W.K.; Zierhut, M.; Chee, S.P.; Gupta, V.; Pavesio, C.E.; et al. Ocular Adverse Events after COVID-19 Vaccination. *Ocul. Immunol. Inflamm.* **2021**, *29*, 1216–1224. [CrossRef]
11. Wang, M.T.M.; Niederer, R.L.; McGhee, C.N.J.; Danesh-Meyer, H.V. COVID-19 Vaccination and The Eye. *Am. J. Ophthalmol.* **2022**, *240*, 79–98. [CrossRef]
12. ElSheikh, R.H.; Haseeb, A.; Eleiwa, T.K.; Elhusseiny, A.M. Acute Uveitis following COVID-19 Vaccination. *Ocul. Immunol. Inflamm.* **2021**, *29*, 1207–1209. [CrossRef] [PubMed]

13. Fujio, K.; Sung, J.; Nakatani, S.; Yamamoto, K.; Iwagami, M.; Fujimoto, K.; Shokirova, H.; Okumura, Y.; Akasaki, Y.; Nagino, K.; et al. Characteristics and Clinical Ocular Manifestations in Patients with Acute Corneal Graft Rejection after Receiving the COVID-19 Vaccine: A Systematic Review. *J. Clin. Med.* **2022**, *11*, 4500. [CrossRef] [PubMed]
14. Elnahry, A.G.; Al-Nawaflh, M.Y.; Gamal Eldin, A.A.; Solyman, O.; Sallam, A.B.; Phillips, P.H.; Elhusseiny, A.M. COVID-19 Vaccine-Associated Optic Neuropathy: A Systematic Review of 45 Patients. *Vaccines* **2022**, *10*, 1758. [CrossRef] [PubMed]
15. Singh, R.B.; Li, J.; Parmar, U.P.S.; Jeng, B.H.; Jhanji, V. Vaccine-associated corneal graft rejection following SARS-CoV-2 vaccination: A CDC-VAERS database analysis. *Br. J. Ophthalmol.* **2022**. [CrossRef] [PubMed]
16. Moher, D.; Shamseer, L.; Clarke, M.; Ghersi, D.; Liberati, A.; Petticrew, M.; Shekelle, P.; Stewart, L.A.; Group, P.-P. Preferred reporting items for systematic review and meta-analysis protocols (PRISMA-P) 2015 statement. *Syst. Rev.* **2015**, *4*, 1. [CrossRef] [PubMed]
17. Kelly, W.N.; Arellano, F.M.; Barnes, J.; Bergman, U.; Edwards, I.R.; Fernandez, A.M.; Freedman, S.B.; Goldsmith, D.I.; Huang, K.; Jones, J.K.; et al. Guidelines for submitting adverse event reports for publication. *Pharmacoepidemiol. Drug Saf.* **2007**, *16*, 581–587. [CrossRef]
18. Abousy, M.; Bohm, K.; Prescott, C.; Bonsack, J.M.; Rowhani-Farid, A.; Eghrari, A.O. Bilateral EK Rejection after COVID-19 Vaccine. *Eye Contact. Lens* **2021**, *47*, 625–628. [CrossRef]
19. Balidis, M.; Mikropoulos, D.; Gatzioufas, Z.; de Politis, P.B.; Sidiropoulos, G.; Vassiliadis, V. Acute corneal graft rejection after anti-severe acute respiratory syndrome-coronavirus-2 vaccination: A report of four cases. *Eur. J. Ophthalmol.* **2021**, 11206721211064033. [CrossRef]
20. Crnej, A.; Khoueir, Z.; Cherfan, G.; Saad, A. Acute corneal endothelial graft rejection following COVID-19 vaccination. *J. Fr. Ophtalmol.* **2021**, *44*, e445–e447. [CrossRef]
21. Eduarda Andrade, E.A.M.; Rodrigues, J.C.; Junior, E.F.; de Lima, M.H.C. Keratoplasty rejection after messenger RNA vaccine (BNT162b2) for COVID-19. *Indian. J. Ophthalmol.* **2022**, *70*, 3134–3136. [CrossRef]
22. Forshaw, T.R.J.; Jorgensen, C.; Kyhn, M.C.; Cabrerizo, J. Acute Bilateral Descemet Membrane Endothelial Keratoplasty Graft Rejection after the BNT162b2 mRNA COVID-19 Vaccine. *Int. Med. Case Rep. J.* **2022**, *15*, 201–204. [CrossRef] [PubMed]
23. Marziali, E.; Pasqualetti, R.; Bacci, G.; de Libero, C.; Caputo, R. Acute Rejection Following COVID-19 Vaccination in Penetrating Keratoplasty in a Young Male—A Case Report and Review of Literature. *Ocul. Immunol. Inflamm.* **2022**, 1–4. [CrossRef] [PubMed]
24. Mohammadzadeh, M.; Hooshmandi, S.; Jafari, M.; Hassanpour, K. Presumably Corneal Graft Rejection after COVID-19 Vaccination. *Case Rep. Ophthalmol.* **2022**, *13*, 562–569. [CrossRef] [PubMed]
25. Molero-Senosiain, M.; Houben, I.; Savant, S.; Savant, V. Five Cases of Corneal Graft Rejection after Recent COVID-19 Vaccinations and a Review of the Literature. *Cornea* **2022**, *41*, 669–672. [CrossRef]
26. Nahata, H.; Nagaraja, H.; Shetty, R. A case of acute endothelial corneal transplant rejection following immunization with ChAdOx1 nCoV-19 coronavirus vaccine. *Indian J. Ophthalmol.* **2022**, *70*, 1817–1818. [CrossRef]
27. Nioi, M.; d'Aloja, E.; Fossarello, M.; Napoli, P.E. Dual Corneal-Graft Rejection after mRNA Vaccine (BNT162b2) for COVID-19 during the First Six Months of Follow-Up: Case Report, State of the Art and Ethical Concerns. *Vaccines* **2021**, *9*, 1274. [CrossRef]
28. Park, J.M.; Lee, J.H.; Hwang, J.H.; Kang, M.J. Corneal Graft Rejection after Vaccination against Coronavirus Disease. *Korean J. Ophthalmol.* **2022**. [CrossRef]
29. Parmar, D.P.; Garde, P.V.; Shah, S.M.; Bhole, P.K. Acute graft rejection in a high-risk corneal transplant following COVID-19 vaccination: A case report. *Indian J. Ophthalmol.* **2021**, *69*, 3757–3758. [CrossRef]
30. Phylactou, M.; Li, J.O.; Larkin, D.F.P. Characteristics of endothelial corneal transplant rejection following immunisation with SARS-CoV-2 messenger RNA vaccine. *Br. J. Ophthalmol.* **2021**, *105*, 893–896. [CrossRef]
31. Rajagopal, R.; Priyanka, T.M. Stromal rejection in penetrating keratoplasty following COVID-19 vector vaccine (Covishield)—A case report and review of literature. *Indian J. Ophthalmol.* **2022**, *70*, 319–321. [CrossRef]
32. Rallis, K.I.; Ting, D.S.J.; Said, D.G.; Dua, H.S. Corneal graft rejection following COVID-19 vaccine. *Eye* **2022**, *36*, 1319–1320. [CrossRef]
33. Ravichandran, S.; Natarajan, R. Corneal graft rejection after COVID-19 vaccination. *Indian J. Ophthalmol.* **2021**, *69*, 1953–1954. [CrossRef]
34. Shah, A.P.; Dzhaber, D.; Kenyon, K.R.; Riaz, K.M.; Ouano, D.P.; Koo, E.H. Acute Corneal Transplant Rejection after COVID-19 Vaccination. *Cornea* **2022**, *41*, 121–124. [CrossRef]
35. Simao, M.F.; Kwitko, S. Corneal Graft Rejection after Inactivated SARS-CoV-2 Vaccine: Case Report. *Cornea* **2022**, *41*, 502–504. [CrossRef] [PubMed]
36. Wasser, L.M.; Roditi, E.; Zadok, D.; Berkowitz, L.; Weill, Y. Keratoplasty Rejection after the BNT162b2 messenger RNA Vaccine. *Cornea* **2021**, *40*, 1070–1072. [CrossRef] [PubMed]
37. Yu, S.; Ritterband, D.C.; Mehta, I. Acute Corneal Transplant Rejection after Severe Acute Respiratory Syndrome Coronavirus 2 mRNA-1273 Vaccination. *Cornea* **2022**, *41*, 257–259. [CrossRef]
38. Al-Dwairi, R.A.; Aleshawi, A.; Adi, S.; Abu-Zreig, L. Reactivation of Herpes Simplex Keratitis on a Corneal Graft Following SARS-CoV-2 mRNA Vaccination. *Med. Arch.* **2022**, *76*, 146–148. [CrossRef]
39. Alkhalifah, M.I.; Alsobki, H.E.; Alwael, H.M.; Al Fawaz, A.M.; Al-Mezaine, H.S. Herpes Simplex Virus Keratitis Reactivation after SARS-CoV-2 BNT162b2 mRNA Vaccination: A Report of Two Cases. *Ocul. Immunol. Inflamm.* **2021**, *29*, 1238–1240. [CrossRef]

40. Alkwikbi, H.; Alenazi, M.; Alanazi, W.; Alruwaili, S. Herpetic Keratitis and Corneal Endothelitis Following COVID-19 Vaccination: A Case Series. *Cureus* **2022**, *14*, e20967. [CrossRef]
41. Bolletta, E.; Iannetta, D.; Mastrofilippo, V.; De Simone, L.; Gozzi, F.; Croci, S.; Bonacini, M.; Belloni, L.; Zerbini, A.; Adani, C.; et al. Uveitis and Other Ocular Complications Following COVID-19 Vaccination. *J. Clin. Med.* **2021**, *10*, 5960. [CrossRef]
42. Cohen, S.; Olshaker, H.; Fischer, N.; Vishnevskia-Dai, V.; Hagin, D.; Rosenblatt, A.; Zur, D.; Habot-Wilner, Z. Herpetic Eye Disease Following the SARS-CoV-2 Vaccinations. *Ocul. Immunol. Inflamm.* **2022**, 1–12. [CrossRef]
43. Fard, A.M.; Desilets, J.; Patel, S. Recurrence of Herpetic Keratitis after COVID-19 Vaccination: A Report of Two Cases. *Case Rep. Ophthalmol. Med.* **2022**, *2022*, 7094893. [CrossRef]
44. Lazzaro, D.R.; Ramachandran, R.; Cohen, E.; Galetta, S.L. COVID-19 vaccination and possible link to Herpes zoster. *Am. J. Ophthalmol. Case Rep.* **2022**, *25*, 101359. [CrossRef]
45. Li, S.; Jia, X.; Yu, F.; Wang, Q.; Zhang, T.; Yuan, J. Herpetic Keratitis Preceded by COVID-19 Vaccination. *Vaccines* **2021**, *9*, 1394. [CrossRef]
46. Mishra, S.B.; Mahendradas, P.; Kawali, A.; Sanjay, S.; Shetty, R. Reactivation of varicella zoster infection presenting as acute retinal necrosis post COVID 19 vaccination in an Asian Indian male. *Eur. J. Ophthalmol.* **2021**, *33*, 11206721211046485. [CrossRef]
47. Mohammadpour, M.; Farrokhpour, H.; Sadeghi, R. Herpetic endotheliitis and stromal keratitis following inactivated COVID-19 vaccination. *Clin. Case Rep.* **2022**, *10*, e6397. [CrossRef]
48. Murgova, S.; Balchev, G. Ophthalmic manifestation after SARS-CoV-2 vaccination: A case series. *J. Ophthalmic. Inflamm. Infect.* **2022**, *12*, 20. [CrossRef]
49. Pang, K.; Pan, L.; Guo, H.; Wu, X. Case Report: Associated Ocular Adverse Reactions With Inactivated COVID-19 Vaccine in China. *Front. Med.* **2021**, *8*, 823346. [CrossRef]
50. Rallis, K.I.; Fausto, R.; Ting, D.S.J.; Al-Aqaba, M.A.; Said, D.G.; Dua, H.S. Manifestation of Herpetic Eye Disease after COVID-19 Vaccine: A UK Case Series. *Ocul. Immunol. Inflamm.* **2022**, *30*, 1136–1141. [CrossRef]
51. Rehman, O.; Arya, S.K.; Jha, U.P.; Nayyar, S.; Goel, I. Herpes Zoster Ophthalmicus after COVID-19 Vaccination: Chance Occurrence or More? *Cornea* **2022**, *41*, 254–256. [CrossRef]
52. Richardson-May, J.; Rothwell, A.; Rashid, M. Reactivation of herpes simplex keratitis following vaccination for COVID-19. *BMJ Case Rep.* **2021**, *14*, e245792. [CrossRef]
53. Ryu, K.J.; Kim, D.H. Recurrence of Varicella-Zoster Virus Keratitis after SARS-CoV-2 Vaccination. *Cornea* **2022**, *41*, 649–650. [CrossRef]
54. Shan, H.; Jia, R.; Liu, W.; Wu, X. Viral keratitis after the second and third doses of inactivated COVID-19 vaccination: A case report. *Hum. Vaccines Immunother.* **2022**, *18*, 2090177. [CrossRef]
55. Song, M.Y.; Koh, K.M.; Hwang, K.Y.; Kwon, Y.A.; Kim, K.Y. Relapsed Disciform Stromal Herpetic Keratitis Following mRNA COVID-19 Vaccination: A Case Report. *Korean J. Ophthalmol.* **2022**, *36*, 80–82. [CrossRef]
56. You, I.C.; Ahn, M.; Cho, N.C. A Case Report of Herpes Zoster Ophthalmicus and Meningitis after COVID-19 Vaccination. *J. Korean Med. Sci.* **2022**, *37*, e165. [CrossRef]
57. De la Presa, M.; Govil, A.; Chamberlain, W.D.; Holland, E.J. Acute Corneal Epithelial Rejection of LR-CLAL after SARS-CoV-2 Vaccination. *Cornea* **2022**, *41*, 252–253. [CrossRef]
58. Farrell, D.A.; Deacon, S.; Mauger, T. "Marginal keratitis following COVID 19 vaccination". *IDCases* **2022**, *29*, e01536. [CrossRef]
59. Gouvea, L.; Slomovic, A.R.; Chan, C.C. "Smoldering" Rejection of Keratolimbal Allograft. *Cornea* **2022**, *41*, 651–653. [CrossRef]
60. Khan, T.A.; Sidhu, N.; Khan, L.; Sen, S.; Hussain, N.; Tandon, R.; Gupta, N. Bilateral Immune-Mediated Keratolysis after Immunization With SARS-CoV-2 Recombinant Viral Vector Vaccine. *Cornea* **2021**, *40*, 1629–1632. [CrossRef]
61. Lee, J.Y.; Han, S.B. Case report of transient corneal edema after immunization with adenovirus-vectored COVID-19 vaccine. *Medicine* **2022**, *101*, e30041. [CrossRef]
62. Penbe, A. Peripheral Ulcerative Keratitis Secondary to the Inactive COVID-19 Vaccine-CoronaVac. *Ocul. Immunol. Inflamm.* **2022**, 1–5. [CrossRef]
63. Qazi, Y.; Hamrah, P. Corneal Allograft Rejection: Immunopathogenesis to Therapeutics. *J. Clin. Cell. Immunol.* **2013**, *2013*. [CrossRef]
64. Lee, E.H.; Li, J.Y. Immunization-Associated Corneal Transplantation Rejection: A Review. *Cornea* **2022**, *41*, 660–663. [CrossRef]
65. Lockington, D.; Lee, B.; Jeng, B.H.; Larkin, D.F.P.; Hjortdal, J. Survey of Corneal Surgeons' Attitudes Regarding Keratoplasty Rejection Risk Associated With Vaccinations. *Cornea* **2021**, *40*, 1541–1547. [CrossRef]
66. Busin, M.; Zauli, G.; Pellegrini, M.; Virgili, G.; Yu, A.C. COVID-19 Vaccination May Not Increase Rates of Corneal Graft Rejection. *Cornea* **2022**, *41*, 1536–1538. [CrossRef]
67. Roberts, H.W.; Wilkins, M.R.; Malik, M.; Talachi-Langroudi, M.; Myerscough, J.; Pellegrini, M.; Yu, A.C.; Busin, M. A lack of an association between COVID-19 vaccination and corneal graft rejection: Results of a large multi-country population based study. *Eye* **2022**, 1–4. [CrossRef]
68. Amouzegar, A.; Chauhan, S.K.; Dana, R. Alloimmunity and Tolerance in Corneal Transplantation. *J. Immunol.* **2016**, *196*, 3983–3991. [CrossRef]
69. Tahvildari, M.; Inomata, T.; Amouzegar, A.; Dana, R. Regulatory T cell modulation of cytokine and cellular networks in corneal graft rejection. *Curr. Ophthalmol. Rep.* **2018**, *6*, 266–274. [CrossRef]
70. Dugan, S.P.; Mian, S.I. Impact of vaccination on keratoplasty. *Curr. Opin. Ophthalmol.* **2022**, *33*, 296–305. [CrossRef]

71. Di Zazzo, A.; Lee, S.M.; Sung, J.; Niutta, M.; Coassin, M.; Mashaghi, A.; Inomata, T. Variable Responses to Corneal Grafts: Insights from Immunology and Systems Biology. *J. Clin. Med.* **2020**, *9*, 586. [CrossRef]
72. Sahin, U.; Muik, A.; Vogler, I.; Derhovanessian, E.; Kranz, L.M.; Vormehr, M.; Quandt, J.; Bidmon, N.; Ulges, A.; Baum, A.; et al. BNT162b2 vaccine induces neutralizing antibodies and poly-specific T cells in humans. *Nature* **2021**, *595*, 572–577. [CrossRef]
73. McMahon, D.E.; Amerson, E.; Rosenbach, M.; Lipoff, J.B.; Moustafa, D.; Tyagi, A.; Desai, S.R.; French, L.E.; Lim, H.W.; Thiers, B.H.; et al. Cutaneous reactions reported after Moderna and Pfizer COVID-19 vaccination: A registry-based study of 414 cases. *J. Am. Acad. Dermatol.* **2021**, *85*, 46–55. [CrossRef]
74. Ozdemir, A.K.; Kayhan, S.; Cakmak, S.K. Herpes zoster after inactivated SARS-CoV-2 vaccine in two healthy young adults. *J. Eur. Acad. Dermatol. Venereol.* **2021**, *35*, e846–e847. [CrossRef]
75. Martinez-Reviejo, R.; Tejada, S.; Adebanjo, G.A.R.; Chello, C.; Machado, M.C.; Parisella, F.R.; Campins, M.; Tammaro, A.; Rello, J. Varicella-Zoster virus reactivation following severe acute respiratory syndrome coronavirus 2 vaccination or infection: New insights. *Eur. J. Intern. Med.* **2022**, *104*, 73–79. [CrossRef]
76. Gringeri, M.; Battini, V.; Cammarata, G.; Mosini, G.; Guarnieri, G.; Leoni, C.; Pozzi, M.; Radice, S.; Clementi, E.; Carnovale, C. Herpes zoster and simplex reactivation following COVID-19 vaccination: New insights from a vaccine adverse event reporting system (VAERS) database analysis. *Expert Rev. Vaccines* **2022**, *21*, 675–684. [CrossRef]
77. Barda, N.; Dagan, N.; Ben-Shlomo, Y.; Kepten, E.; Waxman, J.; Ohana, R.; Hernan, M.A.; Lipsitch, M.; Kohane, I.; Netzer, D.; et al. Safety of the BNT162b2 mRNA COVID-19 Vaccine in a Nationwide Setting. *N. Engl. J. Med.* **2021**, *385*, 1078–1090. [CrossRef]
78. Shasha, D.; Bareket, R.; Sikron, F.H.; Gertel, O.; Tsamir, J.; Dvir, D.; Mossinson, D.; Heymann, A.D.; Zacay, G. Real-world safety data for the Pfizer BNT162b2 SARS-CoV-2 vaccine: Historical cohort study. *Clin. Microbiol. Infect.* **2022**, *28*, 130–134. [CrossRef]
79. Stoeger, T.; Adler, H. "Novel" Triggers of Herpesvirus Reactivation and Their Potential Health Relevance. *Front. Microbiol.* **2018**, *9*, 3207. [CrossRef]
80. Katsikas Triantafyllidis, K.; Giannos, P.; Mian, I.T.; Kyrtsonis, G.; Kechagias, K.S. Varicella Zoster Virus Reactivation Following COVID-19 Vaccination: A Systematic Review of Case Reports. *Vaccines* **2021**, *9*, 1013. [CrossRef]
81. Xu, B.; Fan, C.Y.; Wang, A.L.; Zou, Y.L.; Yu, Y.H.; He, C.; Xia, W.G.; Zhang, J.X.; Miao, Q. Suppressed T cell-mediated immunity in patients with COVID-19: A clinical retrospective study in Wuhan, China. *J. Infect.* **2020**, *81*, e51–e60. [CrossRef]
82. Diez-Domingo, J.; Parikh, R.; Bhavsar, A.B.; Cisneros, E.; McCormick, N.; Lecrenier, N. Can COVID-19 Increase the Risk of Herpes Zoster? A Narrative Review. *Dermatol. Ther.* **2021**, *11*, 1119–1126. [CrossRef] [PubMed]
83. Furer, V.; Zisman, D.; Kibari, A.; Rimar, D.; Paran, Y.; Elkayam, O. Herpes zoster following BNT162b2 mRNA COVID-19 vaccination in patients with autoimmune inflammatory rheumatic diseases: A case series. *Rheumatology* **2021**, *60*, SI90–SI95. [CrossRef] [PubMed]

Disclaimer/Publisher's Note: The statements, opinions and data contained in all publications are solely those of the individual author(s) and contributor(s) and not of MDPI and/or the editor(s). MDPI and/or the editor(s) disclaim responsibility for any injury to people or property resulting from any ideas, methods, instructions or products referred to in the content.

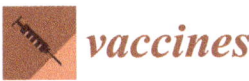

Review

The Characteristics of COVID-19 Vaccine-Associated Uveitis: A Summative Systematic Review

Yasmine Yousra Sadok Cherif [1,†], Chakib Djeffal [1,†], Hashem Abu Serhan [2,3], Ahmed Elnahhas [2,4], Hebatallah Yousef [2,5], Basant E. Katamesh [2,4], Basel Abdelazeem [2,6,7] and Abdelaziz Abdelaal [2,4,8,9,*]

1. Faculty of Medicine, University of Algiers, Algiers 16311, Algeria
2. Tanta Research Team, El-Gharbia 31516, Egypt
3. Department of Ophthalmology, Hamad Medical Corporations, Doha 576214, Qatar
4. Faculty of Medicine, Tanta University, Tanta 31527, Egypt
5. Ophthalmology Department, Kafr Ash Shaykh Ophthalmology Hospital, Kafr Ash Shaykh 33511, Egypt
6. McLaren Health Care, Flint, MI 48532, USA
7. Internal Medicine Department, Michigan State University, East Lansing, Michigan, MI 48824, USA
8. Harvard Medical School, Postgraduate Medical Education, Boston, MA 02115, USA
9. Doheny Eye Institute, University of California, Los Angeles, CA 90033, USA
* Correspondence: tantaresearchteam@gmail.com or drabdoseliem@gmail.com; Tel.: +20-1128608660
† These authors contributed equally to this work.

Abstract: Numerous complications following COVID-19 vaccination has been reported in the literature, with an increasing body of evidence reporting vaccination-associated uveitis (VAU). In this systematic review, we searched six electronic databases for articles reporting the occurrence of VAU following COVID-19 vaccination. Data were synthesized with emphasis on patients' characteristics [age, gender], vaccination characteristics [type, dose], and outcome findings [type, nature, laterality, course, location, onset, underlying cause, and associated findings]. Data are presented as numbers (percentages) for categorical data and as mean (standard deviation) for continuous data. Sixty-five studies were finally included [43 case reports, 16 case series, four cohort, one cross-sectional, and one registry-based study]. VAU occurred in 1526 cases, most commonly in females (68.93%) and middle-aged individuals (41–50 years: 19.71%), following the first dose (49.35%) of vaccination, especially in those who received Pfizer (77.90%). VAU occurred acutely (71.77%) as an inflammatory reaction (88.29%) in unilateral eyes (77.69%), particularly in the anterior portion of the uvea (54.13%). Importantly, most cases had a new onset (69.92%) while only a limited portion of cases had a reactivation of previous uveitis condition. In conclusion, although rare, uveitis following COVID-19 vaccination should be considered in new-onset and recurrent cases presenting with either acute or chronic events.

Keywords: COVID-19; vaccine; uveitis; vaccine-associated uveitis

Citation: Cherif, Y.Y.S.; Djeffal, C.; Abu Serhan, H.; Elnahhas, A.; Yousef, H.; Katamesh, B.E.; Abdelazeem, B.; Abdelaal, A. The Characteristics of COVID-19 Vaccine-Associated Uveitis: A Summative Systematic Review. *Vaccines* 2023, 11, 69. https://doi.org/10.3390/vaccines11010069

Academic Editor: Rohan Bir Singh

Received: 13 November 2022
Revised: 14 December 2022
Accepted: 24 December 2022
Published: 28 December 2022

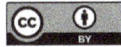

Copyright: © 2022 by the authors. Licensee MDPI, Basel, Switzerland. This article is an open access article distributed under the terms and conditions of the Creative Commons Attribution (CC BY) license (https://creativecommons.org/licenses/by/4.0/).

1. Introduction

Following the declaration of the COVID-19 pandemic, healthcare systems all over the globe were burdened by the increased number of daily diagnosed cases and associated deaths. This urged the need to develop effective vaccines within a short time period. During the past two years, a number of vaccines received emergency authorization and were then disseminated globally. Currently, over 12.6 billion doses have been distributed, including messenger RNA vaccines (the Pfizer-BioNTech and the Moderna), vector vaccines (Johnson & Johnson, AstraZeneca), and protein subunit vaccine (Novavax). Although these vaccines were effective in limiting the spread of the disease and limiting the occurrence of severe forms, several adverse events were reported, particularly those involving the eye [1,2].

Uveitis is a potentially vision-threatening condition that involves intraocular inflammation. It accounts for 10–15% of blindness cases worldwide [3]. It has incidence and prevalence rates of 50.45 and 9–730 per 100,000 cases, respectively. The etiology of uveitis is multifactorial, which can be autoimmune, systemic (60.1%), infectious (30–50%), or idiopathic (20–40%) in origin [3]. That being said, uveitis can occur postvaccination. Vaccination-related uveitis, although uncommon, has been reported during previous Hepatitis B virus (40%), human papillomavirus (15%), hepatitis A virus, influenza virus, Bacille-Calmette-Guerin, varicella virus, and measles-mumps-rubella vaccination programs [4]. In this context, the hypothesis of COVID-19 vaccine-associated uveitis (VAU) has emerged, with several reports highlighting the magnitude of this problem [1,5,6]. For instance, non-infectious uveitis has been reported in 66.8 and 62.7 cases per 100,000 person-years following the first and second doses of the BNT162b2 mRNA vaccine, respectively [7].

In light of COVID-19 VAU, the level of evidence has shifted. Instead of being based solely on case reports, a number of new cohort and cross-sectional studies have been published in this regard, all of which highlight the magnitude of this newly emerging observation. Therefore, we conducted a systematic review to summarize available evidence on COVID-19 vaccine-associated uveitis with a particular focus on vaccines' information [type, dose, duration], patients' characteristics [sociodemographic and clinical], and disease-associated outcomes [origin, type, location, presentation, management, and outcomes].

2. Materials and Methods

2.1. Study Protocol and Database Search

This research was carried out in accordance with the Preferred Reporting for Systematic Review and Meta-Analysis (PRISMA) recommendations. In July 2022, our protocol was registered on PROSPERO [registration number: CRD42022358117]. Meanwhile, on 26–27 July 2022, we searched six electronic databases [PubMed, Scopus, EMBASE, Web of Science, CENTRAL, and Google Scholar] to retrieve all studies that reported the occurrence of VAU following COVID-19 vaccination using the following keywords: COVID-19 AND vaccin* AND uveitis. Medical Subject Headings (MESH) terms were also added whenever applicable to retrieve all relevant studies based on their indexed terms in included databases. Of note, only the first 200 records from Google Scholar were retrieved and screened as per the recent recommendations [8]. The detailed search strategy for each database is provided in Table A1. It is worth noting that an updated database search was carried out on 11 September 2022, to include any newly published studies before the official synthesis of collected data.

Additionally, on 1 September 2022, after finishing the screening process, we conducted a manual search of references to identify any relevant studies that we could not identify through the original database search. This search was conducted through: (1) the reference list of included studies, (2) "similar article" of included papers on PubMed, and (3) Google by using these keywords: "COVID-19" + "uveitis" + "vaccine".

2.2. Eligibility Criteria

We included original research papers that discussed the occurrence of VAU following COVID-19 vaccination. We included all of the following study designs: case reports and series, cohorts, and cross-sectional studies. Studies were included regardless of the type and/or dose of vaccine, history or location of uveitis, or the language of publication. Meanwhile, studies were excluded if they: (1) recruited individuals (healthy or infected with COVID-19) who did not receive COVID-19 vaccines, (2) were not original (reviews, editorials, commentaries, books, etc.), (3) included duplicated records, (4) did not have a full text, or (5) reported other types of ocular/ophthalmic complications other than uveitis.

2.3. Screening and Study Selection

Retrieved records from the database search were exported into EndNote software for duplicate removal before the beginning of the screening phase. Records were then imported into an Excel (Microsoft, Rochester, MN, USA) Sheet for screening. The screening was divided into two steps: title and abstract screening and full-text screening. The full texts of eligible articles were then retrieved for screening before being finally included in the review. Both steps were carried out by three reviewers (HY, HA, AE). Any differences between reviewers were solved through group discussions, and the senior authors (YYSC, CD) were consulted if reviewers could not reach an agreement.

2.4. Data Extraction

The data extraction was performed by three reviewers [HY, HA, AE] through a data extraction sheet that was formatted through Excel (Microsoft, Rochester, MN, USA). This sheet consisted of six parts. The first part included the baseline characteristics of included studies (title, authors' names, year of publication, country, and study design) and patients as well [sample size, age, and gender]—only those with evidence VAU. The second part included data on the administered vaccines (type and dose), while the third part included information regarding VAU cases' medical history (systemic, immunological, and ocular diseases). The fourth part included patients' clinical presentation and examination findings (symptoms, signs, and intraocular pressure (IOP)), while the fifth part included data on the main outcome of interest—VAU (type, location, laterality, interval between vaccination and symptom onset, nature, underlying cause, and associated findings). The final part included the management approach in such cases and reported outcomes (resolution, improvement, complications, recurrence, etc.).

2.5. Data Synthesis

All of the included studies were qualitatively analyzed as per our plan in priori. Additionally, since data were provided on a per-case basis, we performed several descriptive analyses to detect patterns on the occurrence of VAU based on: age, gender, type and dose of vaccination, presenting symptoms, laterality (right, left, unilateral, bilateral), type of uveitis (new-onset, reactivation), longevity (acute, chronic), location (anterior, intermediate, posterior, panuveitis), duration of vaccination to symptom onset, associated findings [macular edema, glaucoma, synechiae], and management outcomes (resolution, improvement, recurrence, complications). Data are presented as mean/standard deviation (SD) for continuous variables and as numbers/percentages for categorical ones.

3. Results

3.1. Search Results

The results of the database search and screening phases are presented in Figure 1. The initial database search yielded 538 articles, of which 209 duplicates were removed through EndNote. Following the screening of 329 articles, the full texts of 65 articles were retrieved for full-text screening, of which 11 articles were excluded. The manual search resulted in 10 articles, and an updated database search revealed one additional article, resulting in a total number of relevant eligible studies of 65.

3.2. Baseline Characteristics of Studies Reporting COVID-19 VAU

A total of 65 studies were both qualitatively and quantitatively analyzed (Table 1) [1,5,7,9–69], out of which 43 were case reports, 16 were case series, four were retrospective cohort, one was cross-sectional, and one was a registry-based study. The sample size of included patients with VAU ranged from 1 to 1094, with an overall sample size of 1526 VAU cases. Most reports were from India ($n = 9$), followed by China ($n = 7$), Israel ($n = 7$), Korea ($n = 6$), Italy ($n = 4$), and USA ($n = 4$), respectively.

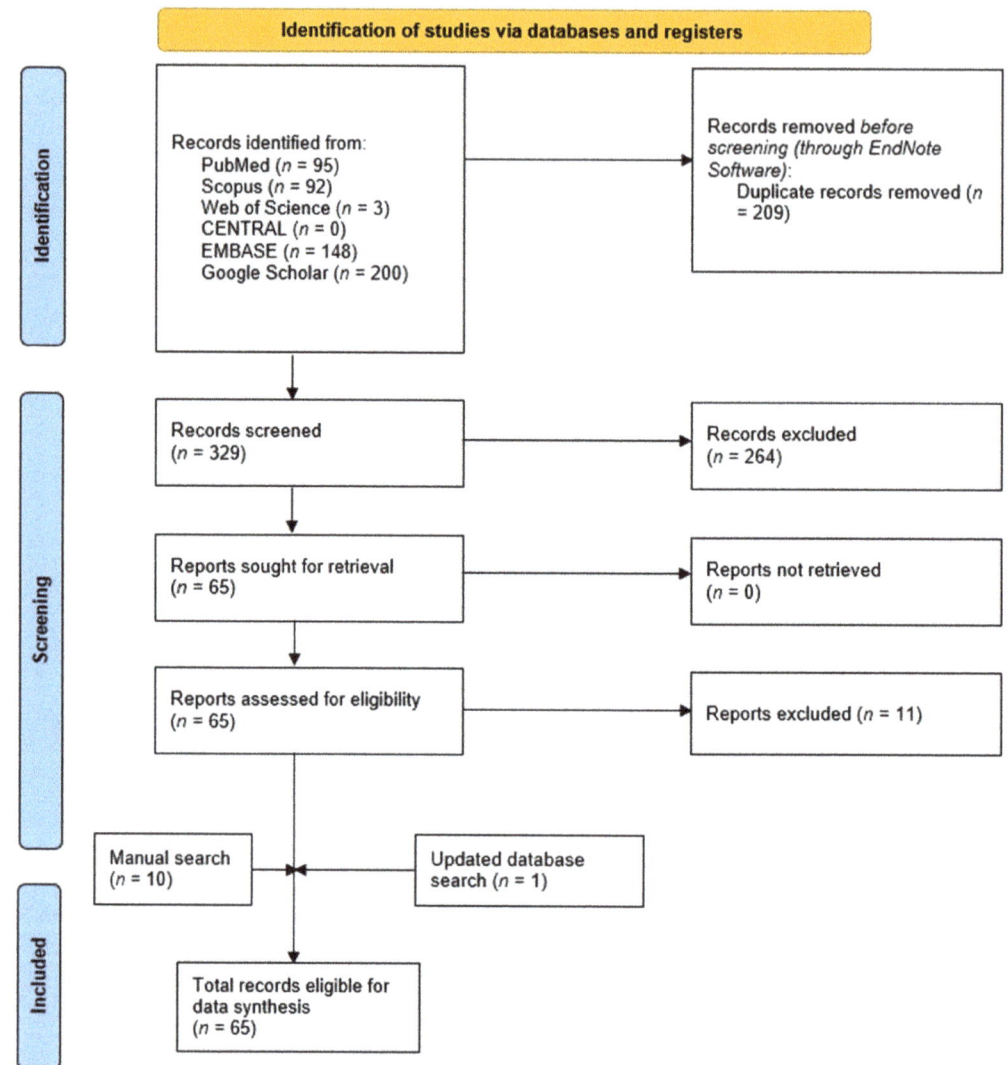

Figure 1. A PRISMA flow diagram showing the database search and screening results.

Table 1. The baseline characteristics of studies reporting COVID-19 vaccine-associated uveitis cases.

Author (YOP)	Country	Design	Gender	Age	Type	Dose
		Case Reports				
Accorinti (2022) [9]	Italy	Case Report	Female	54	Pfizer-BioNTech	First
Achiron (2022) [10]	Finland	Case Report	Male	17	Pfizer-BioNTech	-
Al-Allaf (2022) [11]	Qatar	Case Report	Male	46	Pfizer-BioNTech	First
Alhamazani (2022) [12]	Saudi Arabia	Case Report	Male	37	Pfizer-BioNTech	First
Brunet de Courssou (2022) [16]	France	Case Report	Female	57	Pfizer-BioNTech	First
Chen (2022a) [18]	China	Case Report	Male	19	Sinovac	First

Table 1. Cont.

Author (YOP)	Country	Design	Gender	Age	Type	Dose
De Carvalho (2022) [22]	Brazil	Case Report	Male	51	Oxford/AstraZeneca	First
De Domingo (2022) [23]	Spain	Case Report	Female	46	Pfizer-BioNTech	Second
Ishay (2021) [32]	Israel	Case Report	Male	28	Pfizer-BioNTech	First
Duran (2022) [25]	Israel	Case Report	Female	54	Pfizer-BioNTech	First
ElSheikh (2021) [26]	Egypt	Case Report	Female	18	Sinopharm	First
Lee (2022) [39]	South Korea	Case Report	Female	83	Pfizer-BioNTech	Second
Gedik (2022) [28]	Turkey	Case Report	Male	47	Pfizer-BioNTech	Second
Goyal (2021) [29]	India	Case Report	Male	34	Oxford/AstraZeneca	Second
Hébert (2022) [30]	Canada	Case Report	Male	41	Pfizer-BioNTech	First
Hwang (2022) [31]	South Korea	Case Report	Female	21	Pfizer-BioNTech	Second
Jain (2021) [33]	India	Case Report	Male	27	Oxford/AstraZeneca	First
Joo (2022) [34]	South Korea	Case Report	Female	50	Moderna	First
Kim (2022) [36]	South Korea	Case Report	Female	72	Oxford/AstraZeneca	First
Koong (2021) [37]	Singapore	Case Report	Male	54	Pfizer-BioNTech	First
Papasavvas (2021) [53]	Switzerland	Case Report	Female	73	Moderna	First
Ding (2022) [24]	China	Case Report	Male	33	Sinopharm	First
Lee (2022) [40]	USA	Case Report	Female	25	Moderna	Second
Mahendradas (2022) [42]	India	Case Report	Female	19	Covaxin	Second
Matsuo (2022) [43]	Japan	Case Report	Male	34	Pfizer-BioNTech	Second
Mishra (2021) [44]	India	Case Report	Male	71	Oxford/AstraZeneca	First
Mudie (2021) [45]	Spain	Case Report	Female	43	Pfizer-BioNTech	Second
Pan (2021) [51]	China	Case Report	Female	50	Sinopharm	
Papasavvas (2021) [53]	Switzerland	Case Report	Female	43	Pfizer-BioNTech	Second
Reddy (2021) [57]	India	Case Report	Female	30	Oxford/AstraZeneca	Second
Renisi (2021) [59]	Italy	Case Report	Male	23	Pfizer-BioNTech	Second
Sangoram (2022) [60]	India	Case Report	Female	40	Oxford/AstraZeneca	Second
Santiago (2021) [61]	Puerto Rico	Case Report	Male	32	Pfizer-BioNTech	Second
Saraceno (2021) [62]	Brazil	Case Report	Female	62	Oxford/AstraZeneca	-
Singh (2022a) [64]	India	Case Report	Male	29	Oxford/AstraZeneca	First
Yalçinkaya (2022) [67]	Turkey	Case Report	Male	12	Pfizer-BioNTech	First
Yamaguchi (2022) [68]	Japan	Case Report	Female	30	Pfizer-BioNTech	Second
Shilo (2022) [70]	Israel	Case Report	Male	20	Pfizer-BioNTech	First
Kakarla (2022) [35]	India	Case Report	Female	15	Covaxin	First
Numakura (2022) [48]	Japan	Case Report	Male	61	Pfizer-BioNTech	First
Murgova (2022) [46]	Bulgaria	Case Report	Female	89	Pfizer-BioNTech	Second
Patel (2022) [54]	USA	Case Report	Male	79	Pfizer-BioNTech	Second
Lawson-Tovey (2022) [38]	Italy	Case Report	Female	-	-	Second

| Case Series ||||||||
Author (YOP)	Country	Cases	Gender	Age	Type	Dose
Arora (2022) [13]	India	Case 1	Female	20	Oxford/AstraZeneca	First
		Case 2	Male	26	Oxford/AstraZeneca	First
Choi (2022) [20]	Korea	Case 1	Male	62	Oxford/AstraZeneca	First
		Case 2	Female	79	Pfizer-BioNTech	First
		Case 3	Female	55	Pfizer-BioNTech	First
Ortiz-Egea (2022) [49]	Spain	Case 1	Female	92	Pfizer-BioNTech	First
		Case 2	Female	85	Pfizer-BioNTech	First
Nanji (2022) [47]	USA	Case 1	Female	58	Moderna	First
		Case 2	Female	60	Moderna	First
Pang (2022) [52]	China	Case 1	Female	50	Sinopharm	First
		Case 2	Female	34	Sinopharm	Second
Ren (2022) [58]	China	Case 1	Female	46	Sinovac	First
		Case 2	Female	26	Sinovac	First
Cohen (2022) [21]	Israel	Case 1	Female	81	Pfizer-BioNTech	Second
		Case 2	Female	64	Pfizer-BioNTech	Second
		Case 3	Male	74	Pfizer-BioNTech	Third
		Case 4	Male	63	Pfizer-BioNTech	Third
Aguiar (2022) [17]	Portugal	Case 1	Female	21	Pfizer-BioNTech	First
		Case 2	Male	70	Pfizer-BioNTech	Second
De Queiroz Tavares Ferreira (2022) [5]	Brazil	Case 1	Female	27	Oxford/AstraZeneca	First
		Case 2	Male	39	Oxford/AstraZeneca	First
		Case 3	Female	38	Pfizer-BioNTech	First
		Case 4	Female	32	Sinovac	Second

Table 1. *Cont.*

Author (YOP)	Country	Cases	Gender	Age	Type	Dose
Chen (2022b) [19]	China	Case 1	Male	33	Sinopharm	First
		Case 2	Female	57	Sinovac	Second
		Case 3	Male	21	Sinovac	First
		Case 4	Female	30	Sinovac	Second
		Case 5	Female	28	Sinopharm	First
Chew (2022) [1]	Singapore	Case 1	Female	64	Pfizer-BioNTech	Second
		Case 2	Male	74	Sinopharm	Second
		Case 3	Female	31	Pfizer-BioNTech	Second
		Case 4	Female	71	Pfizer-BioNTech	Second
		Case 5	Female	32	Pfizer-BioNTech	Second
		Case 6	Female	28	Pfizer-BioNTech	Second
Rallis (2022) [56]	UK	Case 1	Female	47	Oxford/AstraZeneca	First
		Case 2	Female	48	Oxford/AstraZeneca	First
		Case 3	Male	44	Oxford/AstraZeneca	First
		Case 4	Female	59	Oxford/AstraZeneca	First
		Case 5	Male	65	Oxford/AstraZeneca	First
		Case 6	Male	95	Pfizer-BioNTech	First
		Case 7	Male	68	Pfizer-BioNTech	First
Li (2022) [41]	China	Case 1	Female	48	Sinovac	First
		Case 2	Male	41	Sinovac	Third
		Case 3	Male	8	Sinovac	First
		Case 4	Female	52	Sinovac	Second
		Case 5	Female	55	Sinovac	First
		Case 6	Female	67	Sinovac	First
		Case 7	Female	46	Sinovac	First
		Case 8	Female	57	Sinovac	First
		Case 9	Male	22	Sinovac	First
Sim (2022) [63]	Korea	Case 1	Female	51	Pfizer-BioNTech	Second
		Case 2	Female	21	Pfizer-BioNTech	Second
		Case 3	Male	50	Pfizer-BioNTech	Second
		Case 4	Female	52	Pfizer-BioNTech	Third
		Case 5	Male	32	Johnson & Johnson	Second
		Case 6	Male	72	Oxford/AstraZeneca	Second
		Case 7	Female	67	Oxford/AstraZeneca	Third
		Case 8	Male	54	Pfizer-BioNTech	Second
		Case 9	Female	61	Pfizer-BioNTech	Third
		Case 10	Female	63	Pfizer-BioNTech	Second
		Case 11	Female	47	Pfizer-BioNTech	Third
Rabinovitch (2021) [55]	Israel	Case 1	Female	43	Pfizer-BioNTech	First
		Case 2	Male	34	Pfizer-BioNTech	First
		Case 3	Female	34	Pfizer-BioNTech	First
		Case 4	Male	78	Pfizer-BioNTech	Second
		Case 5	Male	53	Pfizer-BioNTech	First
		Case 6	Male	64	Pfizer-BioNTech	First
		Case 7	Male	68	Pfizer-BioNTech	First
		Case 8	Female	61	Pfizer-BioNTech	First
		Case 9	Male	59	Pfizer-BioNTech	Second
		Case 10	Male	72	Pfizer-BioNTech	Second
		Case 11	Male	51	Pfizer-BioNTech	Second
		Case 12	Female	42	Pfizer-BioNTech	Second
		Case 13	Male	74	Pfizer-BioNTech	Second
		Case 14	Male	39	Pfizer-BioNTech	Second
		Case 15	Female	64	Pfizer-BioNTech	Second
		Case 16	Female	50	Pfizer-BioNTech	Second
		Case 17	Female	23	Pfizer-BioNTech	Second
		Case 18	Female	65	Pfizer-BioNTech	First
		Case 19	Male	36	Pfizer-BioNTech	Second
		Case 20	Male	41	Pfizer-BioNTech	Second
		Case 21	Female	28	Pfizer-BioNTech	Second

Table 1. Cont.

Author (YOP)	Country	Cases	Gender	Age	Type	Dose
Bolletta (2021) [15]	Italy	Case 1	Male	79	Oxford/AstraZeneca	Second
		Case 2	Female	65	Pfizer-BioNTech	Second
		Case 3	Female	42	Oxford/AstraZeneca	Second
		Case 4	Female	52	Pfizer-BioNTech	Second
		Case 5	Male	44	Pfizer-BioNTech	First
		Case 6	Female	35	Moderna	Second
		Case 7	Male	47	Pfizer-BioNTech	First
		Case 8	Female	58	Pfizer-BioNTech	First
		Case 9	Female	52	Oxford/AstraZeneca	First
		Case 10	Female	44	Pfizer-BioNTech	Second
		Case 11	Female	58	Pfizer-BioNTech	Second
		Case 12	Female	47	Pfizer-BioNTech	First
		Case 13	Female	68	Pfizer-BioNTech	Second

Observational Studies

Author (YOP)	Country	Design	Male/Total	Age Mean (SD)	Type [N]	Dose [N]
Ferrand (2022) [27]	Germany	Retrospective Cohort	6/25	43.2 (13.9)	Pfizer-BioNTech [15]; Oxford/AstraZeneca [6]; Moderna [3]; Covaxin [1]	First [6]; Second [19]
Ozdede (2022) [50]	Istanbul	Cross-Sectional	-/5	-	Sinovac [3]; Pfizer-BioNTech [2]	-
Testi (2022)	UK	Retrospective Cohort	22/50	41.3 (13.9)	Pfizer-BioNTech [24]; Oxford/AstraZeneca [16]; Moderna [8]; Sinopharm [1]; Covaxin [1]	First [28]; Second [22]
Tomkins-Netzer (2022) [7]	Israel	Retrospective Cohort	-	-	Pfizer-BioNTech [188]	First [100]; Second [88]
Barda (2021) [14]	Israel	Retrospective Cohort	-/26	-	Pfizer-BioNTech [26]	-
Singh (2022b) [71]	USA	Retrospective registry-based	322/1094	46.24 (16.93)	Pfizer-BioNTech [853]; Moderna [220]; Johnson & Johnson [21]	First [452]; Second [373]; Third [97]; Fourth [5]

YOP: Year of Publication; UK: United Kingdom; USA: United States of America; N: Number of Cases; SD: Standard Deviation.

3.3. Sociodemographic and Clinical Characteristics of VAU Cases

3.3.1. Age and Gender

COVID-19 vaccine-associated uveitis was twice more likely to occur in females than in males (68.93% vs. 31.06%). Patients' age ranged from 8 to 95 years (mean of 48.18 and standard deviation of 18.94). The peak of vaccine-associated uveitis occurred in middle-aged patients (41–50 years of age) with a declining trend as it comes nearer to both extremes (0–10 or ≥ 91 years) [Table 2].

3.3.2. Medical History

A minority of VAU cases reported having either systemic, ocular, or immunological diseases [Table 3]. SARS-CoV-2 infection occurred in a very limited number of patients (0.93%), while only 0.59% and 0.42% reported having hypertension or diabetes, respectively. More than one-tenth of VAU cases reported having uveitis in the past (13.51%). Although cases reported a wide variety of previous ocular conditions, none of them seems to be correlated with VAU due to their rare occurrence (below 0.50%). In terms of immunological diseases, autoimmune diseases (AIDS) were the most frequent among VAU cases, accounting for 1.19% of cases.

Table 2. Patients' and COVID-19 vaccines' characteristics.

Variable	Subgroup	Number	%
Gender			
	Male	406	31.06
	Female	901	68.93
Age			
	1–10	1	0.73
	11–20	8	5.84
	21–30	20	14.6
	31–40	19	13.87
	41–50	27	19.71
	51–60	23	16.79
	61–70	20	14.6
	71–80	13	9.49
	81–90	4	2.92
	≥91	2	1.46
Vaccine Type			
	Covaxin	4	0.26
	Johnson & Johnson	22	1.44
	Moderna	237	15.54
	Oxford/AstraZeneca	46	3.01
	Pfizer-BioNTech	1188	77.9
	Sinovac	11	0.72
	Sinopharm	17	1.11
Vaccine Dose			
	First	654	49.35
	Second	562	42.41
	Third	104	7.84
	Fourth	5	0.37

Table 3. The systemic, ocular, and immunologic history of vaccine-associated uveitis cases.

Author (YOP)	Systemic [N]	Medical History Ocular [N]	Immunological [N]	Total
Accorinti (2022)	None	-	-	1
Achiron (2022)	-	Uveitis [1]—RVO [1]—Iridis Rubeosis [1]	-	1
Al-Allaf (2022)	HTN	-	-	1
Alhamazani (2022)	-	-	-	1
Brunet de Courssou (2022)	-	-	-	1
Chen (2022a)	None	None	None	1
De Carvalho (2022)	AS	Uveitis [1]	HLA-B27 [1]	1
De Domingo (2022)	-	None	None	1
Ishay (2021)	Bechet's disease	None	Bechet's disease [1]	1
Duran (2022)	DM	None	-	1
ElSheikh (2021)	-	None	JIA [1]	1
Lee (2022)	HTN—Lipidemia	None	-	1
Gedik (2022)	-	-	-	1
Goyal (2021)	None	None	None	1
Hébert (2022)	None	None	None	1
Hwang (2022)	None	None	None	1
Jain (2021)	-	Uveitis [1]	JIA [1]	1
K. Joo (2022)	None	Allergic conjunctivitis [1]	None	1
Kim (2022)	-	-	-	1
Koong (2021)	DM—Lipidemia	None	None	1

Table 3. Cont.

Author (YOP)	Systemic [N]	Medical History Ocular [N]	Immunological [N]	Total
Papasavvas (2021)	None	Cataract [1]	None	1
Ding (2022)	HTN	None	None	1
Lee (2022)	-	-	None	1
Sai (2022)	-	Uveitis [1]	JIA [1]	1
Matsuo (2022)	-	-	-	1
Mishra (2021)	DM—HTN	-	-	1
Mudie (2021)	-	-	-	1
Pan (2021)	-	-	-	1
Papasavvas (2021)	-	VKH [1]	None	1
Reddy (2021)	-	-	-	1
Renisi (2021)	None	None	None	1
Sangoram (2022)	None	None	None	1
Santiago (2021)	None	None	None	1
Saraceno (2021)	None	None	None	1
Singh (2022a)	None	None	None	1
Yalçinkaya (2022)	None	None	None	1
Yamaguchi (2022)	None	None	None	1
Shilo (2022)	None	None	None	1
Kakarla (2022)	None	None	None	1
Numakura (2022)	None	None	None	1
Murgova (2022)	-	CRVO [1]—Cataract [1]—Glaucoma [1]—Herpetic uveitis [1]	-	1
Patel (2022)	None	Cataract [1]—RD [1]—ERM [1]	None	1
Lawson-Tovey (2022)	-	-	-	1
Arora (2022)	-	Uveitis [2]—SLC [1]	-	2
Choi (2022)	HTN [2]—DM [1]—Asthma [1]	Uveitis [2]—BRVO [1]	HLAB51 [1]	3
Ortiz-Egea (2022)	-	AMD [1]	-	2
Nanji (2022)	-	Uveitis [1]—OU [1]	-	2
Pang (2022)	-	-	-	2
Ren (2022)	-	-	-	2
Cohen (2022)	None	HZO [1]—Uveitis [1]	Psoriasis [1]—RA [1]	4
Aguiar (2022)	Epilepsy [1]—Asthma [1]—DM [1]—HTN [1]—Rhinitis [1]	None	None	2
Ferreira (2022)	COVID-19 [2]—HTN [1]	None	None	4
Chen (2022b)	AS [1]	-	-	5
Chew (2022)	None	Uveitis [3]—Cataract [1]—PACG [1]—HSK [4]	HLAB51 [1]	6
Rallis (2022)	-	-	-	7
Li (2022)	-	-	-	9
Sim (2022)	-	-	-	11
Rabinovitch (2021)	AS [3]—Psoriasis [2]—Crohn's disease [1]—Spondylarthritis [1]	Uveitis [8]—HZO [1]	-	21
Bolletta (2021)	Spondylarthritis [1]—Psoriatic arthritis [1]	Uveitis [3]—VKH [2]—Toxoplasma Retinochoroiditis [2]	-	13
Ferrand (2022)	-	Uveitis [19]—VKH [1]	HLAB27 [2]—MS [2]—JIA [1]	25
Ozdede (2022)	-	-	Bechet's syndrome [1]	5
Testi (2022)	-	Uveitis [20]—Glaucomatocyclitic Crisis [3]		50
Tomkins-Netzer (2022)	-	-	-	188
Barda (2021)	-	-	-	26
Singh (2022b)	COVID-19 [9]	Uveitis [106]	AIDs [14]	1094

Table 3. Cont.

Category	Disease	Number	Total	%
	Summary of the History of VAU Cases			
	Systemic Diseases			
	HTN	7	1178	0.59
	DM	5	1178	0.42
	AS	5	1178	0.42
	Lipidemia	2	1178	0.16
	Asthma	2	1178	0.16
	Epilepsy	1	1178	0.08
	Rhinitis	1	1178	0.08
	COVID-19	11	1178	0.93
	Ocular Diseases			
	Uveitis	170	1258	13.51
	VKH	4	1258	0.32
	HZO	2	1258	0.16
	Toxoplasma Retinochoroiditis	2	1258	0.16
	Glaucoma	5	1258	0.39
	Cataract	4	1258	0.32
	HSK	4	1258	0.32
	SLC	1	1258	0.07
	BRVO	1	1258	0.07
	RVO	1	1258	0.07
	Iridis Rubeosis	1	1258	0.07
	OU	1	1258	0.07
	CRVO	1	1258	0.07
	ERM	1	1258	0.07
	RD	1	1258	0.07
	Conjunctivitis	1	1258	0.07
	AMD	1	1258	0.07
	Immunological Diseases			
	HLA-B27	3	1170	0.26
	JIA	4	1170	0.34
	Psoriasis	3	1170	0.26
	HLAB51	2	1170	0.17
	MS	2	1170	0.17
	Bechet's disease	3	1170	0.26
	AIDs	14	1170	1.19
	RA	1	1170	0.08
	Crohn's disease	2	1170	0.17
	Spondylarthritis	1	1170	0.08

AS: Ankylosing Spondylitis; AMD: Age-related Macular Degeneration; BRVO: Branch Retinal Vein Occlusion; CRVO: Central Retinal Vein Occlusion; ERM: Epiretinal Membrane; HTN: Hypertension; HSK: Herpes-Simplex Keratitis; HZO: Herpes-Zoster Ophthalmicus; JIA: Juvenile Idiopathy Arthritis; OU: Optic Disc Vasculitis; PACG: Primary Angle-Closure Glaucoma; RD: Retinal Detachment; SLC: Serpiginous-like Choroiditis; VAU: Vaccine-Associated Uveitis; VKH: Vogt-Koyanagi-Harada.

3.4. Vaccine- and Outcome-Related Characteristics

3.4.1. Type and Dose of COVID-19 Vaccines

The majority of cases were documented in those who took the Pfizer-BioNTech vaccine (77.9%), followed by Moderna (15.54%), and AstraZeneca (3.01%), respectively [Table 2]. Most cases were more likely to occur following the first dose of the vaccine (49.35%), and the occurrence of vaccine-related uveitis was remarkably minimized following the third and fourth booster doses (7.84% and 0.37%), respectively.

3.4.2. Clinical Presentation

The majority of patients presented with redness (72.99%), followed by diminished vision (23.53%), photophobia (10.48%), and blurry vision (5.28%), respectively [Table 4].

Although infrequent, some VAU cases presented with floaters (2.22%) and vision loss (1.07%). The IOP was measured in 38 and 17 right and left eyes of VAU cases, respectively. IOP ranged from 9 to 55 and from 8 to 60 mmHg in the left and right eyes, with a mean IOP of 17.93 (SD = 11.03) and 17.3 (SD = 9.38) mmHg, respectively.

Table 4. The clinical presentation of COVID-19 vaccine-associated uveitis.

Author (YOP)	Eye Symptoms/Signs [N]	Total
Accorinti (2022)	Central scotoma [1]	1
Achiron (2022)	Vision loss [1]	1
Al-Allaf (2022)	Pain [1]—Erythema [1]—Photophobia [1]—Blurry vision [1]	1
Alhamazani (2022)	Pain [1]—Photophobia [1]—Redness [1]—Diminished Vision [1]	1
Brunet de Courssou (2022)	Headache [1]—Blurry vision [1]	1
Chen (2022a)	Headache [1]—Blurry vision [1]—Fatigue [1]	1
De Carvalho (2022)	Pain [1]—Redness [1]—Foreign Body Sensation [1]	1
De Domingo (2022)	Blurry vision [1]	1
Ishay (2021)	Pain [1]—Redness [1]—Blurry vision [1]	1
Duran (2022)	Blurry vision [1]—Redness [1]—Headache [1]	1
ElSheikh (2021)	Blurry vision [1]—Photophobia [1]	1
Lee (2022)	Vision loss [1]	1
Gedik (2022)	Pain [1]—Diminished vision [1]	1
Goyal (2021)	Vision loss [1]	1
Hébert (2022)	Vision loss [1]—Floaters [1]	1
Hwang (2022)	Erythema [1]	1
Jain (2021)	Pain [1]—Redness [1]	1
K. Joo (2022)	Pain [1]—Blurry vision [1]—Headache [1]—Eyelid swelling [1]	1
Kim (2022)	Vision loss [1]—Headache [1]	1
Koong (2021)	Blurry vision [1]	1
Papasavvas (2021)	Pain [1]	1
Ding (2022)	Vision loss [1]	1
Lee (2022)	Pain [1]—Blurry vision [1]	1
Sai (2022)	Blurry vision [1]—Floaters [1]	1
Matsuo (2022)	Blurry vision [1]	1
Mishra (2021)	Pain [1]—Diminished vision [1]	1
Mudie (2021)	Pain [1]—Photophobia [1]—Redness [1]—Vision loss [1]	1
Pan (2021)	Vision loss [1]	1
Papasavvas (2021)	Pain [1]—Diminished vision [1]—Photophobia [1]	1
Reddy (2021)	Blurry vision [1]	1
Renisi (2021)	Pain [1]—Redness [1]—Diminished vision [1]—Photophobia [1]	1
Sangoram (2022)	Blurry vision [1]—Pain [1]	1
Santiago (2021)	Redness [1]	1
Saraceno (2021)	Vision loss [1]	1
Singh (2022a)	Diminished vision [1]	1
Yalçinkaya (2022)	Redness [1]	1
Yamaguchi (2022)	Metamorphopsia [1]—Diminished vision [1]	1
Shilo (2022)	Photophobia [1]—Vision loss [1]	1
Kakarla (2022)	Blurry vision [1]—Headache [1]	1
Numakura (2022)	Blurry vision [1]	1
Murgova (2022)	Metamorphopsia [1]	1
Patel (2022)	Pain [1]—Blurry vision [1]—Floaters [1]	1
Lawson-Tovey (2022)	-	1
Arora (2022)	Diminished vision [1]—Floaters [1]	2
Choi (2022)	Diminished vision [3]	3
Ortiz-Egea (2022)	Pain [2]—Redness [1]	2
Nanji (2022)	Pain [2]—Redness [2]	2
Pang (2022)	Blurry vision [1]	2
Ren (2022)	Diminished vision [1]—Blurry vision [1]—Redness [1]—Pain [1]	2
Cohen (2022)	Pain [1]—Photophobia [1]—Diminished vision [1]—Floaters [1]	4
Aguiar (2022)	Redness [2]—Photophobia [2]—Pain [1]—Diminished vision [1]	2

Table 4. Cont.

Author (YOP)	Eye Symptoms/Signs [N]	Total	
Ferreira (2022)	Vision loss [3]—Headache [4]—Blurry vision [1]—Hyperemia [1]	4	
Chen (2022b)	Blurry vision [5]—Redness [3]	5	
Chew (2022)	Blurry vision [6]—Redness [3]—Pain [1]	6	
Rallis (2022)	Diminished vision [7]—Pain [7]	7	
Li (2022)	-	9	
Sim (2022)	-	11	
Rabinovitch (2021)	Redness [21]—Pain [21]—Blurry vision [21]—Photophobia [21]—Photopsia [2]—Diminished vision [2]	21	
Bolletta (2021)	Blurry vision [12]—Redness [3]—Pain [2]—Photophobia [1]	13	
Ferrand (2022)	-	25	
Ozdede (2022)	-	5	
Testi (2022)	-	50	
Tomkins-Netzer (2022)	-	188	
Barda (2021)	-	26	
Singh (2022b)	Pain [270]—Redness [839]—Diminished vision [262]—Photophobia [95]—Floaters [21]—Lacrimation [22]	1094	
Summary of Symptoms/Signs of VAU			
Presentation	Number	Total	%
Central Scotoma	1	1211	0.08
Vision Loss	13	1211	1.07
Pain	53	1211	4.37
Erythema	2	1211	0.16
Photophobia	127	1211	10.48
Blurry vision	64	1211	5.28
Redness	884	1211	72.99
Diminished vision	285	1211	23.53
Headache	10	1211	0.82
Foreign Body Sensation	1	1211	0.08
Floaters	27	1211	2.22
Eyelid swelling	1	1211	0.08
Photopsia	2	1211	0.16
Metamorphopsia	2	1211	0.16

YOP: Year of Publication; VAU: Vaccine-Associated Uveitis; N: Number.

3.4.3. The Nature of the Reported VAU and Disease Laterality

Out of 1526 VAU cases, only 1476 cases had the type of intraocular inflammation documented [Table 5]. The most common type was uveitis (97.56%), followed by VKH (1.08%) and retinochoroiditis (0.20%), respectively. The mean interval from COVID-19 vaccination to the occurrence of uveitis was 9.61 (SD = 8.07) days, ranging from 1 to 42 days post-vaccination. VAU was twice more likely to occur in one eye/unilaterally (77.69%) than in both eyes/bilaterally (22.05%). The rate of VAU occurrence in the right and left eyes was comparable (32.3% vs. 34.61%), respectively [Table 5].

3.4.4. Disease Course, Location, Nature, and Underlying Cause of VAU

The course of VAU was acute in more than two-thirds of the population (71.77%) as compared to chronic cases (28.22%) [Table 5]. Among VAU cases where the location was determined, the anterior segment of the uveal tract in more than half the population was affected (54.13%). Surprisingly, panuveitis was more likely to occur than posterior uveitis by almost two-fold (10.02% vs. 5.28%). Of note, the majority of VAU cases did not have a history of uveitis and experienced an episode of uveitis for the first time (69.92%), while only one-third of VAU cases had prior episodes of uveitis (30.08%). VAU was inflammatory in nature in most cases (88.29%) and infectious in 8.36% of them. The underlying cause of VAU was idiopathic in almost half the population (43.26%), while VKH (7.34%) accounted for the most commonly reported cause among other causes [Table 5].

Table 5. The type, laterality, course, location, onset, nature, and underlying cause of vaccine-associated uveitis.

Outcome	Category	Number	Total	%
	Type of VAU			
	VKH	16	1476	1.08
	Choroiditis	9	1476	0.6
	Iridocyclitis	1	1476	0.06
	Iritis	2	1476	0.13
	Kerato-uveitis	1	1476	0.06
	Retinitis	2	1476	0.13
	Uveitis	1440	1476	97.56
	Retinochoroiditis	3	1476	0.2
	Pars planitis	2	1476	0.13
	Laterality			
	Right	126	390	32.3
	Left	135	390	34.61
	Unilateral	303	390	77.69
	Bilateral	86	390	22.05
	Course			
	Acute	234	326	71.77
	Chronic	92	326	28.22
	Location			
	Anterior	799	1476	54.13
	Intermediate	14	1476	0.94
	Posterior	78	1476	5.28
	Panuveitis	148	1476	10.02
	Onset			
	New-onset	244	349	69.92
	Reactivation	105	349	30.08
	Nature			
	Autoimmune	4	299	1.34
	Granulomatous	6	299	2.01
	Inflammatory [non-infectious]	264	299	88.29
	Infectious	25	299	8.36
	Underlying Cause			
	Behcet's disease	4	245	1.63
	CMV	1	245	0.4
	HSV-1	9	245	3.67
	HZO	3	245	1.22
	JIA	4	245	1.63
	MIS-C	1	245	0.4
	Retinal vasculitis	1	245	0.4
	Sarcoidosis	3	245	1.22
	Toxoplasma	4	245	1.63
	VKH	18	245	7.34
	VZV	3	245	1.22
	Psoriasis	1	245	0.4
	Spondylarthritis	1	245	0.4
	Idiopathic	106	245	43.26
	HLA B27	12	245	4.89
	Fuchs heterochromic iridocyclitis	2	245	0.81
	Posner–Schlossman syndrome	1	245	0.4
	Duration from vaccination to uveitis attack (days)			
	Mean—SD	9.61	8.07	
	Min—Max	1	42	
	Observations	108		

3.5. Management and Treatment Outcomes

A detailed description of the management plan that was carried out per each patient is provided in Table A2. Of note, the majority (90.15%) of VAU cases showed complete resolution following treatment, while only 9.85% had partial improvement. In studies that assessed complications following the treatment of VAU cases, 21.68% of cases had at least one complication, the most common of which being transient elevation in IOP (non-serious) and nummular corneal lesions in 3.61% of cases [Table 6].

Table 6. The outcomes and complications following the treatment of vaccine-associated uveitis.

Outcome	Category	Number	Total	%	Duration (days)
Complications					
	CME	2	83	2.41	60
	Choroidal depigmentation	2	83	2.41	14
	Inflammatory glaucoma	1	83	1.2	-
	Peripheral neovascularization	1	83	1.2	135
	Retinal necrosis	1	83	1.2	-
	Recurrence of choroidal thickening	1	83	1.2	21
	ME	2	83	2.41	180
	Uveitis exacerbation	1	83	1.2	-
	Vitritis	1	83	1.2	-
	Transient IOP elevation	3	83	3.61	-
	Nummular Corneal Lesions	3	83	3.61	-
Treatment Outcome					
	Complete Resolution	174	193	90.15	-
	Partial Improvement	19	193	9.85	-

CME: Cystoid Macular Edema; ME: Macular Edema; IOP: Intraocular Pressure.

4. Discussion

Since the emergence of COVID-19 vaccines, many adverse events have been recognized globally. Of these adverse events, uveitis was one of the most commonly reported ocular events. Specifically, a recent study, using the CDC-VAERS registry, reported that VAU was evident in 1094 VAU cases across 40 countries with a crude incidence rate of 0.57 cases per million doses of the COVID-19 Pfizer vaccine [71].

The exact pathophysiology of VAU is unclear, but it is believed to be mediated through an autoimmune reaction by the vaccines [72]. Additionally, it could be due to a combination of mechanisms such as molecular mimicry, the production of specific autoantibodies, hypersensitivity reactions, and the role of some vaccine adjuvants [73,74]. Vaccines provoke an inflammatory cascade by expression of type 1 interferon, resulting in a host immune response. On the other hand, they may also induce the production of autoantibodies, which can potentially trigger an autoimmune reaction [73]. Rabinovitch et al. [55] suggested that VAU caused by mRNA vaccines is a type I autoimmune reaction resulting in spiked levels of type 1 interferon. Cunningham et al. [75] attributed VAU to type 4 hypersensitivity reaction due to molecular mimicry between uveal self-peptides and vaccine peptides. Nevertheless, the postulated mechanisms that lead to VAU following COVID-19 vaccinations are mainly hypothetical and warrant additional studies. Due to the autoimmunity nature of VAU, it tends to occur more frequently in females [76]. Although the underlying cause of this trend is uncertain, the latest evidence has shown that sex hormones have an impact on the immune reaction, with estrogen enhancing it and androgens repressing it [77]. Furthermore, recent research has demonstrated that estrogen is essential for the development and function of Th17 cells in addition to IL-17 generation [78]. Our findings coincide with this, showing that COVID-19 VAU was twice more likely to occur in females than in males (68.93% vs. 31.06%). In addition, AIDS was the most frequent among VAU cases, accounting for 1.19% of cases, which strengthens the hypothesis of autoimmunity.

Our study supports the hypothesis that uveitis can occur following COVID-19 vaccination either as new-onset (the majority of cases) or as an exacerbation or reactivation of a previous uveitis. The peak of vaccine-associated uveitis occurred in middle-aged individuals (41–50 years of age), which is parallel to findings made by Darrell et al. [79]. The majority of cases were documented in those who took the Pfizer-BioNTech vaccine (77.9%), followed by Moderna (15.54%), and AstraZeneca (3.01%), respectively. This could be explained by the fact that Pfizer–BioNTech COVID-19 vaccine elicits an additional CD8 T-cell immune response, providing additional protection against SARS-CoV2 infection—however, also triggering autoimmune reactions [80,81]. This could also be attributed to the dominance of Pfizer-BioNTech vaccine over other COVID-19 vaccine type in the number of administered doses. For instance, up to December 2022, 656.90 million Pfizer doses have been administered followed by Moderna (153.82 million), AstraZeneca (67.03 million), Jhonshon&Jhonson (18.93 million), Sinopharm (2.32 million), and Sputnik (1.85 million), respectively. Other vaccines (Sinovac, Novavax, and Covaxin) have been administered at a much lower rate (below 1 million doses) [82]. These findings were also observed in Singh RB et al. [71]'s registry analysis. Most cases were more likely to occur following the first dose of the vaccine (49.35%), and the occurrence of vaccine-related uveitis was remarkedly minimized following the third and fourth booster doses (7.84% and 0.37%, respectively). Oberhardt V et al. [83] found that the first dose of COVID-19 vaccines is associated with inducing a significantly higher level of anti-spike IgG protein, resulting in a proportionately higher number of naive and transitional B cells, as well as functional spike-specific CD8+ T cells, which is parallel to findings observed by Singh RB et al. [71]. The mean interval from COVID-19 vaccination till to the occurrence of uveitis was 9.61 (SD = 8.07) days. This might be explained by the fact that the highest immune response usually occurs during the first ten days [84]. Unfortunately, given the small sample size, we could not determine the interval time from vaccination to symptom onset per each vaccine type. That being said, the previous study [71] indicated that the interval is significantly longer in those who received the Moderna vaccine as compared to those who received either Pfizer or AstraZeneca ($p < 0.0001$). However, no conclusive, clinically applicable evidence can be drawn from such observations given the non-normal distribution of analyzed data (standard deviation was larger than the mean).

Moreover, the occurrence of VAU following COVID-19 vaccination did not follow a specific pattern regarding the location of uveitis or the course of the disease. However, in our study, VAU was more likely to occur as an acute inflammatory (non-infectious) reaction involving mainly the anterior portion of the uveal tract. The majority of VAU cases did not have a history of uveitis and experienced an episode of uveitis for the first time (69.92%), while only one-third of VAU cases had prior episodes of uveitis (30.08%). This necessitates the importance of early recognition of symptoms of uveal tract involvement especially diminished vision, photophobia, and blurry vision. Similar to any uveitis, the management of COVID-19 VAU is an exclusion diagnosis. Therefore, identifying an underlying cause whilst also ruling out infections is critical. In addition to the standard uveitis questionnaires for previous uveitis, medical history, and constitutional health symptoms during the COVID-19 pandemic, clinicians should inquire about COVID-19 vaccination status.

5. Conclusions

Our review summarizes the occurrence of COVID-19 vaccination-associated uveitis, which is more likely to occur among middle-aged females. This event occurs either as a new onset of the disease or a reactivation of previous uveitis, most commonly after vaccination with Pfizer vaccine. Although it commonly occurs after the first and then second doses of the vaccines, it can occur after the first and second booster doses as well. It usually involves the anterior part of the uveal tract as an inflammatory event in an acute form.

Author Contributions: Conceptualization, Y.Y.S.C., C.D. and A.A.; methodology, Y.Y.S.C., C.D., B.A., H.A.S., H.Y. and A.E.; software, A.A.; validation, Y.Y.S.C., C.D. and A.A.; formal analysis, A.A.; investigation, Y.Y.S.C., C.D. and A.A.; resources, A.A.; data curation, Y.Y.S.C., C.D. and A.A.; writing—original draft preparation, A.A., H.A.S., Y.Y.S.C. and C.D.; writing—review and editing, B.A. and B.E.K.; visualization, Y.Y.S.C., C.D. and A.A.; supervision, A.A.; project administration, B.E.K.;

funding acquisition, not applicable. All authors have read and agreed to the published version of the manuscript.

Funding: This research received no external funding.

Institutional Review Board Statement: Not applicable.

Informed Consent Statement: Not applicable.

Data Availability Statement: The data provided in this manuscript can be provided upon reasonable request by contacting the corresponding author.

Conflicts of Interest: The authors declare no conflict of interest.

Appendix A

Table A1. The detailed search strategy used in our review.

Database	No.	Search Query	Results
PubMed [date of search: 27 July 2022]			
	#1	("COVID-19"[Mesh] OR "SARS-CoV-2"[Mesh] OR 2019-ncov*[tiab] OR 2019ncov*[tiab] OR 2019-novel-cov*[tiab] OR coronavirus-2*[tiab] OR coronavirus-disease-19*[tiab] OR corona-virus-disease-19*[tiab] OR coronavirus-disease-20*[tiab] OR corona-virus-disease-20*[tiab] OR COVID-19*[tiab] OR COVID19*[tiab] OR COVID-20*[tiab] OR COVID20*[tiab] OR ncov-2019*[tiab] OR ncov2019*[tiab] OR new-coronavirus[tiab] OR new-corona-virus[tiab] OR novel-coronavirus[tiab] OR novel-corona-virus[tiab] OR SARS-2*[tiab] OR SARS2*[tiab] OR SARS-CoV-19*[tiab] OR SARS-CoV19*[tiab] OR SARSCoV19*[tiab] OR SARSCoV-19*[tiab] OR SARS-CoV-2*[tiab] OR SARS-CoV2*[tiab] OR SARSCoV2*[tiab] OR SARSCoV-2*[tiab] OR (("Coronavirus"[mh] OR "Coronavirus Infections"[mh] OR betacoronavirus[tiab] OR beta-coronavirus[tiab] OR beta-corona-virus[tiab] OR corona-virus[tiab] OR coronavirus[tiab] OR SARS*[tiab] OR severe-acute-respiratory*[tiab]) AND (2019[tiab] OR 2020[tiab] OR wuhan*[tiab] OR hubei*[tiab] OR china*[tiab] OR chinese*[tiab] OR outbreak*[tiab] OR epidemic*[tiab] OR pandemic*[tiab]))) AND 2019/12:3000[dp]	276,477
	#2	Uveiti* OR choroiditis OR iritis OR iridocyclitis OR "Uveitis"[Mesh] OR "Choroiditis"[Mesh] OR "Iritis"[Mesh] OR "Iridocyclitis"[Mesh]	92,380
	#3	Pfizer-BioNTech OR BTN162b2 OR Sinopharm OR Sinovac OR Moderna OR AstraZeneca OR ChAdOx1 OR AZD1222 OR Janssen OR "Johnson & Johnson" OR Novavax OR CoronaVac OR Covaxin OR Convidecia OR Sputnik OR Zifivax OR Corbevax OR COVIran OR SCB-2019 OR vaccin* OR "COVID-19 Vaccines"[Mesh]	564,424
	#4	#1 AND #2 AND #3	95
Scopus [date of search: 27 July 2022]			
	#1	(TITLE-ABS-KEY (COVID-19) OR TITLE-ABS-KEY (SARS-CoV-2) OR TITLE-ABS-KEY (2019-ncov*) OR TITLE-ABS-KEY (2019ncov*) OR TITLE-ABS-KEY (2019-novel-cov*) OR TITLE-ABS-KEY (coronavirus-2*) OR TITLE-ABS-KEY (coronavirus-disease-19*) OR TITLE-ABS-KEY (corona-virus-disease-19*) OR TITLE-ABS-KEY (coronavirus-disease-20*) OR TITLE-ABS-KEY (corona-virus-disease-20*) OR TITLE-ABS-KEY (COVID-19*) OR TITLE-ABS-KEY (COVID19*) OR TITLE-ABS-KEY (COVID-20*) OR TITLE-ABS-KEY (COVID20*) OR TITLE-ABS-KEY (ncov-2019*) OR TITLE-ABS-KEY (ncov2019*) OR TITLE-ABS-KEY (new-coronavirus) OR TITLE-ABS-KEY (new-corona-virus) OR TITLE-ABS-KEY (novel-coronavirus) OR TITLE-ABS-KEY (novel-corona-virus) OR TITLE-ABS-KEY (sars-2*) OR TITLE-ABS-KEY (sars2*) OR TITLE-ABS-KEY (SARS-CoV-19*) OR TITLE-ABS-KEY (SARS-CoV19) OR TITLE-ABS-KEY (SARSCoV19*) OR TITLE-ABS-KEY (SARSCoV-19*) OR TITLE-ABS-KEY (SARS-CoV-2*) OR TITLE-ABS-KEY (SARS-CoV2*) OR TITLE-ABS-KEY (SARSCoV2*) OR TITLE-ABS-KEY (SARSCoV-2*) OR TITLE-ABS-KEY (coronavirus) OR TITLE-ABS-KEY (coronavirus AND infections) OR TITLE-ABS-KEY (betacoronavirus) OR TITLE-ABS-KEY (beta-coronavirus) OR TITLE-ABS-KEY (beta-corona-virus) OR TITLE-ABS-KEY (corona-virus) OR TITLE-ABS-KEY (coronavirus) OR TITLE-ABS-KEY (sars*))	414,003

Table A1. Cont.

Database	No.	Search Query	Results
	#2	(TITLE-ABS-KEY (uveiti) OR TITLE-ABS-KEY (choroiditis) OR TITLE-ABS-KEY (iritis) OR TITLE-ABS-KEY (iridocyclitis))	43,658
	#3	(TITLE-ABS-KEY (pfizer-biontech) OR TITLE-ABS-KEY (btn162b2) OR TITLE-ABS-KEY (sinopharm) OR TITLE-ABS-KEY (sinovac) OR TITLE-ABS-KEY (moderna) OR TITLE-ABS-KEY (astrazeneca) OR TITLE-ABS-KEY (chadox1) OR TITLE-ABS-KEY (azd1222) OR TITLE-ABS-KEY (janssen) OR TITLE-ABS-KEY (johnson AND & AND johnson) OR TITLE-ABS-KEY (novavax) OR TITLE-ABS-KEY (coronavac) OR TITLE-ABS-KEY (covaxin) OR TITLE-ABS-KEY (convidecia) OR TITLE-ABS-KEY (sputnik) OR TITLE-ABS-KEY (zifivax) OR TITLE-ABS-KEY (corbevax) OR TITLE-ABS-KEY (coviran) OR TITLE-ABS-KEY (scb-2019) OR TITLE-ABS-KEY (vaccin*) OR TITLE-ABS-KEY (COVID-19 AND vaccines))	659,050
	#4	#1 AND #2 AND #3	92
EMBASE [date of search: 27 July 2022]			
	#1	COVID 19':ti,ab,kw OR 'SARS CoV 2':ti,ab,kw OR '2019 ncov':ti,ab,kw OR 2019ncov:ti,ab,kw OR '2019 novel cov':ti,ab,kw OR 'coronavirus 2':ti,ab,kw OR 'coronavirus disease 19*':ti,ab,kw OR 'corona virus disease 19*':ti,ab,kw OR 'coronavirus disease 20*':ti,ab,kw OR 'corona virus disease 20*':ti,ab,kw OR 'COVID 19*':ti,ab,kw OR COVID19*:ti,ab,kw OR 'COVID 20*':ti,ab,kw OR COVID20*:ti,ab,kw OR 'ncov 2019*':ti,ab,kw OR ncov2019*:ti,ab,kw OR 'new coronavirus':ti,ab,kw OR 'new coronavirus':ti,ab,kw OR 'novel coronavirus':ti,ab,kw OR 'novel corona virus':ti,ab,kw OR 'sars 2':ti,ab,kw OR sars2*:ti,ab,kw OR 'SARS CoV 19*':ti,ab,kw OR 'SARS CoV19*':ti,ab,kw OR SARSCoV19*:ti,ab,kw OR 'SARSCoV 19*':ti,ab,kw OR 'SARS CoV2*':ti,ab,kw OR SARSCoV2*:ti,ab,kw OR 'SARSCoV 2*':ti,ab,kw OR 'coronavirus infections':ti,ab,kw OR betacoronavirus:ti,ab,kw OR 'beta coronavirus':ti,ab,kw OR 'beta coronavirus':ti,ab,kw OR 'corona virus':ti,ab,kw OR coronavirus:ti,ab,kw	302,489
	#2	coronavirus disease 2019'/exp OR 'severe acute respiratory syndrome coronavirus 2'/exp OR 'coronavirinae'/exp	280,492
	#3	#1 OR #2	333,874
	#4	pfizer biontech':ti,ab,kw OR btn162b2:ti,ab,kw OR sinopharm:ti,ab,kw OR sinovac:ti,ab,kw OR moderna:ti,ab,kw OR astrazeneca:ti,ab,kw OR chadox1:ti,ab,kw OR azd1222:ti,ab,kw OR janssen:ti,ab,kw OR 'johnson & johnson':ti,ab,kw OR novavax:ti,ab,kw OR coronavac:ti,ab,kw OR covaxin:ti,ab,kw OR convidecia:ti,ab,kw OR sputnik:ti,ab,kw OR zifivax:ti,ab,kw OR corbevax:ti,ab,kw OR coviran:ti,ab,kw OR 'scb 2019':ti,ab,kw OR vaccin*:ti,ab,kw OR 'COVID-19 vaccines':ti,ab,kw	492,172
	#5	SARS-CoV-2 vaccine'/exp OR 'pfizer biontech'/exp OR 'covilo'/exp OR 'coronavac'/exp OR 'elasomeran'/exp OR 'vaxzevria'/exp OR 'ad26.cov2.s vaccine'/exp OR 'nvx-cov2373 vaccine'/exp OR 'covaxin'/exp OR 'convidecia'/exp OR 'zifivax'/exp OR 'corbevax'/exp OR 'coviran barekat'/exp	21,790
	#6	#4 OR #5	494,823
	#7	uveiti:ti,ab,kw OR choroiditis:ti,ab,kw OR iridocyclitis:ti,ab,kw OR uveitis:ti,ab,kw	34,836
	#8	uveitis'/exp OR 'choroiditis'/exp OR 'iritis'/exp OR 'iridocyclitis'/exp	71,059
	#9	#7 OR #8	75,142
	#10	#3 AND #6 AND #9	148
Web of Science [date of search: 27 July 2022]			
	#1	COVID-19 (All Fields) or SARS-CoV-2 (All Fields) or 2019-ncov* (All Fields) or 2019ncov* (All Fields) or 2019-novel-cov* (All Fields) or coronavirus-2* (All Fields) or coronavirus-disease-19* (All Fields) or corona-virus-disease-19* (All Fields) or oronavirus-disease-20* (All Fields) or corona-virus-disease-20* (All Fields) or COVID-19* (All Fields) or COVID19* (All Fields) or COVID-20* (All Fields) or COVID20* (All Fields) or ncov-2019* (All Fields) or ncov2019* (All Fields) or new-coronavirus (All Fields) or new-corona-virus (All Fields) or novel-coronavirus (All Fields) or novel-corona-virus (All Fields) or sars-2* (All Fields) or sars2* (All Fields) or SARS-CoV-19* (All Fields) or SARS-CoV19* (All Fields) or SARSCoV19* (All Fields) or SARSCoV-19* (All Fields) or SARS-CoV-2* (All Fields) or SARS-CoV2* (All Fields) or SARSCoV2* (All Fields) or SARSCoV-2* (All Fields) or Coronavirus (All Fields) or Coronavirus Infections (All Fields) or betacoronavirus (All Fields) or beta-coronavirus (All Fields) or beta-corona-virus (All Fields) or corona-virus (All Fields) or coronavirus (All Fields) or sars* (All Fields)	371,351

Table A1. Cont.

Database	No.	Search Query	Results
	#2	PfizerBioNTech (All Fields) or BTN162b2 (All Fields) or Sinopharm (All Fields) or Sinovac (All Fields) or Moderna (All Fields) or AstraZeneca (All Fields) or ChAdOx1 (All Fields) or AZD1222 (All Fields) or Janssen (All Fields) or Johnson Johnson (All Fields) or Novavax (All Fields) or CoronaVac (All Fields) or Covaxin (All Fields) or Convidecia (All Fields) or Sputnik (All Fields) or Zifivax (All Fields) or Corbevax (All Fields) or COVIran (All Fields) or SCB-2019 (All Fields) or vaccin (All Fields) or COVID19 Vaccines (All Fields)	766,301
	#3	Uveiti (All Fields) or choroiditis (All Fields) or iritis (All Fields) or iridocyclitis (All Fields)	3452
	#4	#1 AND #2 AND #3	3
CENTRAL [date of search: 27 July 2022]			
	#1	(COVID-19):ti,ab,kw OR (SARS-CoV-2):ti,ab,kw OR ("coronavirus infection"):ti,ab,kw OR (novel-coronavirus):ti,ab,kw OR (sars-2):ti,ab,kw	11,673
	#2	(Coronavirus Infections):ti,ab,kw OR (betacoronavirus):ti,ab,kw AND (COVID20):ti,ab,kw AND (new-coronavirus):ti,ab,kw AND (SARSCoV2):ti,ab,kw	1291
	#3	#1 OR #2	11,710
	#4	("uveitis"):ti,ab,kw OR (choroiditis):ti,ab,kw OR (iritis):ti,ab,kw OR (iridocyclitis):ti,ab,kw	1596
	#5	(Pfizer-BioNTech):ti,ab,kw OR (BTN162b2):ti,ab,kw OR (Sinopharm):ti,ab,kw OR (Sinovac):ti,ab,kw OR (Moderna):ti,ab,kw	331
	#6	(AstraZeneca):ti,ab,kw OR (ChAdOx1):ti,ab,kw OR (AZD1222):ti,ab,kw OR (Janssen):ti,ab,kw OR (Johnson & Johnson):ti,ab,kw	3752
	#7	(Novavax):ti,ab,kw OR (CoronaVac):ti,ab,kw OR (Covaxin):ti,ab,kw OR (Convidecia):ti,ab,kw OR (Sputnik):ti,ab,kw	104
	#8	(Zifivax):ti,ab,kw OR (Corbevax):ti,ab,kw OR (COVIran):ti,ab,kw OR (SCB-2019):ti,ab,kw OR (COVID-19 Vaccines):ti,ab,kw	663
	#9	#5 OR #6 OR #7 OR #8	4582
	#10	#3 AND #4 AND #9	0
Google Scholar [date of search: 26 July 2022]			
	With all of the words	COVID vaccine	
	With the exact phrase		
	With at least one of the words	Uveitis choroiditis iritis iridocyclitis	
	Total		200

Table A2. The management strategy of COVID-19 vaccine-associated uveitis reported in the literature.

Author (YOP)	N	T	Treatment
Accorinti (2022)	1	1	Oral, IV, and periocular corticosteroids
Achiron (2022)	1	1	Bulbar triamcinolone (40 mg/mL; 1 mL) + systemic prednisolone (starting from 60 mg and tapering down 10 mg every 2–3 days)/topical prednisolone acetate eye drops (10 mg/mL)/cyclopentolate eye drops/prednisolone eye gel
Al-Allaf (2022)	1	1	Triamcinolone drops and Azathioprine (50 mg)
Alhamazani (2022)	1	1	Topical prednisolone acetate 1% + cyclopentolate
Brunet de Courssou (2022)	1	1	Peribulbar injections of dexamethasone 8 mg + 3 intravenous pulses of methylprednisolone 15 mg/kg/day/ + oral prednisone
Chen (2022a)	1	1	Periocular injections of triamcinolone acetonide 40 mg

Table A2. Cont.

Author (YOP)	N	T	Treatment
De Carvalho (2022)	1	1	Steroid
De Domingo (2022)	1	1	Steroid
Ishay (2021)	1	1	Pulse intravenous prednisolone + topical steroid therapy
Duran (2022)	1	1	Topical 0.1% dexamethasone 8 × 1, 1% cycloplegic drops 3 × 1 and 0.1% dexamethasone ointment 1 × 1 nightly were started.
ElSheikh (2021)	1	1	Topical prednisolone acetate 1% every 2 h and cyclopentolate hydrochloride three times daily.
Lee (2022)	1	1	1g of intravenous methylprednisolone daily for 3 days, followed by oral prednisolone with a tapering dosage
Gedik (2022)	1	1	Topical steroid eye drops, cycloplegin eye drops and anti-glaucomata eye drops
Goyal (2021)	1	1	oral prednisolone 100 mg daily
Hébert (2022)	1	1	Prednisolone 1%, cyclopentolate, timolol, dexamethasone ointment, oral prednisone
Hwang (2022)	1	1	Topical dexamethasone, atropine sulfate eye drops, and systemic prednisone
Jain (2021)	1	1	Topical steroids and cycloplegics.
K. Joo (2022)	1	1	Oral prednisolone
Kim (2022)	1	1	Installation of 0.5%loteprednol etabonate + steroid pulse therapy
Koong (2021)	1	1	Pulsed intravenous methylprednisolone
Papasavvas (2021)	1	1	Capsaicin
Ding (2022)	1	1	Steroid
Lee (2022)	1	1	Systemic prednisone and mycophenolate mofetil
Sai (2022)	1	1	Topical difluprednate four times a day with gradual taper over 6 weeks with continued bimonthly dose of 40 mg adalimumab and weekly dose of 25 mg methotrexate
Matsuo (2022)	1	1	0.1% betamethasone eye drops + oral prednisolone 20 mg daily
Mishra (2021)	1	1	Oral corticosteroids Tablets. Prednisolone 40 mg/day and was added then Table Prednisolone was tapered over a period of 6 weeks.
Mudie (2021)	1	1	50 mg/day of oral prednisone and her difluprednate was increased to every 2 h
Pan (2021)	1	1	Triamcinolone acetonide (40 mg, periocular injection) and oral prednisone (20 mg once a day).
Papasavvas (2021)	1	1	5 days of oral prednisone (1 mg/kg) and Infliximab was administered following again a loading dose scheme with positive short-term evolution
Reddy (2021)	1	1	High-dose oral steroids of 70 mg per day which was tapered gradually. After reactivation: ongoing steroids of 20 mg per day. Her systemic steroid dosage is stepped up with the addition of topical steroids and cycloplegic
Renisi (2021)	1	1	Dexamethasone eye drops with a cycloplegic agent (atropine 1%)
Sangoram (2022)	1	1	Topical steroids and a cycloplegic agent.
Santiago (2021)	1	1	Prednisone and azathioprine
Saraceno (2021)	1	1	oral systemic prednisone (1.5 mg/kg/day)
Singh (2022a)	1	1	Oral steroids (prednisolone 1 mg/kg/day) with slow tapering over 6 weeks.
Yalçinkaya (2022)	1	1	IVIG (2 g/kg) and methylprednisolone (2 mg/kg)
Yamaguchi (2022)	1	1	IV methylprednisolone (1000 mg/day) for 3 days followed by oral prednisolone (60 mg/day)
Shilo (2022)	1	1	Oral prednisone which was tapered to a lower dose, and azathioprine treatment was initiated for a long-term effect.
Kakarla (2022)	1	1	Topical prednisolone
Numakura (2022)	1	1	Subcapsular injection of steroids
Murgova (2022)	1	1	Steroids, and anti-glaucoma therapy
Patel (2022)	3	3	Oral prednisone and topical difluorinated steroid therapy
Lawson-Tovey (2022)	2	2	Intravitreal injection dexamethasone
Arora (2022)	-	1	-
Choi (2022)	3	3	Steroid and methotrexate
Ortiz-Egea (2022)	2	2	Topical acyclovir, oral valaciclovir, cycloplegic, and moxifloxacin
Nanji (2022)	1	2	Topical prednisolone acetate 1% and cyclogyl 1%
Pang (2022)	1	2	One-time periocular triamcinolone acetonide injection and oral prednisone
	1	2	Topical application of prednisolone acetate and oral prednisone

Table A2. Cont.

Author (YOP)	N	T	Treatment
Ren (2022)	1	2	Systemic corticosteroid administered orally at a dose of 1 mg/kg per day
	1	2	Topical steroid (prednisolone acetate), tropicamide and pirprofen eye drops
Cohen (2022)	1	4	Oral valacyclovir, topical dexamethasone eye
	2	4	Topical dexamethasone and tropicamide
	1	4	Systemic corticosteroids (prednisone), topical dexamethasone and cycloplegic eye drops (0.5% tropicamide)
Aguiar (2022)	2	2	Dexamethasone, prednisolone ointment and cycloplegic agent (cyclopentolate)
Ferreira (2022)	1	4	Systemic corticosteroid/methotrexate
	3	4	Systemic corticosteroid/azathioprine
Chen (2022b)	1	5	Topical and periocular steroid
	2	5	Systemic steroids
	2	5	Periocular steroids
Chew (2022)	4	6	Steroid
	2	6	Sulfadiazine, Folinic acid, Pyrimethamine, Clindamycin
Rallis (2022)	7	7	Topical ganciclovir, oral acyclovir, and topical steroids
Li (2022)	-	9	-
Sim (2022)	11	11	Topical 1% prednisolone acetate eye drops and systemic prednisolone
Rabinovitch (2021)	-	21	-
Bolletta (2021)	4	13	Dexamethasone eye drops 2 mg/mL
	1	13	Ganciclovir ophthalmic gel 0.15%, dexamethasone eye drops 2 mg/mL
	3	13	Sulfadiazine and pyrimethamine tablets, and oral prednisone
	5	13	Oral prednisone
Ferrand (2022)	14	25	Topical steroid
	12	25	Systemic steroid
	2	25	Acyclovir
	1	25	Azathioprine
	3	25	Methotrexate
	4	25	Tocilizumab/natalizumab/Ixekizumab
	1	25	Dimethyl fumarate
Ozdede (2022)	-	5	-
Testi (2022)	37	50	Topical Corticosteroids
	8	50	Systemic Corticosteroids
	5	50	Antivirals
	0	50	NSAID
	4	50	Antibiotics
Tomkins-Netzer (2022)	-	188	-
Barda (2021)	-	26	-
Singh (2022b)	-	1094	-

IV: Intravenous; YOP: Year of Publication; NSAID: Non-steroidal anti-inflammatory drug; IVIG: Intravenous Immunoglobulins.

References

1. Chew, M.C.; Wiryasaputra, S.; Wu, M.; Khor, W.B.; Chan, A.S.Y. Incidence of COVID-19 Vaccination-Related Uveitis and Effects of Booster Dose in a Tertiary Uveitis Referral Center. *Front. Med.* **2022**, *9*, 925683. [CrossRef] [PubMed]
2. Nyankerh, C.N.A.; Boateng, A.K.; Appah, M. Ocular Complications after COVID-19 Vaccination, Vaccine Adverse Event Reporting System. *Vaccines* **2022**, *10*, 941. [CrossRef] [PubMed]
3. Wang, L.; Guo, Z.; Zheng, Y.; Li, Q.; Yuan, X.; Hua, X. Analysis of the clinical diagnosis and treatment of uveitis. *Ann. Palliat. Med.* **2021**, *10*, 12782–12788. [CrossRef] [PubMed]
4. Benage, M.; Fraunfelder, F.W. Vaccine-Associated Uveitis. *Mo. Med.* **2016**, *113*, 48–52.
5. de Queiroz Tavares Ferreira, F.; Araújo, D.C.; de Albuquerque, L.M.; Bianchini, P.M.; Holanda, E.C.; Pugliesi, A. Possible Association between Vogt-Koyanagi-Harada Disease and Coronavirus Disease Vaccine: A Report of Four Cases. *Ocul. Immunol. Inflamm.* **2022**, 1–7. [CrossRef] [PubMed]
6. Ritchie, H.; Mathieu, E.; Rodés-Guirao, L.; Appel, C.; Giattino, C.; Ortiz-Ospina, E.; Hasell, J.; Macdonald, B.; Beltekian, D.; Roser, M. Coronavirus pandemic (COVID-19). *Our World Data* **2020**.
7. Tomkins-Netzer, O.; Sar, S.; Barnett-Griness, O.; Friedman, B.; Shyriaieva, H.; Saliba, W. Association between vaccination with the BNT162b2 mRNA COVID-19 vaccine and non-infectious uveitis: A population-based study. *Ophthalmology* **2022**, *129*, 1087–1095. [CrossRef]

8. Muka, T.; Glisic, M.; Milic, J.; Verhoog, S.; Bohlius, J.; Bramer, W.; Chowdhury, R.; Franco, O.H. A 24-step guide on how to design, conduct, and successfully publish a systematic review and meta-analysis in medical research. *Eur. J. Epidemiol.* **2020**, *35*, 49–60. [CrossRef]
9. Accorinti, M.; Saturno, M.C.; Manni, P. Vogt-Koyanagi-Harada Relapse after COVID-19 Vaccination. *Ocul Immunol Inflamm* **2022**, *30*, 1228–1233. [CrossRef]
10. Achiron, A.; Tuuminen, R. Severe panuveitis with iridis rubeosis activation and cystoid macular edema after BioNTech-Pfizer COVID-19 vaccination in a 17-year-old. *Am. J. Ophthalmol. Case Rep.* **2022**, *25*, 101380. [CrossRef]
11. Al-Allaf, A.W.; Razok, A.; Al-Allaf, Y.; Aker, L. Post-COVID-19 vaccine medium-vessel vasculitis and acute anterior uveitis, causation vs temporal relation; case report and literature review. *Ann. Med. Surg.* **2022**, *75*, 103407. [CrossRef] [PubMed]
12. Alhamazani, M.A.; Alruwaili, W.S.; Alshammri, B.; Alrashidi, S.; Almasaud, J. A Case of Recurrent Acute Anterior Uveitis After the Administration of COVID-19 Vaccine. *Cureus* **2022**, *14*, e22911. [CrossRef] [PubMed]
13. Arora, A.; Handa, S.; Singh, S.R.; Sharma, R.; Bansal, R.; Agrawal, R.; Gupta, V. Recurrence of tubercular choroiditis following anti-SARS-CoV-2 vaccination. *Eur. J. Ophthalmol.* **2022**, 11206721221088439. [CrossRef] [PubMed]
14. Barda, N.; Dagan, N.; Ben-Shlomo, Y.; Kepten, E.; Waxman, J.; Ohana, R.; Hernán, M.A.; Lipsitch, M.; Kohane, I.; Netzer, D.; et al. Safety of the BNT162b2 mRNA COVID-19 Vaccine in a Nationwide Setting. *N. Engl. J. Med.* **2021**, *385*, 1078–1090. [CrossRef] [PubMed]
15. Bolletta, E.; Iannetta, D.; Mastrofilippo, V.; De Simone, L.; Gozzi, F.; Croci, S.; Bonacini, M.; Belloni, L.; Zerbini, A.; Adani, C.; et al. Uveitis and Other Ocular Complications Following COVID-19 Vaccination. *J. Clin. Med.* **2021**, *10*, 5960. [CrossRef]
16. Brunet de Coursou, J.B.; Tisseyre, M.; Hadjadj, J.; Chouchana, L.; Broca, F.; Terrier, B.; Duraffour, P.; Henriquez, S. De Novo Vogt-Koyanagi-Harada Disease following COVID-19 Vaccine: A Case Report and Literature Overview. *Ocul. Immunol. Inflamm.* **2022**, *30*, 1292–1295. [CrossRef]
17. Catarina Pestana Aguiar, L.F.; Costa, J.; Matias, M.J.; Miranda, V.; Chibante-Pedro, J.; Ruão, M. Acute Bilateral Uveitis Following COVID-19 Vaccination: Case Reports. *Acta Sci. Ophthalmol.* **2022**, *5*, 8–11. [CrossRef]
18. Chen, X.; Li, X.; Li, H.; Li, M.; Gong, S. Ocular Adverse Events after Inactivated COVID-19 Vaccination in Xiamen. *Vaccines* **2022**, *10*, 482. [CrossRef]
19. Chen, X.; Wang, B.; Li, X. Acute-onset Vogt-Koyanagi-Harada like uveitis following COVID-19 inactivated virus vaccination. *Am. J. Ophthalmol. Case Rep.* **2022**, *26*, 101404. [CrossRef]
20. Choi, M.; Seo, M.H.; Choi, K.E.; Lee, S.; Choi, B.; Yun, C.; Kim, S.W.; Kim, Y.Y. Vision-Threatening Ocular Adverse Events after Vaccination against Coronavirus Disease 2019. *J. Clin. Med.* **2022**, *11*, 3318. [CrossRef]
21. Cohen, S.; Olshaker, H.; Fischer, N.; Vishnevskia-Dai, V.; Hagin, D.; Rosenblatt, A.; Zur, D.; Habot-Wilner, Z. Herpetic Eye Disease Following the SARS-CoV-2 Vaccinations. *Ocul. Immunol. Inflamm.* **2022**, 1–12. [CrossRef] [PubMed]
22. De Carvalho, J.; Catunda, J.V.; Rodrigues, C.M. Uveitis following COVID-19 Vaccination: A Case Report and a Literature Review. *Beyond Rheumatol.* **2022**, *4*, e379.
23. De Domingo, B.; López, B.; Lopez-Valladares, M.; Ortegon-Aguilar, E.; Sopeña-Perez-Argüelles, B.; Gonzalez, F. Vogt-Koyanagi-Harada Disease Exacerbation Associated with COVID-19 Vaccine. *Cells* **2022**, *11*, 1012. [CrossRef] [PubMed]
24. Ding, X.; Chang, Q. Probable Vogt-Koyanagi-Harada Disease after COVID-19 Vaccination: Case Report and Literature Review. *Vaccines* **2022**, *10*, 783. [CrossRef]
25. Duran, M. Bilateral anterior uveitis after BNT162b2 mRNA vaccine: Case report. *J. Fr. Ophtalmol.* **2022**, *45*, e311–e313. [CrossRef]
26. ElSheikh, R.H.; Haseeb, A.; Eleiwa, T.K.; Elhusseiny, A.M. Acute Uveitis following COVID-19 Vaccination. *Ocul. Immunol. Inflamm.* **2021**, *29*, 1207–1209. [CrossRef]
27. Ferrand, N.; Accorinti, M.; Agarwal, M.; Spartalis, C.; Manni, P.; Stuebiger, N.; Zierhut, M. COVID-19 Vaccination and Uveitis: Epidemiology, Clinical Features and Visual Prognosis. *Ocul. Immunol. Inflamm.* **2022**, *30*, 1265–1273. [CrossRef]
28. Gedik, B.; Erol, M.K.; Bulut, M.; Suren, E.; Bozdogan, Y.C.; Seymen, B. Two doses of the Pfizer-BioNTech vaccine, two different side effects: Skin and eye. *J. Fr. Ophtalmol.* **2022**, *45*, 767–770. [CrossRef]
29. Goyal, M.; Murthy, S.I.; Annum, S. Bilateral Multifocal Choroiditis following COVID-19 Vaccination. *Ocul. Immuno.l Inflamm.* **2021**, *29*, 753–757. [CrossRef]
30. Hébert, M.; Couture, S.; Schmit, I. Bilateral Panuveitis with Occlusive Vasculitis following Coronavirus Disease 2019 Vaccination. *Ocul. Immunol. Inflamm.* **2022**, 1–5. [CrossRef]
31. Hwang, J.H. Uveitis after COVID-19 Vaccination. *Case Rep. Ophthalmol.* **2022**, *13*, 124–127. [CrossRef] [PubMed]
32. Ishay, Y.; Kenig, A.; Tsemach-Toren, T.; Amer, R.; Rubin, L.; Hershkovitz, Y.; Kharouf, F. Autoimmune phenomena following SARS-CoV-2 vaccination. *Int. Immunopharmacol.* **2021**, *99*, 107970. [CrossRef] [PubMed]
33. Jain, A.; Kalamkar, C. COVID-19 vaccine-associated reactivation of uveitis. *Indian J. Ophthalmol.* **2021**, *69*, 2899–2900. [CrossRef] [PubMed]
34. Joo, C.W.; Kim, Y.K.; Park, S.P. Vogt-Koyanagi-Harada Disease following mRNA-1273 (Moderna) COVID-19 Vaccination. *Ocul. Immunol. Inflamm.* **2022**, *30*, 1250–1254. [CrossRef]
35. Kakarla, P.D.; Venugopal, R.Y.C.; Manechala, U.B.; Rijey, J.; Anthwal, D. Bilateral multifocal choroiditis with disc edema in a 15-year-old girl following COVID-19 vaccination. *Indian J. Ophthalmol.* **2022**, *70*, 3420–3422. [CrossRef]
36. Kim, S.Y.; Kang, M.S.; Kwon, H.J. Bilateral Panuveitis Mimicking Vogt-Koyanagi-Harada Disease following the First Dose of ChAdOx1 nCoV-19 Vaccine. *Ocul. Immunol. Inflamm.* **2022**, *30*, 1218–1221. [CrossRef]

37. Koong, L.R.; Chee, W.K.; Toh, Z.H.; Ng, X.L.; Agrawal, R.; Ho, S.L. Vogt-Koyanagi-Harada Disease Associated with COVID-19 mRNA Vaccine. *Ocul. Immunol. Inflamm.* **2021**, *29*, 1212–1215. [CrossRef]
38. Lawson-Tovey, S.; Machado, P.M.; Strangfeld, A.; Mateus, E.; Gossec, L.; Carmona, L.; Raffeiner, B.; Bulina, I.; Clemente, D.; Zepa, J.; et al. SARS-CoV-2 vaccine safety in adolescents with inflammatory rheumatic and musculoskeletal diseases and adults with juvenile idiopathic arthritis: Data from the EULAR COVAX physician-reported registry. *RMD Open* **2022**, *8*, e002322. [CrossRef]
39. Lee, B.A.; Alsberge, J.B.; Biggee, K.; Lin, H.; Lo, W.R. Presumed panuveitis following COVID-19 vaccination in a patient with granulomatous tattoo inflammation. *Retin. Cases Brief Rep.* **2022**. [CrossRef]
40. Lee, C.; Park, K.A.; Ham, D.I.; Seong, M.; Kim, H.J.; Lee, G.I.; Oh, S.Y. Neuroretinitis after the second injection of a SARS-CoV-2-vaccine: A case report. *Am. J. Ophthalmol. Case Rep.* **2022**, *27*, 101592. [CrossRef]
41. Li, Z.; Hu, F.; Li, Q.; Wang, S.; Chen, C.; Zhang, Y.; Mao, Y.; Shi, X.; Zhou, H.; Cao, X.; et al. Ocular Adverse Events after Inactivated COVID-19 Vaccination. *Vaccines* **2022**, *10*, 918. [CrossRef]
42. Mahendradas, P.; Mishra, S.B.; Mangla, R.; Sanjay, S.; Kawali, A.; Shetty, R.; Dharmanand, B. Reactivation of juvenile idiopathic arthritis associated uveitis with posterior segment manifestations following anti-SARS-CoV-2 vaccination. *J. Ophthalmic Inflamm. Infect.* **2022**, *12*, 15. [CrossRef] [PubMed]
43. Matsuo, T.; Honda, H.; Tanaka, T.; Uraguchi, K.; Kawahara, M.; Hagiya, H. COVID-19 mRNA Vaccine-Associated Uveitis Leading to Diagnosis of Sarcoidosis: Case Report and Review of Literature. *J. Investig. Med. High Impact Case Rep.* **2022**, *10*, 23247096221086450. [CrossRef] [PubMed]
44. Mishra, S.B.; Mahendradas, P.; Kawali, A.; Sanjay, S.; Shetty, R. Reactivation of varicella zoster infection presenting as acute retinal necrosis post COVID 19 vaccination in an Asian Indian male. *Eur. J. Ophthalmol.* **2021**, 11206721211046485. [CrossRef] [PubMed]
45. Mudie, L.I.; Zick, J.D.; Dacey, M.S.; Palestine, A.G. Panuveitis following Vaccination for COVID-19. *Ocul. Immunol. Inflamm.* **2021**, *29*, 741–742. [CrossRef] [PubMed]
46. Murgova, S.; Balchev, G. Ophthalmic manifestation after SARS-CoV-2 vaccination: A case series. *J. Ophthalmic Inflamm. Infect.* **2022**, *12*, 20. [CrossRef] [PubMed]
47. Nanji, A.A.; Fraunfelder, F.T. Anterior Uveitis following COVID Vaccination: A Summary of Cases from Global Reporting Systems. *Ocul. Immunol. Inflamm.* **2022**, *30*, 1244–1246. [CrossRef]
48. Numakura, T.; Murakami, K.; Tamada, T.; Yamaguchi, C.; Inoue, C.; Ohkouchi, S.; Tode, N.; Sano, H.; Aizawa, H.; Sato, K.; et al. A Novel Development of Sarcoidosis Following COVID-19 Vaccination and a Literature Review. *Intern. Med.* **2022**, *61*, 3101–3106. [CrossRef]
49. Ortiz-Egea, J.M.; Sánchez, C.G.; López-Jiménez, A.; Navarro, O.D. Herpetic anterior uveitis following Pfizer-BioNTech coronavirus disease 2019 vaccine: Two case reports. *J. Med. Case Rep.* **2022**, *16*, 127. [CrossRef]
50. Ozdede, A.; Guner, S.; Ozcifci, G.; Yurttas, B.; Toker Dincer, Z.; Atli, Z.; Uygunoğlu, U.; Durmaz, E.; Uçar, D.; Uğurlu, S.; et al. Safety of SARS-CoV-2 vaccination in patients with Behcet's syndrome and familial Mediterranean fever: A cross-sectional comparative study on the effects of M-RNA based and inactivated vaccine. *Rheumatol. Int.* **2022**, *42*, 973–987. [CrossRef]
51. Pan, L.; Zhang, Y.; Cui, Y.; Wu, X. Bilateral uveitis after inoculation with COVID-19 vaccine: A case report. *Int. J. Infect. Dis.* **2021**, *113*, 116–118. [CrossRef] [PubMed]
52. Pang, K.; Pan, L.; Guo, H.; Wu, X. Case Report: Associated Ocular Adverse Reactions With Inactivated COVID-19 Vaccine in China. *Front. Med.* **2021**, *8*, 823346. [CrossRef] [PubMed]
53. Papasavvas, I.; Herbort, C.P., Jr. Reactivation of Vogt-Koyanagi-Harada disease under control for more than 6 years, following anti-SARS-CoV-2 vaccination. *J. Ophthalmic Inflamm. Infect.* **2021**, *11*, 21. [CrossRef] [PubMed]
54. Patel, K.G.; Hilton, T.; Choi, R.Y.; Abbey, A.M. Uveitis and Posterior Ophthalmic Manifestations Following the SARS-CoV-2 (COVID-19) Vaccine. *Ocul. Immunol. Inflamm.* **2022**, *30*, 1142–1148. [CrossRef]
55. Rabinovitch, T.; Ben-Arie-Weintrob, Y.; Hareuveni-Blum, T.; Shaer, B.; Vishnevskia-Dai, V.; Shulman, S.; Newman, H.; Biadsy, M.; Masarwa, D.; Fischer, N.; et al. UVEITIS AFTER THE BNT162b2 mRNA VACCINATION AGAINST SARS-CoV-2 INFECTION. *Retin.* **2021**, *41*, 2462–2471. [CrossRef]
56. Rallis, K.I.; Fausto, R.; Ting, D.S.J.; Al-Aqaba, M.A.; Said, D.G.; Dua, H.S. Manifestation of Herpetic Eye Disease after COVID-19 Vaccine: A UK Case Series. *Ocul. Immunol. Inflamm.* **2022**, *30*, 1136–1141. [CrossRef]
57. Reddy, Y.; Pandey, A.; Ojha, A.; Ramchandani, S. Harada-like syndrome post-Covishield vaccination: A rare adverse effect. *Indian J. Ophthalmol.* **2022**, *70*, 321–323. [CrossRef] [PubMed]
58. Ren, J.; Zhang, T.; Li, X.; Liu, G. Ocular Inflammatory Reactions following an Inactivated SARS-CoV-2 Vaccine: A Four Case Series. *Ocul. Immunol. Inflamm.* **2022**, 1–6. [CrossRef]
59. Renisi, G.; Lombardi, A.; Stanzione, M.; Invernizzi, A.; Bandera, A.; Gori, A. Anterior uveitis onset after bnt162b2 vaccination: Is this just a coincidence? *Int. J. Infect. Dis.* **2021**, *110*, 95–97. [CrossRef]
60. Sangoram, R.; Mahendradas, P.; Bhakti Mishra, S.; Kawali, A.; Sanjay, S.; Shetty, R. Herpes Simplex Virus 1 Anterior Uveitis following Coronavirus Disease 2019 (COVID-19) Vaccination in an Asian Indian Female. *Ocul. Immunol. Inflamm.* **2022**, *30*, 1260–1264. [CrossRef]
61. Santiago, J.; Negron-Ocasio, G.; Ortiz-Troche, S.; Rodriguez, K.P.; Ramirez-Marquez, J.; Velazquez, L.; Lugo, I.D.S.; Feliciano-FIgueroa, J.; Colon-Marquez, J. RARE EXPRESSION OF SYSTEMIC SARCOIDOSIS AFTER A NOVEL RNA VACCINE. *Chest* **2021**, *160*, A1233–A1234. [CrossRef]

62. Saraceno, J.J.F.; Souza, G.M.; dos Santos Finamor, L.P.; Nascimento, H.M.; Belfort, R. Vogt-Koyanagi-Harada syndrome following COVID-19 and ChAdOx1 nCoV-19 (AZD1222) vaccine. *Int. J. Retin. Vitr.* **2021**, *7*, 49. [CrossRef] [PubMed]
63. Sim, H.E.; Hwang, J.H. New onset of acute uveitis following COVID-19 vaccination. *Graefes Arch. Clin. Exp. Ophthalmol.* **2022**, 1–6. [CrossRef]
64. Singh, J.; More, A.; Shetty, S.B.; Chaskar, P.; Sen, A. Herpes simplex virus retinitis following ChAdOx1 nCoV-19 (Covishield) vaccination for SARS-CoV-2: A case report. *Ocul. Immunol. Inflamm.* **2022**, *30*, 1282–1285. [CrossRef] [PubMed]
65. Singh, R.B.; Parmar, U.P.S.; Cho, W.; Ichhpujani, P. Glaucoma Cases Following SARS-CoV-2 Vaccination: A VAERS Database Analysis. *Vaccines* **2022**, *10*, 1630. [CrossRef]
66. Testi, I.; Brandão-de-Resende, C.; Agrawal, R.; Pavesio, C.; Steeples, L.; Balasubramaniam, B.; McCluskey, P.; Pichi, F.; Agarwal, A.; Herbort, C.; et al. Ocular inflammatory events following COVID-19 vaccination: A multinational case series. *J. Ophthalmic Inflamm. Infect.* **2022**, *12*, 4. [CrossRef] [PubMed]
67. Yalçinkaya, R.; Öz, F.N.; Polat, M.; Uçan, B.; Teke, T.A.; Kaman, A.; Özdem, S.; Savaş Şen, Z.; Cinni, R.G.; Tanir, G. A Case of Multisystem Inflammatory Syndrome in a 12-Year-old Male After COVID-19 mRNA Vaccine. *Pediatr. Infect. Dis. J.* **2022**, *41*, e87–e89. [CrossRef]
68. Yamaguchi, C.; Kunikata, H.; Hashimoto, K.; Yoshida, M.; Ninomiya, T.; Hariya, T.; Abe, T.; Nakazawa, T. De novo Vogt-Koyanagi-Harada disease after vaccination for COVID-19, successfully treated with systemic steroid therapy and monitored with laser speckle flowgraphy. *Am. J. Ophthalmol. Case Rep.* **2022**, *27*, 101616. [CrossRef]
69. Yasuda, E.; Matsumiya, W.; Maeda, Y.; Kusuhara, S.; Nguyen, Q.D.; Nakamura, M.; Hara, R. Multiple evanescent white dot syndrome following BNT162b2 mRNA COVID-19 vaccination. *Am. J. Ophthalmol. Case Rep.* **2022**, *26*, 101532. [CrossRef]
70. Shilo, V.; Boaz, S. Ocular Presentation of Behcet's Syndrome Associated with COVID-19 Vaccination. *Am. J. Biomed. Sci. Res.* **2022**, *15*, 649–652. [CrossRef]
71. Singh, R.B.; Parmar, U.P.S.; Kahale, F.; Agarwal, A.; Tsui, E. Vaccine-Associated Uveitis after COVID-19 Vaccination: Vaccine Adverse Event Reporting System Database Analysis. *Ophthalmology*, 2022; in press. [CrossRef] [PubMed]
72. Sachinidis, A.; Garyfallos, A. COVID-19 vaccination can occasionally trigger autoimmune phenomena, probably via inducing age-associated B cells. *Int. J. Rheum. Dis.* **2022**, *25*, 83–85. [CrossRef] [PubMed]
73. Chen, Y.; Xu, Z.; Wang, P.; Li, X.M.; Shuai, Z.W.; Ye, D.Q.; Pan, H.F. New-onset autoimmune phenomena post-COVID-19 vaccination. *Immunology* **2022**, *165*, 386–401. [CrossRef] [PubMed]
74. Teijaro, J.R.; Farber, D.L. COVID-19 vaccines: Modes of immune activation and future challenges. *Nat. Reviews. Immunol.* **2021**, *21*, 195–197. [CrossRef]
75. Cunningham, E.T., Jr.; Moorthy, R.S.; Fraunfelder, F.W.; Zierhut, M. Vaccine-Associated Uveitis. *Ocul. Immunol. Inflamm.* **2019**, *27*, 517–520. [CrossRef]
76. Yeung, I.Y.; Popp, N.A.; Chan, C.C. The role of sex in uveitis and ocular inflammation. *Int. Ophthalmol. Clin.* **2015**, *55*, 111–131. [CrossRef]
77. Choudhary, M.M.; Hajj-Ali, R.A.; Lowder, C.Y. Gender and ocular manifestations of connective tissue diseases and systemic vasculitides. *J. Ophthalmol.* **2014**, *2014*, 403042. [CrossRef]
78. Singh, R.P.; Hasan, S.; Sharma, S.; Nagra, S.; Yamaguchi, D.T.; Wong, D.T.; Hahn, B.H.; Hossain, A. Th17 cells in inflammation and autoimmunity. *Autoimmun. Rev.* **2014**, *13*, 1174–1181. [CrossRef]
79. Darrell, R.W.; Wagener, H.P.; Kurland, L.T. Epidemiology of uveitis. Incidence and prevalence in a small urban community. *Arch. Ophthalmol.* **1962**, *68*, 502–514. [CrossRef]
80. Sahin, U.; Muik, A.; Derhovanessian, E.; Vogler, I.; Kranz, L.M.; Vormehr, M.; Baum, A.; Pascal, K.; Quandt, J.; Maurus, D.; et al. COVID-19 vaccine BNT162b1 elicits human antibody and T(H)1 T cell responses. *Nature* **2020**, *586*, 594–599. [CrossRef]
81. Walter, R.; Hartmann, K.; Fleisch, F.; Reinhart, W.H.; Kuhn, M. Reactivation of herpesvirus infections after vaccinations? *Lancet* **1999**, *353*, 810. [CrossRef] [PubMed]
82. Our World in Data. COVID-19 vaccine doses administered by manufacturer, European Union. Available online: https://ourworldindata.org/grapher/COVID-vaccine-doses-by-manufacturer (accessed on 14 December 2022).
83. Oberhardt, V.; Luxenburger, H.; Kemming, J.; Schulien, I.; Ciminski, K.; Giese, S.; Csernalabics, B.; Lang-Meli, J.; Janowska, I.; Staniek, J.; et al. Rapid and stable mobilization of CD8+ T cells by SARS-CoV-2 mRNA vaccine. *Nature* **2021**, *597*, 268–273. [CrossRef] [PubMed]
84. Polack, F.P.; Thomas, S.J.; Kitchin, N.; Absalon, J.; Gurtman, A.; Lockhart, S.; Perez, J.L.; Marc, G.P.; Moreira, E.D.; Zerbini, C. Safety and efficacy of the BNT162b2 mRNA COVID-19 vaccine. *N. Engl. J. Med.* **2020**, *383*, 2603–2615. [CrossRef] [PubMed]

Disclaimer/Publisher's Note: The statements, opinions and data contained in all publications are solely those of the individual author(s) and contributor(s) and not of MDPI and/or the editor(s). MDPI and/or the editor(s) disclaim responsibility for any injury to people or property resulting from any ideas, methods, instructions or products referred to in the content.

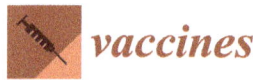

Review

Ocular Vascular Events following COVID-19 Vaccines: A Systematic Review

Hashem Abu Serhan [1,2,*], Abdelaziz Abdelaal [2,3,4], Mohammad T. Abuawwad [5], Mohammad J. J. Taha [5], Sara Irshaidat [6], Leen Abu Serhan [7], Luai Abu-Ismail [8], Qusai Faisal Abu Salim [9], Basel Abdelazeem [2,10] and Ayman G. Elnahry [11,12]

1. Department of Ophthalmology, Hamad Medical Corporations, Doha 3050, Qatar
2. Tanta Research Team, El-Gharbia 31511, Egypt
3. Harvard Medical School, Postgraduate Medical Education, Boston, MA 02115, USA
4. Doheny Eye Institute, University of California, Los Angeles, CA 94720, USA
5. Department of Clinical Medicine, Kasr Alainy Faculty of Medicine, Cairo University, Cairo 11562, Egypt
6. Department of Pediatrics, King Hussein Cancer Centre, Amman 11941, Jordan
7. Faculty of Medicine, Hashemite University, Zarqa 13133, Jordan
8. Department of Ophthalmology, Islamic Hospital, Amman 11190, Jordan
9. Department of Ophthalmology, The Eye Specialty Hospital, Amman 11118, Jordan
10. Department of Internal Medicine, Michigan State University, East Lansing, MI 48824, USA
11. Department of Ophthalmology, Faculty of Medicine, Cairo University, Cairo 11591, Egypt
12. Division of Epidemiology and Clinical Applications, National Eye Institute, National Institutes of Health, Bethesda, MD 20892, USA
* Correspondence: habuserhan@hamad.qa; Tel.: +974-77912335

Abstract: The main aim of this study is to investigate the current evidence regarding the association between COVID-19 vaccination and ocular vascular events. The protocol is registered on PROSPERO (CRD42022358133). On 18 August 2022, an electronic search was conducted through five databases. All original articles reporting individuals who were vaccinated with COVID-19 vaccines and developed ophthalmic vascular events were included. The methodological quality of the included studies was assessed using the NIH tool. A total of 49 studies with 130 ocular vascular cases were included. Venous occlusive events were the most common events (54.3%), which mostly occurred following the first dose (46.2%) and within the first five days following vaccination (46.2%). Vascular events occurred more with the Pfizer and AstraZeneca vaccines (81.6%), and mostly presented unilaterally (73.8%). The most frequently reported treatment was intravitreal anti-VEGF (n = 39, 30.4%). The majority of patients (90.1%) demonstrated either improvement ($p = 0.321$) or persistence ($p = 0.414$) in the final BCVA. Ophthalmic vascular events are serious vision-threatening side effects that have been associated with COVID-19 vaccination. Clinicians should be aware of the possible association between COVID-19 vaccines and ocular vascular events to provide early diagnosis and treatment.

Keywords: vaccination; SARS-CoV-2; ophthalmic adverse events; adverse events; COVID-19 vaccination; vascular events; central artery occlusion; ischemic optic neuropathy

1. Introduction

Vaccines against the SARS-CoV-2 infection are the primary modality to prevent the disease from spreading. In 2020, an international race to develop vaccines against SARS-CoV-2 started [1], and by May 2022, a total of nine vaccines had been listed for emergency use by the World Health Organization (WHO): AstraZeneca (recombinant vaccine), Johnson & Johnson/Janssen (recombinant), Pfizer-BioNTech (mRNA), Moderna (mRNA), Sinopharm (inactivated), CoronaVac (inactivated), Novavax (recombinant, adjuvanted), Convidecia (recombinant), and Baharat (inactivated) [2]. Despite substantial protection against severe outcomes following vaccination, and the boosting maintained for most of the population, multiple side effects were reported to occur following vaccination [3]. Generally, WHO defined Adverse Events Following Immunization (AEFI) as any undesirable medical circumstances that occur after vaccination but do not necessarily have a direct link to the use of the vaccine [4]. Regarding COVID-19-vaccine-related complications, vascular complications were the most serious to happen. Many vascular complications of the COVID-19 vaccine were reported including many serious vaccine-related thrombo-embolic events, resulting in cerebral venous thrombosis, thrombocytopenia, and coagulation disorders [5].

Although COVID-19 vaccination can be complicated by several ocular events such as abducens nerve palsy, acute macular neuro-retinopathy, and multiple evanescent white dot syndrome, vascular events remain the most serious group of complications that needs higher medical attention, due to their high association with vision loss and blindness [6]. Despite their rarity, ocular vascular events were indeed reported following COVID-19 vaccines. For example, retinal artery occlusions (RAO), venous stasis retinopathy, and non-arteritic anterior ischemic optic neuropathy (NAAION) were reported in the literature [7]. In early May 2021, The Royal College of Ophthalmologists in the United Kingdom reported an increased incidence of central venous sinus thrombosis (CVST) and retinal vein occlusion (RVO) subsequent to COVID-19 vaccination [8].

Nevertheless, vaccination against COVID-19 is now being conducted on a large scale worldwide due to its proven benefit of preventing severe COVID-19 infection, which is also known to cause vascular events including in the eye [9]. Thus, more light should be shed on the ocular complications generally and vascular events specifically associated with COVID-19 vaccination. In this systematic review, we collect and analyze all observational studies to date that reported cases of ocular vascular events following COVID-19 vaccination, to summarize the current evidence regarding their association. To our knowledge, this is the first systematic review that specifically tackles ocular vascular events occurring after COVID-19 vaccination.

2. Materials and Methods

2.1. Study Design

This research was conducted in accordance with the Preferred Reporting Items for Systematic Reviews and Meta-Analyses (PRISMA) guidelines, and the protocol was pre-registered on PROSPERO [CRD42022358133]. The design of this research followed the PICOS framework as follows: population (healthy individuals with no prior ocular pathologies), intervention (COVID-19 vaccines of different types and/or doses), comparison (none), outcomes (occurrence of ophthalmic vascular events), and study design (observational and/or experimental studies).

2.2. Search Strategy

On 18 August 2022, PubMed, Scopus, Web of Science (WoS), EMBASE, Cochrane Central Register of Controlled Trials (CENTRAL), and Google Scholar were searched for studies reporting the occurrence of ophthalmic vascular events after receiving COVID-19 vaccines. It should be noted that, based on recent recommendations [10], only the first 200 records of Google Scholar were searched, after which their relevance significantly dropped. The following keywords were used to identify relevant articles: (COVID-19 OR SARS-CoV-2) AND (vaccine *) AND ("ophthalmic vascular event *"). Additionally, Medical Subject Headings (MeSH) terms were used to identify all potentially relevant articles based on these indexed terms. The detailed search criteria, adjusted per each searched database, is provided in [Supplementary Table S1].

A manual search was also conducted following the screening of articles to identify any potentially missing relevant articles through three approaches: (a) screening the reference list of included articles, (b) screening "similar articles" to the included ones, through the "similar articles" options on PubMed, and (c) manually searching for articles on Google with the use of following keywords: "COVID" + "vaccine" + "ophthalmic". The key ophthalmic vascular events that we looked for included choroidal ischemia, retinal artery occlusions (RAO), retinal vein occlusion (RVO), ophthalmic artery occlusion (OAO), ophthalmic vein occlusion (OVO), ophthalmic artery spasm, vitreous hemorrhage, or ischemic optic neuropathy. An updated search was conducted right before the analysis to include any recently published studies in the time between our original and updated search.

2.3. Study Outcomes

The primary outcome of this review is to summarize the available evidence on the occurrence of any ophthalmic vascular events following COVID-19 vaccination while providing an emphasis on the association between these events and the type, dose, and time interval from vaccination until their occurrence.

2.4. Eligibility Criteria

Studies were included if they recruited individuals who were vaccinated with any of the COVID-19 vaccines and developed an ophthalmic vascular event following vaccination. No limitations were set on language, country, or study design. Of note, case reports, case series, case–control, cohort, cross-sectional, and experimental studies were eligible for inclusion.

On the other hand, studies were excluded if they had one of the following criteria: (1) non-original research (i.e., reviews, commentaries, guidelines, editorials, correspondence, letters to editors, etc.), (2) unavailable full texts, (3) duplicated records or records with overlapping datasets, (4) studies reporting adverse events other than ophthalmic vascular events, and (5) studies that discuss non-COVID-19 vaccines.

2.5. Study Selection

Following the retrieval of the studies from the database search, citations were imported into EndNote for duplicate removal, after which, the citations were exported into an Excel Sheet for screening. First, the titles and abstracts of the retrieved articles were screened against our prespecified eligibility criteria. Then, studies that were potentially relevant underwent full-text screenings. This process was carried out by two sets of two reviewers [S.I. and L.A.S.; L.A.I. and Q.A.S.] who resolved their differences through discussions. Meanwhile, the senior author was consulted when an agreement could not be reached.

2.6. Data Extraction

A pilot extraction was carried out to design the data extraction sheet using Microsoft Excel. The data extraction sheet consisted of four main parts. The first part includes the baseline characteristics of the included studies (name of the first author, year of publication, country, name of the journal, and study design) and included participants (sample size, age, and gender). The second part includes data on the reported ophthalmic vascular event (name, type, number, and laterality [right or left eye or both]) and COVID-19 vaccines (type, dose, time from vaccination to symptom onset, and COVID-19 infection status). The third part summarizes the medical history of the reported cases with ophthalmic vascular events (i.e., systemic diseases, cardiovascular diseases, cerebrovascular diseases, immunological diseases, history of eye trauma, previous eye diseases, and previous ocular surgeries). The fourth part included a thorough assessment of the reported event in terms of presenting symptoms, diagnostic methods, examination findings, initial best-corrected visual acuity (BCVA), investigations (blood and eye investigations), management (either medical or surgical), the follow-up period, and management outcomes and associated complications if present. The data extraction process was carried out by two sets of two reviewers [S.I. and L.A.S.; L.A.I. and Q.A.S.], and any discrepancies were resolved by discussion or consultation with the senior author.

2.7. Quality Assessment

The methodological quality of the included studies was assessed using the National Institute of Health (NIH) tool (https://www.nhlbi.nih.gov/health-topics/study-quality-assessment-tools, accessed on 17 October 2022) for each respective study design included (no quality assessment was done for case reports). This process was carried out by two sets of two reviewers [S.I. and L.A.S.; L.A.I. and Q.A.S.], and any discrepancies were resolved by discussion or consultation with a senior author.

2.8. Data Synthesis

Retrieved data from the included studies were qualitatively synthesized. No quantitative analyses were carried out. Frequencies and proportions were used to summarize the data. Comparisons between categorical variables were analyzed using the Pearson Chi-square test. At a *p*-value of 0.05, statistical significance was deemed to exist. The Social Sciences Statistical Program was used to conduct the statistical analysis (IBM SPSS Corp, Statistical Product and Service Solutions (SPSS) Statistics version 26, Chicago, USA). The qualitative synthesis included summarizing the occurrence of ophthalmic vascular events following COVID-19 vaccination, where data were categorized based on the study design and type and dose of the COVID-19 vaccine. Then, our outcome of interest (the occurrence of ophthalmic vascular events) was analyzed in terms of baseline characteristics (age, gender, vaccine type and dose, presenting symptoms, and time interval from vaccination to symptom onset). Such data were stratified by the type and location of the vascular event. Finally, the outcomes of the management of each vascular event were summarized, including complete resolution, partial resolution, recurrence, and complications.

3. Results

3.1. Search Results

We retrieved 360 records from our searches, 120 duplicates were removed, and the remaining 242 titles and abstracts were screened. Then, 58 potential full texts were assessed and only 49 studies were included (Figure 1). It should be noted that both the manual and updated database search did not yield any additional studies.

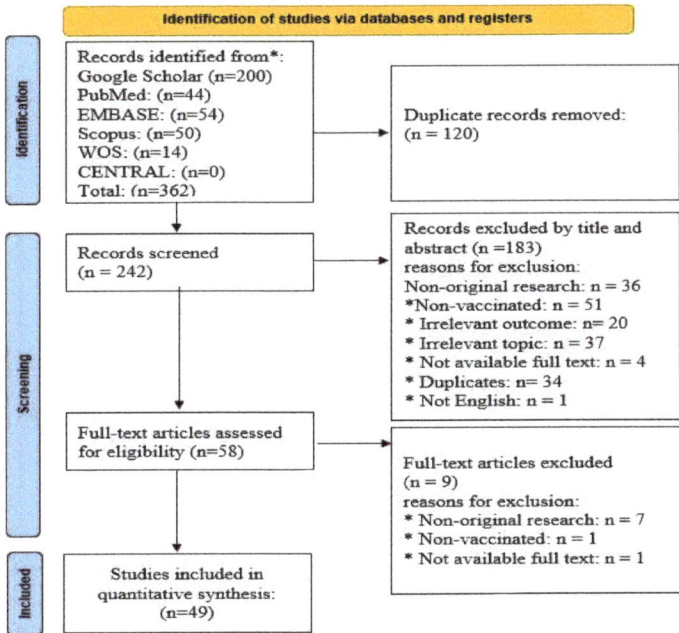

Figure 1. PRISMA chart for article selection. *: the following different databases.

3.2. Baseline Characteristics of Studies Reporting COVID-19-Vaccine-Associated Vascular Events

In this systematic review, a total of 49 case reports and series with 130 cases of ocular vascular events following COVID-19 vaccination from 23 countries around the world were identified. The included papers are summarized in Table 1.

Table 1. Summary of papers reviewed in this systematic review.

No.	Author	Country	Type of Study	No. of Cases	Mean Age	Gender	Diagnosis
1	Abdallah & Hamzah [11]	USA	Case Report	1	51	M	CRAO
2	Abdin et al. [12]	Germany	Case Report	1	76	F	CRAO
3	Amin et al. [13]	Bangladesh	Case Report	1	41	M	VH
4	Bialasiewicz et al. [14]	Qatar	Case Report	1	50	M	CRVO
5	Bolletta et al. [15]	Italy	Case Series	6	49.5	3 M, 3 F	1 CRVO, 5 BRVO
6	Cackett et al. [16]	UK	Case Report	2	45	2 F	2 CRVO
7	Casarini et al. [17]	Italy	Case Report	1	60	M	VH
8	Che et al. [18]	South Korea	Case Report	1	87	F	AAION
9	Chen et al. [19]	Taiwan	Case Report	1	48	F	BRAO
10	Choi et al. [20]	Korea	Case Series	9	60.8	3 M, 6 F	4 CRVO, 5 BRVO
11	Chow et al. [21]	Taiwan	Case Report	1	70	M	CRAO
12	Chung et al. [22]	Korea	Case Report	1	65	F	NAAION
13	Da Silva et al. [23]	Brazil	Case Series	11	57	3 M, 8 F	5 CRAO, 4 CRVO, 2 Intraretinal Hemorrhage
14	Majumder & Prakash [24]	India	Case Report	1	28	M	CRVO
15	Elhusseiny et al. [25]	USA	Case Report	1	51	M	NAAION
16	Endo et al. [26]	Spain	Case Report	1	52	M	CRVO
17	Franco & Fonollosa [27]	Spain	Case Report	2	59	2 M	2 NAAION
18	Girbardt et al. [7]	India	Case Series	6	46.5	4 M, 2 F	BRAO, CRVO, Venous Stasis Retinopathy, NAAION, CRAO, AMN
19	Goyal et al. [28]	Japan	Case Report	1	28	M	CRVO
20	Ikegami et al. [29]	Japan	Case Report	1	54	F	CRAO
21	Ishibashi et al. [30]	Japan	Case Series	6	59.3	3 M, 3 F	4 BRAO, PAMM, AMN
22	Kang et al. [31]	Korea	Case Report	1	64	M	BRAO
23	Lee et al. [32]	USA	Case Report	1	34	M	CRVO
24	Chen et al. [33]	China	Case Series	5	54.2	4 M, 1 F	BRAO, BRVO, CRAO, CRVO, VH
25	Lin et al. [34]	Taiwan	Case Report	1	61	F	NAAION
26	Maleki et al. [35]	US	Case Series	2	56	2 F	AAION, AZOOR
27	Murgova & Balchev [36]	Bulgaria	Case Series	1	58.4	3 M, 2 F	NAAION
28	Nachbor et al. [37]	Nepal	Case Report	1	64	F	NAAION
29	Nusanti et al. [38]	Indonesia	Case Report	1	50	M	N/A
30	Park et al. [39]	Korea	Case Series	21	77	11 M, 19 F	11 AMD, 10 RVO
31	Peters et al. [40]	Australia	Case Series	5	57	3 M, 2 F	3 BRVO, RVO, CRVO
32	Priluck et al. [41]	USA	Case Report	2	38.5	2 F	BRVO, AMN
33	Pur et al. [42]	Canada	Case Report	1	34	M	BRVO
34	Romano et al. [43]	Italy	Case Report	1	54	F	CRVO
35	Sacconi et al. [44]	Italy	Case Report	1	74	F	RVO
36	Sanjay et al. [45]	India	Case Report	1	50	F	N/A
37	Shah et al. [46]	USA	Case Report	1	27	M	CRVO
38	Sodhi et al. [47]	India	Case Report	1	43	M	CRVO
39	Sonawane et al. [48]	India	Case Report	2	46.5	M	2 CRVO
40	Sugihara et al. [49]	Japan	Case Report	1	38	M	BRVO
41	Takacs et al. [50]	Hungary	Case Report	1	35	M	CRVO
42	Tanaka et al. [51]	Japan	Case Report	2	71.5	M	2 BRVO
43	Suphachaiprasert & Thammakumpee [52]	Thailand	Case Report	1	41	M	CRAO
44	Tsukii et al. [53]	Japan	Case Report	1	55	F	NAAION
45	Vinzamuri et al. [54]	India	Case Report	1	35	M	N/A
46	Vujosevic et al. [55]	Italy	Case Series	14	77	5 M, 9 F	6 BRVO, 6 CRVO, 2 RVO
47	Wang et al. [56]	Taiwan	Case Series	1	47.7	4 M, 7 F	CRAO
48	Elnahry et al. [57]	USA	Case Series	2	50.5	F	NAAION
49	Haseeb et al. [58]	Egypt	Case Report	1	40	M	NAAION

Abbreviations: AAION: Arteritic Anterior Ischemic Optic Neuropathy, AMN: Acute Macular Neuroretinopathy, AZOOR: Acute Zonal Occult Outer Retinopathy, BRVO: Branch Retinal Venous Occlusion, CRAO: Central Retinal Arterial Occlusion, CRVO: Central Retinal Venous Occlusion, NAAION: Non-Arteritic Anterior Ischemic Optic Neuropathy, PAMM: Paracentral Acute Middle Maculopathy, RVO: Retinal Venous Occlusion, VH: Vitreous Hemorrhage.

The patients' ages ranged between 20 and 96, with a mean (±SD) of 58.92 (±17.57), and the population was nearly equally distributed between males and females (51.5%). Pfizer-BioNTech was the most reported vaccine (n = 56, 43.1%), while AstraZeneca was the second most reported with 50 cases (38.5%). The remaining 24 cases (18.6%) were associated with other types of vaccines, namely Moderna, CoronaVac, Johnson & Johnson, one case of non-available data on the vaccine, and one case with a non-specific mRNA vaccine (Figure 2). Regarding the doses, most ocular vascular events occurred after the administration of the first dose (46.2%).

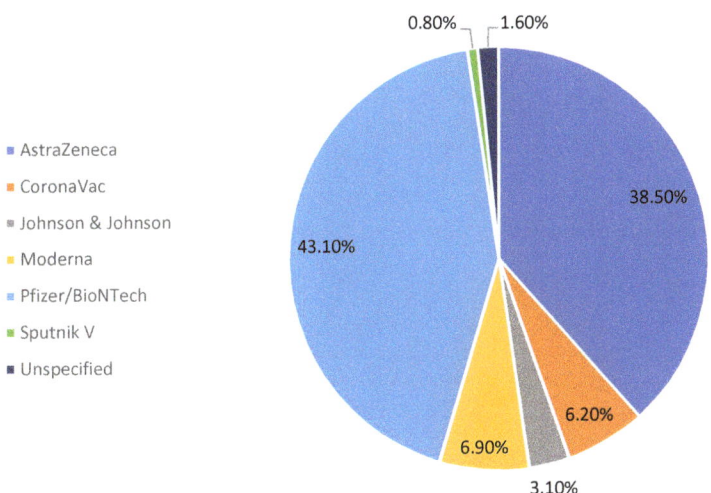

Figure 2. Types of COVID-19 vaccine used in patients with ophthalmic vascular event.

Table 2 shows the demographic characteristics of the included cases, categorized into five main categories: arterial events (CRAO, NAAION, etc.), venous events CRVO/BRVO, etc.), simultaneous arterial and venous together, hemorrhagic events, and other events. Venous events were the most reported events with 69 cases (53%), followed by arterial events with 36 cases (27.7%). There was no significant difference in the five categories regarding age (p = 0.692). However, hemorrhagic events were associated mainly with older age (74.15 ± 9.11), while the arterial and venous events were associated with similar age groups (57.86 ± 16.89 and 59.36 ± 16.84 respectively). Regarding gender, all the events were distributed equally in the five categories and we found no statistical difference between them (p = 0.804). The AstraZeneca vaccine was associated the most with venous complications (n = 33, 25.4%) compared to the other vaccines, followed by the Pfizer vaccine (n = 27, 20.8%), which was reported the most with arterial complications (p = 0.38). The dosage effect was most commonly associated with the first and second doses (88.5%); however, events were evenly distributed between the first and second dosage, except in the dual arterial and venous category, which was mainly associated with the second dose only. The booster dose was reported only in three cases of venous complications (2.3%) (p = 0.429).

Table 2. Demographic characteristics of the included cases.

Characteristic		Nature of Ocular Event					Total	p-Value
		Arterial n (%)	Venous n (%)	Venous & Arterial n (%)	Hemorrhagic n (%)	Others n (%)		
Demographics								
Age		57.86 ± 16.89	59.39 ± 16.84	56.33 ± 23.58	74.15 ± 9.11	38.33 ± 13.89	58.92 ± 17.57	0.692
Sex								0.804
	Female	17 (13.1%)	35 (26.9%)	2 (1.5%)	7 (5.4%)	6 (4.6%)	67 (51.5%)	
	Male	19 (14.6%)	34 (26.2%)	1 (0.8%)	6 (4.6%)	3 (2.3%)	63 (48.5%)	
COVID-19 Vaccine								0.380
	AstraZeneca	10 (7.7%)	33 (25.4%)	0 (0%)	3 (2.3%)	4 (3.1%)	50 (38.5%)	
	CoronaVac	4 (3.1%)	2 (1.5%)	0 (0%)	1 (0.8%)	1 (0.8%)	8 (6.2%)	
	Johnson & Johnson	1 (0.8%)	2 (1.5%)	0 (0%)	0 (0%)	1 (0.8%)	4 (3.1%)	
	Moderna	4 (3.1%)	3 (2.3%)	1 (0.8%)	0 (0%)	1 (0.8%)	9 (6.9%)	
	Pfizer-BioNTech	17 (13.1%)	27 (20.8%)	2 (1.5%)	8 (6.2%)	2 (1.5%)	56 (43.1%)	
	Sputnik V	0 (0%)	1 (0.8%)	0 (0%)	0 (0%)	0 (0%)	1 (0.8%)	
	Unspecified	0 (0%)	1 (0.8%)	0 (0%)	1 (0.8%)	0 (0%)	2 (1.6%)	
Dose								0.429
	First	17 (13.1%)	29 (22.3%)	0 (0%)	10 (7.7%)	4 (3.1%)	60 (46.2%)	
	Second	15 (11.5%)	30 (23.1%)	3 (2.3%)	3 (2.3%)	4 (3.1%)	55 (42.3%)	
	Booster	0 (0%)	3 (2.3%)	0 (0%)	0 (0%)	0 (0%)	3 (2.3%)	
	Unspecified	4 (3.1%)	7 (5.4%)	0 (0%)	0 (0%)	1 (0.8%)	12 (9.2%)	
Total		36 (27.7%)	69 (53%)	3 (2.3%)	13 (1%)	9 (4.6%)	130 (100%)	

Table 3 shows the clinical characteristics of the cases with underlying systemic and ocular diseases. Hypertension was more frequently associated with ocular vascular events compared to diabetes in most of the categories. Furthermore, old vascular events were reported in eight cases, while previous ocular surgeries were reported in 18 cases, and six cases had a history of treatment with anti-vascular endothelial growth factor (VEGF) injections, five of which were associated with hemorrhagic events. In addition, only one case with a history of glaucoma secondary to epiretinal membrane was reported. Regarding the laterality, most cases were unilateral (96 cases, 73.8%) and affected the right eye ($p = 0.002$). As to the duration between vaccination and the ocular events, we classified the durations into five-day categories (Table 3). An inverse relationship was observed between the duration following vaccination and the incidence of ocular vascular events, indicating that most ocular vascular events in this review occurred in the first five days following vaccination (46.2%), which, however, was not statistically significant ($p = 0.095$) (Figure 3). Patients' complaints were classified into three categories: visual disturbances, non-available data, and others (proptosis, red eye, scalp tenderness, temporal headache, ophthalmoplegia, retrobulbar pain, uveitis, etc.). Visual disturbances included decreased visual acuity, floaters, light flashes, photopsia, curtains obstructing vision, visual field defects, and greyish spots, which represented 68.5% of the total patients' presenting complaints.

Table 4 shows the interventions that were used in the cases; we classified them into two main groups, medical and surgical. The medical treatment was also subdivided into four groups. Medical treatment was much more common than surgical intervention, as the most frequent treatment used as the first-line therapy following the events was intravitreal anti-VEGF (n = 39, 30.7%), followed by corticosteroids, which were given in 18 (14.2%) of the cases. Nine patients (6.92%) had received some type of thrombolytic, antiplatelet, or anticoagulant, of whom four (3.07%) had received Aspirin, two (1.5%) received Apixaban, one received Clopidogrel, one received Fondaparinux, and one case received a nonspecific anti-platelet. On the other hand, vitrectomy was the most commonly performed surgery (60% of total performed surgeries) ($p < 0.001$). In addition, the use of both intravitreal anti-VEGF and vitrectomy reached a statistically significant point ($p < 0.001$) while other interventions did not. Furthermore, vitrectomy was done almost exclusively for hemorrhagic events (five out of six total), while 76.92% of the total intravitreal anti-VEGF was given after venous vascular complications.

Table 3. Clinical characteristics of included cases.

Characteristic		Nature of Ocular Event					Total	p-Value
		Arterial n (%)	Venous n (%)	Venous & Arterial n (%)	Hemorrhagic n (%)	Others n (%)		
No. of Patients		36 (27.7%)	69 (53%)	3 (2.3%)	13 (1%)	9 (4.6%)	130 (100%)	
Clinical Characteristics								
Underlying Systemic Disease								
	Hypertension	11 (8.7%)	21 (16.5%)	1 (0.8%)	5 (3.9%)	2 (1.6%)	40 (31.5%)	0.964
	Diabetes Mellitus	8 (6.2%)	12 (9.2%)	0 (0%)	6 (4.6%)	0 (0%)	26 (20%)	0.062
	Other	9 (7.2%)	17 (13.6%)	1 (0.8%)	8 (6.4%)	2 (1.6%)	37 (29.6%)	N/A
Underlying Ocular Condition								
	Old Vascular Event	1 (0.8%)	6 (4.8%)	0 (0%)	1 (0.8%)	0 (0%)	8 (6.4%)	0.953
	Old Ocular Surgery/Procedure	4 (3.2%)	9 (7.2%)	0 (0%)	5 (4%)	0 (0%)	18 (14.4%)	0.862
	Anti-VEGF Injections	0 (0%)	1 (0.8%)	0 (0%)	5 (4%)	0 (0%)	6 (4.8%)	0.004
	Other	2 (1.6%)	5 (4%)	0 (0%)	6 (4.7%)	0 (0%)	13 (10.3%)	N/A
Laterality								0.002
	Right	15 (11.5%)	32 (24.6%)	2 (1.5%)	8 (6.2%)	1 (0.8%)	58 (44.6%)	
	Left	11 (8.5%)	19 (14.6%)	1 (0.8%)	4 (3.1%)	3 (2.3%)	38 (29.2%)	
	Bilateral	3 (2.3%)	1 (0.8%)	0 (0%)	1 (0.8%)	4 (3.1%)	9 (6.9%)	
	Not reported	7 (5.4%)	17 (13.1%)	0 (0%)	0 (0%)	1 (0.8%)	25 (19.2%)	
Duration between Vaccination and Ocular Event (days)								0.095
	≤5	17 (13.1%)	33 (25.4%)	1 (0.8%)	6 (4.6%)	3 (2.3%)	60 (46.2%)	
	6–10	6 (4.6%)	16 (12.3%)	0 (0%)	2 (1.5%)	4 (3.1%)	28 (21.5%)	
	11–15	5 (3.8%)	11 (8.5%)	2 (1.5%)	1 (0.8%)	0 (0%)	19 (14.6%)	
	16–20	2 (1.5%)	1 (0.8%)	0 (0%)	1 (0.8%)	0 (0%)	4 (3.1%)	
	21–25	1 (0.8%)	5 (3.8%)	0 (0%)	0 (0%)	0 (0%)	6 (4.6%)	
	26–30	1 (0.8%)	3 (2.3%)	0 (0%)	3 (2.3%)	1 (0.8%)	8 (6.2%)	
	>30	4 (3.1%)	0 (0%)	0 (0%)	0 (0%)	1 (0.8%)	5 (3.8%)	
Main Presenting Complaint								
	Visual Disturbances	26 (20%)	50 (38.5%)	3 (2.3%)	2 (1.5%)	8 (6.2%)	89 (68.5%)	
	Other	2 (1.6%)	2 (1.6%)	0 (0%)	0 (0%)	3 (2.4%)	7 (5.3%)	
	Not reported	10 (7.9%)	19 (15%)	0 (0%)	11 (8.7%)	1 (0.8%)	41 (31.5%)	

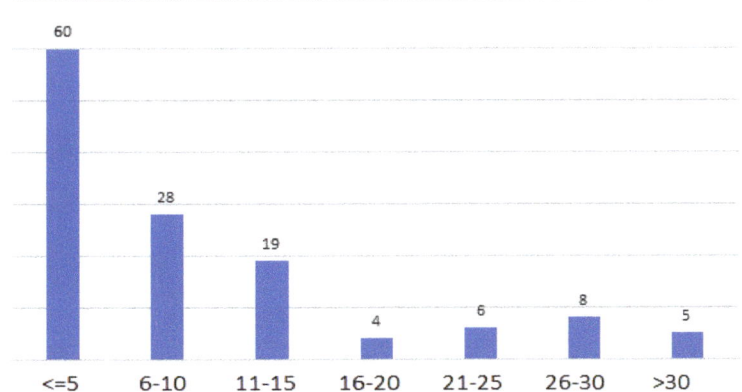

Figure 3. Day of onset of vascular ocular event divided into segments of five days.

Table 4. Medical & surgical interventions for included cases.

Management		Nature of Ocular Event					Total	p-Value
		Arterial n (%)	Venous n (%)	Venous & Arterial n (%)	Hemorrhagic n (%)	Others n (%)		
Medical								
	Intravitreal anti-VEGF	1 (0.8%)	30 (23.6%)	2 (1.6%)	6 (4.7%)	0 (0%)	39 (30.7%)	<0.001
	Corticosteroid	6 (4.6%)	12 (9.2%)	1 (0.8%)	0 (0%)	1 (0.8%)	20 (15.4%)	0.43
	Observation	3 (2.4%)	9 (7.1%)	1 (0.8%)	2 (1.6%)	1 (0.8%)	16 (12.6%)	0.798
	Other Intervention	7 (5.4%)	4 (3.1%)	0 (0%)	0 (0%)	2 (1.5%)	13 (10%)	0.116
	Unavailable Data	18 (14.2%)	16 (12.6%)	0 (0%)	2 (1.6%)	5 (3.9%)	41 (32.3%)	N/A
Surgical/Procedural								
	Vitrectomy	0 (0%)	1 (0.8%)	0 (0%)	5 (3.9%)	0 (0%)	6 (4.7%)	<0.001
	Laser Procedure	0 (0%)	3 (2.4%)	0 (0%)	0 (0%)	0 (0%)	3 (2.4%)	0.63
	Other Interventions	1 (0.8%)	0 (0%)	0 (0%)	0 (0%)	0 (0%)	1 (0.8%)	0.58
Total		36 (27.7%)	69 (53%)	3 (2.3%)	13 (1%)	9 (4.6%)	130 (100%)	

The outcome and degree of improvement of the cases are shown in Table 5 based on the difference between the final BCVA and the initial BCVA, which was calculated using the formula (Final BCVA-Initial BCVA), with any (+) value denoting improvement, any (−) value denoting worsening, and "0" or no change denoting persistence. The improvement was grouped into three categories: improved, persisted, and deteriorated. Among the data that were available, the majority of patients (91.3%) demonstrated either improvement or persistence in the final BCVA. There were no significant differences between improvement, persistence, or worsening between the groups ($p = 0.369$, $p = 0.516$, and $p = 0.34$, respectively). Persistence in venous events was marginally higher than the number of patients who improved, whereas among arterial issues, persistence was more than twice as great as improvement.

Table 5. The overall outcome for included cases.

Outcome	Nature of Ocular Event					Total	p-Value
	Arterial n (%)	Venous n (%)	Venous & Arterial n (%)	Hemorrhagic n (%)	Others n (%)		
Improved	6 (16.7%)	17 (24.6%)	1 (33.3%)	3 (23.1%)	1 (11.1%)	28 (21.5%)	0.369
Persisted	8 (22.2%)	22 (31.9%)	0 (0%)	4 (30.8%)	1 (11.1%)	35 (26.9%)	0.516
Worsened	2 (5.6%)	2 (2.9%)	0 (0%)	2 (15.4%)	0 (0%)	6 (4.6%)	0.34
Unavailable Data	20 (55.6%)	28 (40.6%)	2 (66.7%)	4 (30.8%)	7 (77.8%)	61 (46.9%)	N/A
Total	36 (20%)	69 (41.77%)	3 (1.85%)	13 (7.85%)	9 (5.46%)	130 (100%)	

Supplementary Table S2 provides an aggregation for all case characteristics and information.

4. Discussion

In the present systematic review, 49 reports describing 130 cases of ocular vascular events in close proximity to COVID-19 vaccination were described. This occurred after the first dose or second dose of their Pfizer-BioNTech (n = 56 (43.1%)) or AstraZeneca (n = 50, 38.5%) vaccines. The exact mechanism by which these pathologies occur remains unclear; nevertheless, a few hypotheses were suggested to explain these adverse events. Immune-mediated mechanisms are thought to cause thrombosis through an activation of platelets, immune cells, and hypercoagulability factors [59]. Other potential mechanisms also have been suggested, like molecular mimicry, protein contaminants, and adenovirus vector proteins [60,61]. Since these vascular events are likely brought about by immune-medicated mechanisms, they are more likely to happen after the administration of the first dose due to higher spikes of immunoglobulins after the first exposure, with the risk decreasing with the second and third doses [62]. However, we still identified a relatively large number of cases after the second dose. Although a higher risk of adverse events was attributed to the AstraZeneca vaccine [63], it is hard to validate this information with regards to vascular ocular events since data on vaccine type per population is difficult to acquire. The AstraZeneca vaccine is also reported to be one of the most commonly administered COVID-19 vaccines which may explain its frequent association with adverse events (REF). Most events occurred within five days of vaccination ($p = 0.095$), and 67.8% of events occurred within 10 days post-vaccination. In the literature, retinal vascular events were observed within 3.1 ± 2.4 days of vaccination, and other ocular adverse effects of COVID-19 vaccines generally occurred during the first 10 days after vaccination [64]. This temporal association may be attributed to vaccine-related antibodies that induce hypercoagulability, as they appear within the first 5–10 days after vaccination, and disappear within 100 days [59].

Our cohort had a mean age of 58.92 ± 17.57, falling within the older age group. Age above 50 years was linked to COVID vaccine-related adverse events [39,65], and ocular vascular events were recorded in the same age group in [64]. This was also true when comparing ischemic optic neuropathy versus optic neuritis in patients that developed optic neuropathy after COVID-19 vaccination [61]. Ocular hemorrhagic events were also specifically linked to advanced age [66], which is the case in our population. Older patients (74.2 ± 9.11) had a higher incidence of hemorrhagic vascular complications. This could be attributed to age-related degeneration of macular and choroidal tissues, which may involve neovascularization (NS) and pathologic angiogenesis [67]. Vascular occlusive events of veins (central or branch) were observed with a higher frequency compared to arterial occlusions: 69 venous cases (53%) compared to 36 arterial cases (27.7%). This goes in accordance with observations in the literature, where retinal venous events were observed more than arterial events [68–71]. The venous involvement in the adverse effects of vaccines is thought to be due to the relation between cerebral veins, including retinal veins, and the clearance of toxins from nasal sinuses, which could lead to higher immunogenicity, hence a higher risk of thrombosis, especially in the setting of immune activation post vaccination [60]. Most patients suffered from a unilateral vascular event, with only nine (6.9%, $p = 0.002$) patients presenting with bilateral ocular affection, as previously observed in literature [70] . The anatomical variations between the right and left retinal veins and arteries can help explain the preferences of retinal vascular events [70]. Given that the majority of cases in this review were of venous occlusion, right eye involvement was higher (n = 58, 44.6%, $p = 0.002$). This can be due to the anatomical relations between the venous system or the right heart and the right eye.

The history of prior underlying systemic diseases was also collected in this study. Hypertension and diabetes were reported more commonly. Overall, hypertension was frequently associated with ocular vascular events in the current review. This is described in the literature as "hypertensive eye disease," associating chronic and acute elevations in systemic blood pressure with the incidence of ocular vascular events [72]. However, a recent study from Japan suggests that the relationship can be multifactorial and occurs only in females [73]. Changes in systemic blood pressure are directly linked to several ocular complications, since the vasculature of the retina and the optic nerve are vulnerable to fluctuations in blood flow due to limited autoregulation [72]. On the other hand, diabetes compromises retinal blood flow, which in turn predisposes patients to vascular complications [74]. A link between prior intravitreal anti-VEGF injection and hemorrhagic ocular events was also suspected in the current study, since five patients with a history of anti-VEGF treatment presented with hemorrhagic events. This, however, could be a complication of the underlying condition for which the anti-VEGF agent was administered in the first place, or, less likely, a complication related to the anti-VEGF agent's vascular and inflammatory effects [75,76] . More studies are needed to further evaluate this risk.

In the reviewed cases, a clear management criterion was often not mentioned. Nevertheless, 39 (30.7%, $p < 0.001$) patients received intravitreal anti-VEGF injections of various types, likely because many patients are expected to develop exudative maculopathy following the retinal venous events [77]. The management of vascular ocular events varies between anti-VEGF injections, surgical procedures, steroid therapy, and other medications according to the type of event. In exudative and ischemic events, intravitreal anti-VEGF injections are mostly used [78].

The patients' improvement was assessed by comparing the patient's presenting BCVA with the patient's final BCVA after follow-up and management. Unfortunately, most case reports did not include sufficient data on their management and outcome. The available data showed persisting symptoms in most patients, which is a known feature of most ocular vascular events, although new research suggests long-term improvement [79].

The issue of ocular vascular events as a consequence of COVID-19 vaccination is therefore, arguably, an important cause of blindness for patients that deserves more attention. However, these adverse events are still considered rare based on the millions of vaccine doses administered worldwide. Individuals particularly at risk should be counselled regarding this risk before receiving COVID-19 vaccines particularly because the visual prognosis appears to be guarded. In addition, further research targeting the underlying pathophysiology of these events is required, especially with respect to their risk factors and possible methods of prevention and treatment. Nevertheless, the benefits of COVID-19 vaccination still far outweigh the associated risks. Future case reporting with detailed descriptions of management criteria is needed in order to provide researchers and ophthalmologists with insight on how to treat similar cases.

The limitations of our study include the lack of diagnostic information in many cases, the lack of outcome assessment for the affected eyes in many cases, and the inability to perform relative risk statistical analysis due to insufficient data.

5. Conclusions

Ophthalmic vascular events are serious vision-threatening side effects that have been associated with COVID-19 vaccination. We provided the first systematic review dedicated to these events. Luckily, venous occlusive events that are currently most amenable to treatment were the most common among other vascular events. These events occurred after the first and second doses mostly within the first five days following vaccination. Moreover, most events tended to occur in older patients. Further studies are needed to better determine the incidence, risk factors, prognosis, and management of ocular vascular events following COVID-19 vaccination.

Supplementary Materials: The following supporting information can be downloaded at https://www.mdpi.com/article/10.3390/vaccines10122143/s1, Table S1: The detailed search strategy used in each of the search databases. Table S2: The characteristics and detailed information of all included cases.

Author Contributions: Conceptualization: H.A.S., A.A., L.A.-I., and Q.F.A.S.; methodology: H.A.S., A.A., L.A.S., and S.I.; software: A.G.E., and A.A.; validation: H.A.S., A.A., A.G.E., M.T.A., and M.J.J.T.; formal analysis, A.A.; investigation: H.A.S., and A.A.; resources: S.I., and L.A.S.; data curation: B.A., L.A.-I., and Q.F.A.S.; writing—original draft preparation: H.A.S., A.A., A.G.E., M.T.A., and M.J.J.T.; writing—review and editing: H.A.S., A.A., and A.G.E.; visualization: B.A., S.I., and L.A.S.; supervision: H.A.S., A.G.E., and A.A.; project administration: N/A; funding acquisition: N/A. All authors have read and agreed to the published version of the manuscript.

Funding: This research received no external funding.

Institutional Review Board Statement: Not applicable.

Informed Consent Statement: Not applicable.

Data Availability Statement: The data provided in this manuscript can be provided upon reasonable request by contacting the corresponding author.

Conflicts of Interest: The authors declare no conflict of interest.

References

1. Karpiński, T.M.; Ożarowski, M.; Seremak-Mrozikiewicz, A.; Wolski, H.; Wlodkowic, D. The 2020 race towards SARS-CoV-2 specific vaccines. *Theranostics* **2021**, *11*, 1690. [CrossRef]
2. WHO. *COVID-19 Vaccines with WHO Emergency Use Listing. WHO—Prequalification of Medical Products (IVDs, Medicines, Vaccines and Immunization Devices, Vector Control)*; WHO: Geneva, Switzerland, 2021.
3. Feikin, D.R.; Higdon, M.M.; Abu-Raddad, L.J.; Andrews, N.; Araos, R.; Goldberg, Y.; Groome, M.; Huppert, A.; O'Brien, K.; Smith, P.G.; et al. Duration of effectiveness of vaccines against SARS-CoV-2 infection and COVID-19 disease: Results of a systematic review and meta-regression. *Lancet* **2022**, *399*, 924–944. [CrossRef]
4. WHO. *Adverse Events Following Immunization (AEFI)*. WHO: Geneva, Switzerland, 2021.
5. Pottegård, A.; Lund, L.C.; Karlstad, Ø.; Dahl, J.; Andersen, M.; Hallas, J.; Lidegaard, Ø.; Tapia, G.; Gulseth, H.L.; Ruiz, P.L.-D.; et al. Arterial events, venous thromboembolism, thrombocytopenia, and bleeding after vaccination with Oxford-AstraZeneca ChAdOx1-S in Denmark and Norway: Population based cohort study. *BMJ* **2021**, *373*, n1114. [CrossRef]
6. Taha, M.J.J.; Abuawwad, M.T.; Alrubasy, W.A.; Sameer, S.K.; Alsafi, T.; Al-Bustanji, Y.; Abu-Ismail, L.; Nashwan, A.J. Ocular manifestations of recent viral pandemics: A literature review. *Front. Med.* **2022**, *9*, 1011335. [CrossRef]
7. Girbardt, C.; Busch, C.; Al-Sheikh, M.; Gunzinger, J.M.; Invernizzi, A.; Xhepa, A.; Unterlauft, J.D.; Rehak, M. Retinal Vascular Events after mRNA and Adenoviral-Vectored COVID-19 Vaccines—A Case Series. *Vaccines* **2021**, *9*, 1349. [CrossRef]
8. Dean, A.G.; Arner, T.G.; Sunki, G.G.; Friedman, R.; Lantinga, M.; Sangam, S.; Zubieta, J.C.; Sullivan, K.M.; Brendel, K.A.; Gao, Z.; et al. *Epi Info™, a Database and Statistics Program for Public Health Professionals*; CDC: Atlanta, GA, USA, 2011.
9. Ritchie, H.; Mathieu, E.; Rodés-Guirao, L.; Appel, C.; Giattino, C.; Ortiz-Ospina, E.; Hasell, J.; Macdonald, B.; Beltekian, D.; Roser, M. Coronavirus pandemic (COVID-19). In *Our World in Data*. 2020. Available online: https://ourworldindata.org/coronavirus (accessed on 26 October 2022).
10. Muka, T.; Glisic, M.; Milic, J.; Verhoog, S.; Bohlius, J.; Bramer, W.; Chowdhury, R.; Franco, O.H. A 24-step guide on how to design, conduct, and successfully publish a systematic review and meta-analysis in medical research. *Eur. J. Epidemiol.* **2020**, *35*, 49–60. [CrossRef]
11. Abdallah, S.; Hamzah, K. Case Report—Central Retinal Artery Occlusion After Ad26.COV2.S COVID-19 Vaccine. *Biomed. J. Sci. Tech. Res.* **2022**, *43*, 34720–34724.
12. Abdin, A.D.; Gärtner, B.C.; Seitz, B. Central retinal artery occlusion following COVID-19 vaccine administration. *Am. J. Ophthalmol. Case Rep.* **2022**, *26*, 101430. [CrossRef]
13. Amin, M.A.; Nahin, S.; Dola, T.A.; Afrin, S.; Hawlader, M.D.H. Retinal hemorrhage of late post-COVID-19 and post-vaccine-related pathogenic mechanisms: A new challenge for ophthalmologist in COVID era. *Clin. Case Rep.* **2022**, *10*, e05471. [CrossRef]
14. Bialasiewicz, A.A.; Farah-Diab, M.S.; Mebarki, H.T. Central retinal vein occlusion occurring immediately after 2nd dose of mRNA SARS-CoV-2 vaccine. *Int. Ophthalmol.* **2021**, *41*, 3889–3892. [CrossRef]
15. Bolletta, E.; Iannetta, D.; Mastrofilippo, V.; De Simone, L.; Gozzi, F.; Croci, S.; Bonacini, M.; Belloni, L.; Zerbini, A.; Adani, C.; et al. Uveitis and other ocular complications following COVID-19 vaccination. *J. Clin. Med.* **2021**, *10*, 5960. [CrossRef]
16. Cackett, P.; Ali, A.; Young, S.L.; Pavilion, N.L.P.A.E. Phenotypic appearance of central retinal vein occlusion post AstraZeneca vaccine. *Int. J. Ophthalmol.* **2022**, *15*, 672–673. [CrossRef]
17. Casarini, B.; Bruni, F.; Rubino, P.; Mora, P. Vitreous Hemorrhage and Long-Lasting Priapism After COVID-19 m-RNA Based Vaccine: A Case Report. *Eur. J. Ophthalmol.* **2022**, *0*, 11206721221098880. [CrossRef]
18. Che, S.A.; Lee, K.Y.; Yoo, Y.J. Bilateral Ischemic Optic Neuropathy from Giant Cell Arteritis Following COVID-19 Vaccination. *J. Neuro-Ophthalmol.* **2022**, 1–2, 10–1097. [CrossRef]
19. Chen, P.-J.; Chang, Y.-S.; Lim, C.-C.; Lee, Y.-K. Susac Syndrome Following COVID-19 Vaccination: A Case Report. *Vaccines* **2022**, *10*, 363. [CrossRef]
20. Choi, M.; Seo, M.-H.; Choi, K.-E.; Lee, S.; Choi, B.; Yun, C.; Kim, S.-W.; Kim, Y.Y. Vision-Threatening Ocular Adverse Events after Vaccination against Coronavirus Disease 2019. *J. Clin. Med.* **2022**, *11*, 3318. [CrossRef]
21. Chow, S.Y.; Hsu, Y.-R.; Fong, V.H. Central retinal artery occlusion after Moderna mRNA-1273 vaccination. *J. Formos. Med. Assoc.* **2022**, *121*, 2369–2370. [CrossRef]
22. Chung, S.A.; Yeo, S.; Sohn, S.-Y. Nonarteritic Anterior Ischemic Optic Neuropathy Following COVID-19 Vaccination: A Case Report. *Korean J. Ophthalmol.* **2022**, *36*, 168–170. [CrossRef]
23. Da Silva, L.S.; Finamor, L.P.; Andrade, G.C.; Lima, L.H.; Zett, C.; Muccioli, C.; Sarraf, E.P.; Marinho, P.M.; Peruchi, J.; Oliveira, R.D.D.L.; et al. Vascular retinal findings after COVID-19 vaccination in 11 cases: A coincidence or consequence? *Arq. Bras. Oftalmol.* **2022**, *85*, 158–165. [CrossRef]
24. Majumder, P.D.; Prakash, V.J. Retinal venous occlusion following COVID-19 vaccination: Report of a case after third dose and review of the literature. *Indian J. Ophthalmol.* **2022**, *70*, 2191. [CrossRef]
25. Elhusseiny, A.M.; Sanders, R.N.; Siddiqui, M.Z.; Sallam, A.B. Non-arteritic Anterior Ischemic Optic Neuropathy with Macular Star following COVID-19 Vaccination. *Ocul. Immunol. Inflamm.* **2022**, *30*, 1274–1277. [CrossRef]
26. Endo, B.; Bahamon, S.; Martínez-Pulgarín, D.F. Central retinal vein occlusion after mRNA SARS-CoV-2 vaccination: A case report. *Indian J. Ophthalmol.* **2021**, *69*, 2865. [CrossRef]
27. Franco, S.V.; Fonollosa, A. Ischemic Optic Neuropathy After Administration of a SARS-CoV-2 Vaccine: A Report of 2 Cases. *Am. J. Case Rep.* **2022**, *23*, e935095.

28. Goyal, M.; Murthy, S.; Srinivas, Y. Unilateral retinal vein occlusion in a young, healthy male following Sputnik V vaccination. *Indian J. Ophthalmol.* **2021**, *69*, 3793. [CrossRef]
29. Ikegami, Y.; Numaga, J.; Okano, N.; Fukuda, S.; Yamamoto, H.; Terada, Y. Combined central retinal artery and vein occlusion shortly after mRNA-SARS-CoV-2 vaccination. *QJM Int. J. Med.* **2022**, *114*, 884–885. [CrossRef]
30. Ishibashi, K.; Yatsuka, H.; Haruta, M.; Kimoto, K.; Yoshida, S.; Kubota, T. Branch Retinal Artery Occlusions, Paracentral Acute Middle Maculopathy and Acute Macular Neuroretinopathy After COVID-19 Vaccinations. *Clin. Ophthalmol.* **2022**, *16*, 987–992. [CrossRef]
31. Kang, M.S.; Kim, S.Y.; Kwon, H.J. Case Report: Recanalization of Branch Retinal Artery Occlusion Due to Microthrombi Following the First Dose of SARS-CoV-2 mRNA Vaccination. *Front. Pharmacol.* **2022**, *13*, 845615. [CrossRef]
32. Lee, S.; Sankhala, K.K.; Bose, S.; Gallemore, R.P. Combined Central Retinal Artery and Vein Occlusion with Ischemic Optic Neuropathy After COVID-19 Vaccination. *Int. Med. Case Rep. J.* **2022**, *15*, 7–14. [CrossRef]
33. Chen, X.; Li, X.; Li, H.; Li, M.; Gong, S. Ocular Adverse Events after Inactivated COVID-19 Vaccination in Xiamen. *Vaccines* **2022**, *10*, 482. [CrossRef]
34. Lin, W.-Y.; Wang, J.-J.; Lai, C.-H. Non-Arteritic Anterior Ischemic Optic Neuropathy Following COVID-19 Vaccination. *Vaccines* **2022**, *10*, 931. [CrossRef]
35. Maleki, A.; Look-Why, S.; Manhapra, A.; Foster, C.S. COVID-19 recombinant mRNA vaccines and serious ocular inflammatory side effects: Real or coincidence? *J. Ophthalmic Vis. Res.* **2021**, *16*, 490–501. [CrossRef]
36. Murgova, S.; Balchev, G. Ophthalmic manifestation after SARS-CoV-2 vaccination: A case series. *J. Ophthalmic Inflamm. Infect.* **2022**, *12*, 1–4. [CrossRef]
37. Nachbor, K.M.; Naravane, A.V.; Adams, O.E.; Abel, A.S. Nonarteritic anterior ischemic optic neuropathy associated with COVID-19 vaccination. *J. Neuroophthalmol.* **2021**, 1–3. [CrossRef]
38. Nusanti, S.; Putera, I.; Sidik, M.; Edwar, L.; Koesnoe, S.; Rachman, A.; Kurniawan, M.; Tarigan, T.J.E.; Yunus, R.E.; Saraswati, I.; et al. A case of aseptic bilateral cavernous sinus thrombosis following a recent inactivated SARS-CoV-2 vaccination. *Taiwan J. Ophthalmol.* **2022**, *12*, 334–338. [CrossRef]
39. Park, H.S.; Byun, Y.; Byeon, S.H.; Kim, S.S.; Kim, Y.J.; Lee, C.S. Retinal hemorrhage after SARS-CoV-2 vaccination. *J. Clin. Med.* **2021**, *10*, 5705. [CrossRef]
40. Peters, M.C.; Cheng, S.S.H.; Sharma, A.; Moloney, T.P.; Franzco, S.S.H.C.; Franzco, A.S.; Franzco, T.P.M. Retinal vein occlusion following COVID-19 vaccination. *Clin. Exp. Ophthalmol.* **2022**, *50*, 459–461. [CrossRef]
41. Priluck, A.Z.; Arevalo, J.F.; Pandit, R.R. Ischemic retinal events after COVID-19 vaccination. *Am. J. Ophthalmol. Case Rep.* **2022**, *26*, 101540. [CrossRef]
42. Pur, D.R.; Bursztyn, L.L.C.D.; Iordanous, Y. Branch retinal vein occlusion in a healthy young man following mRNA COVID-19 vaccination. *Am. J. Ophthalmol. Case Rep.* **2022**, *26*, 101445. [CrossRef]
43. Romano, D.; Morescalchi, F.; Romano, V.; Semeraro, F. COVID-19 AdenoviralVector Vaccine and Central Retinal Vein Occlusion. *Ocul. Immunol. Inflamm.* **2022**, *30*, 1286–1288. [CrossRef]
44. Sacconi, R.; Simona, F.; Forte, P.; Querques, G. Retinal vein occlusion following two doses of mRNA-1237 (moderna) immunization for SARS-CoV-2: A case report. *Ophthalmol. Ther.* **2022**, *11*, 453–458. [CrossRef]
45. Sanjay, S.; Acharya, I.; Rawoof, A.; Shetty, R. Non-arteritic anterior ischaemic optic neuropathy (NA-AION) and COVID-19 vaccination. *BMJ Case Rep.* **2022**, *15*, e248415. [CrossRef] [PubMed]
46. Shah, P.P.; Gelnick, S.; Jonisch, J.; Verma, R. Central Retinal Vein Occlusion Following BNT162b2 (Pfizer-BioNTech) COVID-19 Messenger RNA Vaccine. *Retin. Cases Brief Rep.* **2021**, *0*. [CrossRef] [PubMed]
47. Sodhi, P.K.; Yadav, A.; Sharma, B.; Sharma, A.; Kumar, P. Central Retinal Vein Occlusion Following the First Dose of COVID Vaccine. *Cureus* **2022**, *14*, e25842. [CrossRef] [PubMed]
48. Sonawane, N.; Yadav, D.; Kota, A.; Singh, H. Central retinal vein occlusion post-COVID-19 vaccination. *Indian J. Ophthalmol.* **2022**, *70*, 308. [CrossRef] [PubMed]
49. Sugihara, K.; Kono, M.; Tanito, M. Branch Retinal Vein Occlusion after Messenger RNA-Based COVID-19 Vaccine. *Case Rep. Ophthalmol.* **2022**, *13*, 28–32. [CrossRef] [PubMed]
50. Takacs, A.; Ecsedy, M.; Nagy, Z.Z. Possible COVID-19 MRNA Vaccine-Induced Case of Unilateral Central Retinal Vein Occlusion. *Ocul. Immunol. Inflamm.* **2022**, 1–6. [CrossRef]
51. Tanaka, H.; Nagasato, D.; Nakakura, S.; Tanabe, H.; Nagasawa, T.; Wakuda, H.; Imada, Y.; Mitamura, Y.; Tabuchi, H. Exacerbation of branch retinal vein occlusion post SARS-CoV-2 vaccination. *Medicine* **2021**, *100*, e28236. [CrossRef]
52. Suphachaiprasert, K.T.; Thammakumpee, K. A Cilioretinal Artery Occlusion (CLRAO) Associated with Optic Disc Edema after Viral Vector SARS-CoV-2 Vaccination: Case Report. *J. Med. Assoc. Thail.* **2022**, *105*, 565–568.
53. Tsukii, R.; Kasuya, Y.; Makino, S. Nonarteritic anterior ischemic optic neuropathy following COVID-19 vaccination: Consequence or coincidence. *Case Rep. Ophthalmol. Med.* **2021**, *2021*, 5126254. [CrossRef]
54. Kotian, R.; Vinzamuri, S.; Pradeep, T. Bilateral paracentral acute middle maculopathy and acute macular neuroretinopathy following COVID-19 vaccination. *Indian J. Ophthalmol.* **2021**, *69*, 2862–2864. [CrossRef]
55. Vujosevic, S.; Limoli, C.; Romano, S.; Vitale, L.; Villani, E.; Nucci, P. Retinal vascular occlusion and SARS-CoV-2 vaccination. *Graefe's Arch. Clin. Exp. Ophthalmol.* **2022**, *260*, 3455–3464. [CrossRef]

56. Hsu, Y.-R.; Wang, L.-U.; Chen, F.-T.; Wang, J.-K.; Huang, T.-L.; Chang, P.-Y.; Chen, Y.-J. Ocular inflammatory manifestations following COVID-19 vaccinations in Taiwan: A case series. *Taiwan J. Ophthalmol.* **2022**, *12*, 465. [CrossRef]
57. Elnahry, A.G.; Asal, Z.B.; Shaikh, N.; Dennett, K.; Abd Elmohsen, M.N.; Elnahry, G.A.; Shehab, A.; Vytopil, M.; Ghaffari, L.; Athappilly, G.K.; et al. Optic neuropathy after COVID-19 vaccination: A report of two cases. *Int. J. Neurosci.* **2021**, 1–7. [CrossRef]
58. Haseeb, A.; Elhusseiny, A.M.; Chauhan, M.Z.; Elnahry, A.G. Optic neuropathy after COVID-19 vaccination: Case report and systematic review. *Neuroimmunol. Rep.* **2022**, *2*, 100121. [CrossRef]
59. Bilotta, C.; Perrone, G.; Adelfio, V.; Spatola, G.F.; Uzzo, M.L.; Argo, A.; Zerbo, S. COVID-19 Vaccine-Related Thrombosis: A Systematic Review and Exploratory Analysis. *Front. Immunol.* **2021**, *12*, 729251. [CrossRef]
60. McGonagle, D.; De Marco, G.; Bridgewood, C. Mechanisms of immunothrombosis in vaccine-induced thrombotic thrombocytopenia (VITT) compared to natural SARS-CoV-2 infection. *J. Autoimmun.* **2021**, *121*, 102662. [CrossRef]
61. Elnahry, A.G.; Al-Nawaflh, M.Y.; Eldin, A.A.G.; Solyman, O.; Sallam, A.B.; Phillips, P.H.; Elhusseiny, A.M. COVID-19 Vaccine-Associated Optic Neuropathy: A Systematic Review of 45 Patients. *Vaccines* **2022**, *10*, 1758. [CrossRef]
62. Simpson, C.R.; Shi, T.; Vasileiou, E.; Katikireddi, S.V.; Kerr, S.; Moore, E.; McCowan, C.; Agrawal, U.; Shah, S.A.; Ritchie, L.D.; et al. First-dose ChAdOx1 and BNT162b2 COVID-19 vaccines and thrombocytopenic, thromboembolic and hemorrhagic events in Scotland. *Nat. Med.* **2021**, *27*, 1290–1297. [CrossRef]
63. Ostrowski, S.R.; Søgaard, O.S.; Tolstrup, M.; Stærke, N.B.; Lundgren, J.; Østergaard, L.; Hvas, A.M. Inflammation and platelet activation after COVID-19 vaccines-possible mechanisms behind vaccine-induced immune thrombocytopenia and thrombosis. *Front. Immunol.* **2021**, *12*, 779453. [CrossRef]
64. Haseeb, A.A.; Solyman, O.; Abushanab, M.M.; Obaia, A.S.A.; Elhusseiny, A.M. Ocular Complications Following Vaccination for COVID-19: A One-Year Retrospective. *Vaccines* **2022**, *10*, 342. [CrossRef]
65. Vo, A.D.; La, J.; Wu, J.T.Y.; Strymish, J.M.; Ronan, M.; Brophy, M.; Do, N.V.; Branch-Elliman, W.; Fillmore, N.R.; Monach, P.A. Factors Associated with Severe COVID-19 Among Vaccinated Adults Treated in US Veterans Affairs Hospitals. *JAMA Netw. Open* **2022**, *5*, e2240037. [CrossRef] [PubMed]
66. Jiang, H.; Gao, Y.; Fu, W.; Xu, H. Risk Factors and Treatments of Suprachoroidal Hemorrhage. *BioMed Res. Int.* **2022**, *2022*, 6539917. [CrossRef] [PubMed]
67. Thomas, C.J.; Mirza, R.G.; Gill, M.K. Age-Related Macular Degeneration. *Med. Clin. N. Am.* **2021**, *105*, 473–491. [CrossRef] [PubMed]
68. Chang, Y.-S.; Ho, C.-H.; Chu, C.-C.; Wang, J.-J.; Tseng, S.-H.; Jan, R.-L. Risk of retinal artery occlusion in patients with diabetes mellitus: A retrospective large-scale cohort study. *PLoS ONE* **2018**, *13*, e0201627. [CrossRef] [PubMed]
69. Chang, Y.S.; Jan, R.L.; Weng, S.F.; Wang, J.J.; Chio, C.C.; Wei, F.T.; Chu, C.C. Retinal artery occlusion and the 3-year risk of stroke in Taiwan: A nationwide population-based study. *Am. J. Ophthalmol.* **2012**, *154*, 645–652.e1. [CrossRef]
70. Li, Y.; Hall, N.E.; Pershing, S.; Hyman, L.; Haller, J.A.; Lee, A.Y.; Lee, C.S.; Chiang, M.; Lum, F.; Miller, J.W.; et al. Age, Gender, and Laterality of Retinal Vascular Occlusion: A Retrospective Study from the IRIS® Registry. *Ophthalmol. Retin.* **2021**, *6*, 161–171. [CrossRef]
71. Song, P.; Xu, Y.; Zha, M.; Zhang, Y.; Rudan, I. Global epidemiology of retinal vein occlusion: A systematic review and meta-analysis of prevalence, incidence, and risk factors. *J. Glob. Health* **2019**, *9*, 010427. [CrossRef]
72. Cheung, C.Y.; Biousse, V.; Keane, P.A.; Schiffrin, E.L.; Wong, T.Y. Hypertensive eye disease. *Nat. Rev. Dis. Prim.* **2022**, *8*, 1–18. [CrossRef]
73. Kinouchi, R.; Ishiko, S.; Hanada, K.; Hayashi, H.; Mikami, D.; Yoshida, A. Identification of risk factors for retinal vascular events in a population-based cross-sectional study in Rumoi, Japan. *Sci. Rep.* **2021**, *11*, 6340. [CrossRef]
74. Campochiaro, P.A. Molecular pathogenesis of retinal and choroidal vascular diseases. *Prog. Retin. Eye Res.* **2015**, *49*, 67–81. [CrossRef]
75. Porta, M.; Striglia, E. Intravitreal anti-VEGF agents and cardiovascular risk. *Intern. Emerg. Med.* **2019**, *15*, 199–210. [CrossRef]
76. Anderson, W.J.; da Cruz, N.F.S.; Lima, L.H.; Emerson, G.G.; Rodrigues, E.B.; Melo, G.B. Mechanisms of sterile inflammation after intravitreal injection of antiangiogenic drugs: A narrative review. *Int. J. Retin. Vitr.* **2021**, *7*, 37. [CrossRef]
77. Marín-Lambíes, C.; Gallego-Pinazo, R.; Salom, D.; Navarrete-Sanchis, J.; Díaz-Llopis, M. Rapid Regression of Exudative Maculopathy in Idiopathic Retinitis, Vasculitis, Aneurysms and Neuroretinitis Syndrome after Intravitreal Ranibizumab. *Case Rep. Ophthalmol.* **2012**, *3*, 251–257. [CrossRef]
78. Schmidt-Erfurth, U.; Garcia-Arumi, J.; Gerendas, B.S.; Midena, E.; Sivaprasad, S.; Tadayoni, R.; Wolf, S.; Loewenstein, A. Guidelines for the Management of Retinal Vein Occlusion by the European Society of Retina Specialists (EURETINA). *Ophthalmologica* **2019**, *242*, 123–162. [CrossRef]
79. Scott, I.U.; VanVeldhuisen, P.C.; Oden, N.L.; Ip, M.S.; Blodi, B.A. Month 60 Outcomes After Treatment Initiation with Anti-Vascular Endothelial Growth Factor Therapy for Macular Edema Due to Central Retinal or Hemiretinal Vein Occlusion. *Am. J. Ophthalmol.* **2022**, *240*, 330–341. [CrossRef]

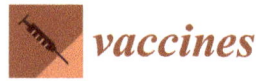 *vaccines*

Review

COVID-19 Vaccine-Associated Ocular Adverse Effects: An Overview

Parul Ichhpujani *, Uday Pratap Singh Parmar, Siddharth Duggal and Suresh Kumar

Department of Ophthalmology, Government Medical College and Hospital, Sector-32, Chandigarh 160030, India
* Correspondence: parul77@rediffmail.com

Abstract: Background: To address the pandemic caused by severe acute respiratory syndrome coronavirus 2 (SARS-CoV-2), vaccination efforts were initiated across the globe in December 2020 and are continuing. We report the onset interval and clinical presentations of ocular adverse effects following SARS-CoV-2 vaccination. Methods: For this narrative review, articles in the English language, published between 1 January 2020 to 1 September 2022, were included to formulate a list of the reported ocular adverse effects of different COVID-19 vaccines. Results: During this period, ocular adverse effects have been reported with BNT162b2 (Pfizer), mRNA-1273 (Moderna), AZD-1222 (AstraZeneca), and Ad26.COV2.S (Johnson & Johnson) vaccines. Endothelial graft rejection, herpes simplex virus keratitis, herpes zoster ophthalmicus, anterior uveitis, eyelid edema, purpuric rashes, ischemic optic neuropathy, and cranial nerve palsies were the most reported with BNT163b2. Retinal hemorrhages, vascular occlusions, and angle closure glaucoma were the most reported with AZD-1222. Most of the ocular adverse effects reported in the literature had a good to fair prognosis with appropriate management. Conclusions: Evidence regarding the ocular adverse effects does not outweigh the benefits of SARS-CoV-2 vaccination in patients with pre-existing systemic or ophthalmic diseases. This review provides insights into the possible temporal association between reported ocular adverse events and SARS-CoV-2 vaccines; however, further investigations are required to identify the link between potential causality and pathological mechanisms.

Keywords: COVID-19 vaccine; booster; molecular mimicry; ocular adverse effects

Citation: Ichhpujani, P.; Parmar, U.P.S.; Duggal, S.; Kumar, S. COVID-19 Vaccine-Associated Ocular Adverse Effects: An Overview. *Vaccines* **2022**, *10*, 1879. https://doi.org/10.3390/vaccines10111879

Academic Editor: Pedro Plans-Rubió

Received: 6 October 2022
Accepted: 1 November 2022
Published: 7 November 2022

Publisher's Note: MDPI stays neutral with regard to jurisdictional claims in published maps and institutional affiliations.

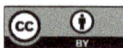

Copyright: © 2022 by the authors. Licensee MDPI, Basel, Switzerland. This article is an open access article distributed under the terms and conditions of the Creative Commons Attribution (CC BY) license (https://creativecommons.org/licenses/by/4.0/).

1. Introduction:

The coronaviruses are positive sense, single-stranded ribonucleic acid (RNA), enveloped medium-sized viruses. Coronaviruses are classified as a family within the order Nidovirales with a spike (S) glycoprotein which mediates receptor binding and cell entry. S protein is the site of the major antigens that stimulate neutralizing antibodies and target cytotoxic lymphocytes, thus making it an important vaccine antigen. Seven different strains of coronaviruses that infect humans include the common cold coronavirus strains; 229E, NL63, OC43, and HKU1 and the more pathogenic strains include Middle East respiratory syndrome (MERS)-CoV, severe acute respiratory syndrome (SARS)-CoV, and SARS-CoV-2. Since the structure and function of pathogenic strains of coronaviruses causing diseases like SARS and MERS were known it helped in the early development of various vaccine platforms across the globe.

A stepwise approach for developing any new vaccine involves vaccine development, clinical trials, U.S. Food and Drug Administration (FDA) approval or authorization, manufacturing, and distribution. The COVID-19 vaccines were developed at an unprecedented pace and were given Emergency Use Authorizations (EUAs) [1]. As of 19 September 2022, a total of 12,640,866,343 vaccine doses have been administered. COVID-19 vaccines and updated/bivalent COVID-19 boosters are effective at protecting people from being hospitalized, serious illness, and death [2].

Currently, 11 COVID-19 vaccines have been approved for EUA, which can be subdivided into four types: mRNA vaccines (BNT162b2, Pfizer-BioNTech14; mRNA-1273, Moderna15), protein subunit vaccines (NVX-CoV2373, Novavax16), vector vaccines (Ad26.COV2, Janssen Johnson & Johnson17; ChAdOx1 nCoV-19/AZD1222, Oxford-AstraZeneca18), and whole virus vaccines (PiCoVacc, Sinovac19; BBIBP-CorV, Sinopharm20) (Table 1) [3]. Individual vaccine trials report vaccine safety with rare ocular adverse effects but given the massive scale of the current vaccination drive, the possible adverse effects are a cause for concern. Since the widespread administration of COVID-19 vaccinations, multiple reports of ocular adverse effects after COVID-19 vaccinations and boosters have emerged [4,5].

Table 1. List of WHO-approved vaccines for COVID-19.

SNo	Name	Type of Vaccine	Country Where Vaccine Was Developed	Countries That Have Used It	Route of Admin	VVM	Preservatives	Diluents
1	Covovax (Novavax formulation)	Protein Subunit (Recombinant Nanoparticle)	India (Serum Institute of India)	6 countries	IM	N/A	N/A	N/A
2	Nuvaxovid (Novavax)	Protein Subunit	Czech Republic	40 countries	IM	N/A	N/A	N/A
3	mRNA-1273 Moderna: Spikevax	RNA (modified nucleoside)	Spain (Moderna Biotech)	88 countries	IM	N/A	N/A	N/A
4	BNT163b2 Pfizer BioNTech: Comirnaty	RNA (Modified nucleoside)	Germany (BioNTech Manufacturing GmbH)	149 countries	IM	N/A	N/A	Sodium Chloride Inj USP 0.9%
5	Convidecia: CanSino (Ad5.CoV2-S)	Non replicating viral vector	People's Republic of China (CanSino Biologics Inc.)	10 countries	IM	None	None	None
6	Jcovden: Janssen (Johnson & Johnson)	Non-replicating viral vector	Belgium (JCINV)	113 countries	IM	None	None	None
7	Vaxzevria (Oxford AstraZeneca)	Non replicating viral vector	Republic of Korea (AstraZeneca/SK Bioscience Co., Ltd.)	149 countries	IM	None	None	None
8	Covidshield (ChAdOx1 nCoV-19 (AZD1222) (Oxford AstraZeneca formulation)	Non-replicating viral vector	India (Serum Institute of India)	49 countries	IM	None	None	None
9	Covaxin	Inactivated (Whole virion)	India (Bharat Biotech)	14 countries	IM	N/A	Phenoxy ethanol	N/A
10	Sinopharm: Covilo/BBIBP-CorV	Inactivated (Antigen is purified and absorbed with aluminium hydroxide)	China (BIBP)	93 countries	IM	VVM7	None	N/A
11	Sinovac: Coronavac	Inactivated (Antigen is purified and absorbed with aluminium hydroxide)	China (Sinovac Biotech)	56 countries	IM	N/A	None	N/A

(IM: Intramuscular; RNA: Ribonucleic acid; VVM: Vaccine Vial Monitor Type).

To develop methods for closely observing 'at risk' patients, reporting of adverse effects must be conducted on a regular basis. This narrative review summarizes ocular adverse effects that are possibly associated with COVID-19 vaccination. The aim is to encourage early recognition of adverse effects not only by ophthalmologists but also by treating physicians.

2. Methodology

A literature search was performed in PubMed for 'COVID-19 vaccine', 'ocular inflammation', 'ophthalmic manifestations', 'adverse effects', 'graft failure', 'retinal hemorrhage', 'uveitis', 'neuro-ophthalmology', 'nerve palsy', and 'vascular occlusion'. Articles of interest were searched using Boolean operators. Each synonymous word was separated by a Boolean operator, "OR", phrases were enclosed within quotation marks, and groups of synonymous words were enclosed within parenthesis. Articles in the English language, published between 1 January 2020 to 1 September 2022, were included to formulate the list of the reported ocular adverse effects of different COVID-19 vaccines. The search, although not exhaustive, includes important and relevant articles. Search results were screened by two authors (PI and SD) for relevance. References cited within the identified articles were also used to further augment the search. We characterized our results into an anterior segment, posterior segment, and neurophthalmic adverse effects.

3. Results

Ocular complications reported post-COVID-19 vaccination included abducens nerve palsy, oculomotor nerve palsy, facial nerve palsy/Bell's palsy, multiple cranial nerve palsies, acute macular neuroretinopathy (AMN), paracentral acute middle maculopathy (PAMM), superior ophthalmic vein thrombosis (SOVT), corneal graft rejection, anterior uveitis, panuveitis, central serous chorioretinopathy(CSCR), Vogt–Koyanagi–Harada (VKH) reactivation, acute zonal occult outer retinopathy (AZOOR) and multifocal choroiditis. The reported ocular adverse effects following vaccination appear to overlap with the ocular manifestations of COVID-19 itself, suggesting a common pathway between virus- and vaccine-mediated immune response in humans. Aggregated information on the reviewed cases is elucidated in Tables 2 and 3.

Table 2. Anterior segment manifestations following COVID-19 vaccines.

Manifestation		Vaccine	Time of Onset	Symptoms	Case/Case Series Age/Age Range	Mechanism	Treatment and Outcome	Article Reference No.
	1	BNT162b2	7 days 3 weeks	Painless decrease in vision Red eye	66 yrs 83 yrs Case report	Allogenic response, generated by the host antibodies and immune system	Treated successfully with topical steroids	(Phylactou, M et al., 2021) [6]
	2	BNT162b2	7 days	Sudden painless decrease in vision, conjunctival injection; diffuse corneal edema	71 yrs Case report	Disruption of immune regulation and upregulation of cytokines like TNF α, chemokines, and pro inflammatory molecules	Treated with topical Dexamethasone sodium phosphate 1 mg/mL/2 hourly Resolution after 2 weeks	(Crnej, A et al., 2021) [7]
	3	BNT162b2	14 days	Painless worsening of vision Corneal thickness increased, OCT Descemet membrane folds	94 yrs Case report	Changes in antibody-mediated immune signalling response following vaccination	Dexamethasone/tobramycin Horshaw, T et al., With hypertonic saline	(Forshaw, T et al., 2022) [8]
Endothelial Graft Rejection	4	BNT162b2 (8 patients)	17 days 3 weeks × 2 13 days 14 days 7 days 3 days 4 days 4 days 9 days 13 days	Conjunctival hyperemia, diffuse corneal edema, KPs, flare and cells, corneal thickness, stromal edema reported in 1 patient	Systematic review Median age 68 (27–83) IQR	Increased anti-spike-neutralizing antibodies, antigen-specific CD4+ T-cell responses, and inflammatory cytokines, including interferon (IFN-γ and interleukin-2 IFN-γ plays a central role in the acute rejection process and the resultant T helper type 1-dominant immune response may have evoked corneal allograft rejection	Dexamethasone eye drops 0.2% hourly, combined oral methyl prednisone, hypertonic saline, intracameral fortecortin injections	(Fujio, K et al., 2022) [9]
		mRNA-1273 (8 patients)	1 week 1 week 2 week 1 week 15 days 3 days 1 week 1 week					
		ChAdOx1 (4 patients)	5 days 10 days 2 days 6 weeks					
		CoronaVac	1 day		63 yrs			

Table 2. Cont.

Manifestation		Vaccine	Time of Onset	Symptoms	Case/Case Series Age/Age Range	Mechanism	Treatment and Outcome	Article Reference No.
Endothelial Graft Rejection	5	BNT163b2 (3 cases) AZD1222 (2 cases)	16.86 ± 6.96 days (mean) 17 ± 11.89 days	Painless loss of VA and conjunctival suffusion	Case series		Topical Steroids	(Molero-Senosiain, M et al., 2022) [10]
	6	BNT163b2	2 weeks	Decreased VA, ocular pain, photophobia	73 yrs Case report		Prednisone acetate every 1–2 h, with Muro ointment	(Abousy, M et al., 2021) [11]
	7	CoronaVac Biotech	24 h		63 yrs Case report	Hyperstimulation of the immune system	Partially resolved by topical corticosteroids and polydimethylsiloxane	(Simão, M.F et al., 2022) [12]
	8	ChAdOx1 COVIDSHIELD, AstraZeneca	2 weeks	Blurring of vision, stromal edema	28 yrs Case report		Hourly topical steroids, cycloplegics and oral steroids	(Nahata, H et al., 2022) [13]
	9	mRNA-1273 (4 cases)	3 weeks 9 days 2 weeks 2 weeks		Case report		Topical steroids Complete resolution	(Shah, A.P et al., 2022) [14]
Herpes zoster Ophthalmicus (HZO)	1	mRNA-1273	6 days	Itchy tender lesions on the right thigh, eruption of vesicles with an erythematous base	79 yrs Case report		Complete resolution after systemic antiviral treatment	(Eid, E et al., 2021) [15]
	2	BNT163b2 (Tozinameran) (2 cases)	15 days 13 days	Painful grouped vesicles in the left lateral of the ox coccyges (S3 dermatome) Painful and swollen inguinal lymph nodes along with a rash on the right leg	29 yrs 34 yrs Case report	Lymphopenia along with any functional impairment of T lymphocytes could trigger herpes zoster reactivation	Self-limiting Valacyclovir 1 g 3×/day for 10 days, complete resolution	(van Dam, C.S et al., 2021) [16]
	3	AZD-1222 (Covidshield)	4 days	Multiple grouped fluid filled lesions on an erythematous base, present on the knee and the anterior aspect of the thigh; biopsy showed acantholytic cells and dyskeratotic cells	60 yrs Case report		Valacyclovir 1 g 3×/day for 7 days Topical Fusidic acid 2×/day	(Arora, P et al., 2021) [17]

Table 2. Cont.

Manifestation		Vaccine	Time of Onset	Symptoms	Case/Case Series Age/Age Range	Mechanism	Treatment and Outcome	Article Reference No.
	4	mRNA-1273 (14 cases)	2, 0, 4, 4, 14, 12, 2, 0, 12, 12, 26, 5, 4, 5–6 days, respectively	Unilateral dermatological skin eruptions, with itching, pain, arm soreness, altered skin sensation	77, 56, 54, 69, 42, 47, 39, 68, 60, 43, 65, 37, 69, 72 yrs, respectively		Valacyclovir Gabapentin LMX, Terrasil Shingles cream	(Lee, C et al., 2021) [18]
		BNT163b2 (6 cases)	38, 5, 3, 12, 9, 5 days, respectively		65, 43, 74, 48, 46, 44 yrs, respectively Case series			
	5	BNT163b2 (5 cases)	1, 5, 3, 2, 16 days, respectively	Umbilicated vesicles, lymphadenopathy, dysesthesias, fever, vesicles and rash in dermatomal pattern	58, 47, 39, 56, 41 yrs, respectively Case series	Immunomodulation due to decrease in lymphocytes, monocytes, eosinophils, CD4/CD8 T cells	Valacyclovir 1 g 3×/day for 7 days	(Rodriguez-Jiménez, P et al., 2021) [19]
Herpes zoster Ophthalmicus (HZO)	6	RNA vaccine	5 days	Painful pimple-like lesions with stinging in the left mammary region, crusted haemorrhagic vesicles upon an erythematous base	78 yrs Case report		Valacyclovir 3×/day for 7 days	(Bostan, E et al., 2021) [20]
	7	Inactivated COVID 19 vaccine	5 days	Multiple pinhead vesicular lesions with an erythematous base occupying right mammary region and back along with stinging sensation and pain	68 yrs Case report		Valacyclovir 3×/day for 7 days Codeine for pain management	(Aksu, S.B et al., 2021) [21]
	8	BNT163b2 (7 cases)	9, 14, 8, 7, 9, 7, 10	Unilateral dermatomal rash in different dermatomes (lumbar, thoracic, 5th cranial nerve) malaise, headache	51, 56, 89, 86, 90, 91, 94 yrs Case series		Valacyclovir for 7 days after symptoms onset	(Psichogiou, M et al., 2021) [22]
Herpes Simplex Virus (HSV) Keratitis	1	ChAdOx1n	1 day	Corneal hyperaemia, reduced corneal sensation, multiple corneal dendrites, reduced VA (6/9)	82 yrs Case report	Molecular mimicry, autoinflammation triggered by the vaccine and lymphopenia	Acyclovir 5×/day, doxycycline 50 mg orally once a day, prednisone phosphate 0.5% Atropine 1% 1×/day	(Richardson-May et al., 2021) [23]

Table 2. Cont.

Manifestation		Vaccine	Time of Onset	Symptoms	Case/Case Series Age/Age Range	Mechanism	Treatment and Outcome	Article Reference No.
	2	Sinovac (2 cases)	2 days 4 days	Tearing, redness, photophobia, decreased visual acuity, dendritic lesions on slit lamp examination	60 yrs 51 yrs Case report	Lymphopenia, insufficient cellular immunity	Topical steroids, topical and oral ganciclovir	(Rallis et al., 2022) [24]
	3	BNT163b2	2 days	Blurry vision, 20/40 VA, patchy stromal haze and confluent punctate epithelial erosions along inferior cornea	52 yrs	Activation of the proinflammatory cytokines like INF gamma post vaccination, can have a role in reactivation	Acyclovir 5×/day Topical trifluride 5×/day Prednisolone acetate 1% 5×/day	(Fard et al., 2022) [25]
		mRNA-1273	2 weeks	Blurry vision, redness, abnormal sensation in OS, corneal epithelial defect	67 yrs		Bandage contact lens, Oral Valacyclovir 1 gm 2×/day Ofloxacin 0.3% drops 4×/day	
	4	BNT163b2 (3 cases)	1 week 1 week 1 week	Pain, Photophobia, Lacrimation Typical dendritic ulcer of the peripheral cornea Stromal infiltration and diffuse conjunctival injection AC trace	18 yrs 40 yrs 29 yrs	Vaccine triggered cytokine release and upregulation of natural killer cells group D ligand, causing reactivation	Lubrication, ganciclovir ophthalmic gel 0.15% 5×/day Oral acyclovir 400 mg 5×/day for 10 days	(Alkwikbi, H et al., 2022) [26]
		AZD1222	1 week	Pain, redness, blurry vision; epithelial dendritic ulcers were noted on the cornea	32 yrs Case report		Prednisone 1 mg/kg/day for 4 weeks	
	5	BNT163b2 (2 cases)	4 days 4 weeks	Necrotizing stromal keratitis Endothelitis and epithelial keratitis	42 yrs 29 yrs Case report	Potential immunological dysregulation	Systemic acyclovir	(Alkhalifah, M.I et al., 2021) [27]

Table 2. *Cont.*

Manifestation		Vaccine	Time of Onset	Symptoms	Case/Case Series Age/Age Range	Mechanism	Treatment and Outcome	Article Reference No.
	6	BNT163b2	5 days	Conjunctival hyperaemia, pseudodendrite in peripheral cornea Along with vesicular skin rash on forehead, scalp, nose, eyelid, meningitis	74 yrs Case report	Temporal association due to immunological upregulation of cellular immunity	Therapeutic contact lens, recombinant human epithelial growth factor, Ofloxacin ointment	(You et al., 2022) [28]
	7	BNT163b2	2 days	OS redness, tearing, and pain	50 yrs Case report	mRNA vaccines dysregulate T cell latency mechanisms in the sensory nerve ganglion	400 mg oral acyclovir + Topical fluorometholone	(Al-Dwairi et al., 2022) [29]
	8	ChAdOx1n	7 days	Pain, photophobia, blurred vision, Examination—peri corneal injection, hazy cornea with paracentral thinning	56 yrs Case report	Potential immune response triggered by molecular mimicry	Topical and systemic acyclovir	(Murgova et al., 2022) [30]
		BNT163b2 (4 cases)	3 weeks 8 days 2 weeks 10 days	Blurred vision and irritation in OS, KP's seen in the anterior segment Moderate vitritis and exudates	89 yrs 50 yrs 52 yrs 45 yrs		Acyclovir Steroids (1 mg/kg methylprednisone)	
	9	BNT163b2	2 days	Sudden visual impairment, diffuse corneal stromal edema, nasal stromal infiltration	87 yrs Case report	T cells activation by the host cell response after vaccination may have caused the recurrance	Oral Valacyclovir and topical corticosteroids	(Ryu et al., 2022) [31]
	10	BNT163b2	7 days	Decreased VA and foreign body sensation	30 yrs Case report	Unknown immunological response or general systemic reactogenicity to the vaccine-causing reactivation	Topical eye drops (Ganciclovir 0.25%) Loteprednol etabonate 0.5%	(Song et al., 2022) [32]
Anterior Uveitis	1	BNT163b2 (3 cases)	6 days 6 days 8 days	Photophobia Blurred vision	44 yrs 47 yrs 44 yrs	Immunological hyperstimulation by the vaccine	Dexamethasone eye drops 2 mg/mL leading to complete resolution	(Bolletta et al., 2022) [33]
		AZD1222	30 days	Redness, pain, blurred vision	66 yrs			
		mRNA-1273	1 day	Redness, pain, blurred vision	35 yrs Case report			

Table 2. Cont.

Manifestation	Vaccine	Time of Onset	Symptoms	Case/Case Series Age/Age Range	Mechanism	Treatment and Outcome	Article Reference No.
2	BNT163b2	14 days	Pain, photophobia and red eye. Conjunctival hyperaemia, posterior synechiae and AC cells, KPs in the lower quadrants	23 yrs	Molecular mimicry	10-day course of topical steroids and cycloplegics	(Renisi et al., 2022) [34]
3	Sinopharm	5 days	Reduced VA, hyperreflective dots in the AC, fine endothelial granularities	18 yrs Case report	Potential immunological mechanisms	Topical steroids leading to complete resolution	(ElSheikh et al., 2021) [35]
4	BNT163b2	3 weeks	Acute onset pain, photophobia, erythema, blurring of vision	46 yrs Case report	Autoantibodies production post vaccination as a component of the hyper-stimulated immune system reacting with self peptides	Topical triamcinolone drops, azathioprine 50mg once daily as a steroid-sparing agent	(Al-Allaf et al., 2022) [36]
5	BNT163b2	3 days	Redness, blurred vision, headache Corneal epithelial edema, KPs in the lower quadrant	54 yrs Case report	Secondary molecular mimicry due to similarity between the vaccine fragments and the peptides of the uvea, adjuvants such as aluminium cause inflammatory damage, delayed hypersensitivity response	0.1% Dexamethasone, 1% Cycloplegic drugs, 0.1% dexamethasone ointment	(Duran 2022) [37]
6	BNT163b2	2 months	Photophobia, redness, decreased vision, pain Intense ciliary flush and posterior synechiae	37 yrs Case report	mRNA vaccine-induced cellular and humoral immune responses, which can lead to molecular mimicry and immunological cross-reactivity	Topical prednisone acetate 1% and cyclopentolate	(Alhamazani et al., 2022) [38]
7	BNT163b2	3 days 3 days	Ocular pain, redness, hemicranial headache	92 yrs 85 yrs Case report	Molecular mimicry and antigen specific cell and antibody-mediated hypersensitivity reactions	Cycloplegic every 8 h and moxifloxacin eye drops every 4 h	(Ortiz Egea et al., 2022) [39]

Table 2. Cont.

Manifestation		Vaccine	Time of Onset	Symptoms	Case/Case Series Age/Age Range	Mechanism	Treatment and Outcome	Article Reference No.
	8	BNT163b2	2 days	Decreased VA and conjunctival injection Hypopyon and flares in the AC	21 yrs Case report	Vaccine-induced molecular mimicry	Topical dexamethasone (0.1%) hourly and systemic prednisone (50 mg/day) for 7 days	(Hwang JH. 2022) [40]
	9	AZD-1222	1 day	Greater vitreous opacity, KPs, increase in inflammatory cells in the AC	62 yrs	Molecular mimicry between vaccine and ocular structures leading to autoreactivity	Topical steroids	(Choi et al., 2022) [41]
		BNT163b2 (2 cases)	3 days / 2 days		79 yrs / 55 yrs		Topical steroids	
Episcleritis and Anterior Scleritis	1	AZD1222		Anterior non-necrotising scleritis				(Hernanz I et al., 2022) [42]
	2	Sinopharm (3 cases)	1 week / 15 days / 15 days	Diffuse scleral hyperemia	33 to 55 yrs Case series	Molecular mimicry and antigen-specific cell and antibody-mediated hypersensitivity reactions	Resolved in 2 weeks after topical steroids	(Pichi F et al., 2022) [43]
Angle closure glaucoma	1	AZD-1222	2 weeks	Ocular pain, acute visual loss, corneal microscopic cystic edema, conjunctival injection, shallow AC, peripheral AC collapse	71 yrs	Swelling of ciliary body after vaccination, that led to zonule laxity accompanied by phacodonesis, causing a closed-angle attack	Phacoemulsification with goniosynechiolysis	(Choi M et al., 2022) [41]
	2	AZD-1222			83 yrs		Trabeculectomy with laser peripheral iridoplasty	
	3	AZD-1222			59 yrs		Phacoemulsification with posterior chamber lens implantation	
	4	AZD-1222			64 yrs		Vitrectomy with IOL scleral fixation	
	5	BNT163b2	3 days	Blurry vision, headache, corneal edema,	54 yrs	Not mentioned	20% Mannitol, acetazolamide 250 mg, timolol, dorzolamide, 0.15% brimonidine	(Duran M 2022) [37]
Eyelid edema	1	BNT162b2	1 day	Transient eyelid edema	39.3 mean age (32–43) Case series	Complement activation that increased complement mediators within the plasma and tear film, resulting in eyelid edema	Observation, Antihistamine, Corticosteroid	(Austria QM et al., 2021) [44]

Table 2. *Cont.*

Manifestation		Vaccine	Time of Onset	Symptoms	Case/Case Series Age/Age Range	Mechanism	Treatment and Outcome	Article Reference No.
Purpuric eyelid rash	1	BNT162b2	Median of 18 days	Purpuric rashes on the upper lids associated with mild itching	44 yrs 63 yrs 67 yrs	Mild and localized form of vaccine-induced microangiopathy	Self-resolving	(Mazzatenta et al., 2021) [45]
Bell's palsy	1	BNT162b2	3 days	Latero-cervical pain in left side, irradiating to the mastoid ipsilaterally, monolateral muscle weakness; flattening of the forehead skin and nasolabial fold	37 yrs	Possible autoimmune reaction	Corticosteroids (prednisone, 50 mg/day), artificial tears eye drops and eye dressing at night Helped resolve systemic symptoms, facial mobility partially improved and pain sensation still persists	(Colella et al., 2022) [46]

(AC: anterior chamber; KP: keratic precipitates; OCT: optical coherence tomography, OS: oculus sinistrum; VA: visual acuity).

Table 3. Posterior segment and neurophthalmic manifestations following COVID-19 vaccines.

	Manifestation	Vaccine	Time of Onset (Days)	Symptoms	Case/Case Series Age/Age Range	Mechanism	Visual Prognosis	Article Reference No.
				Vitreo-Retina:				
1.	Acute Macular Neuroretinopathy (AMN)	AZD1222	3 days	Bilateral paracentral scotomas with underlying bilateral circumscribed paracentral dark lesions on ophthalmoscopy, OCT with outer plexiform layer thickening and discontinuity	21 yrs	Hypoperfusion of the retina might account for the peripheral visual loss, which self-corrected rapidly. Reduction in central acuity is less straight forward to explain, but can result from transient hypoperfusion of retina, optic nerves, or any part of the visual pathways extending to the visual cortices. [7]	Self-limiting	(Book et al., 2021) [47]
		AZD1222	2 days	Unilateral paracentral scotoma with a teardrop-shaped macular lesion nasal to the fovea	27 yrs		Symptoms only lasted for 24 h	(Mambretti et al., 2022) [48]
		AZD1222	2 days	Unilateral presentation with paracentral scotoma	22 yrs		Self-limiting	(Mambretti et al., 2021) [48]
		AZD1222	2 days	Unilateral presentation with paracentral scotoma	28 yrs			(Mambretti et al., 2021) [48]
		BBIBP-CorV Sinopharm	5.2 days (range, 1–10 days)	Previous ocular history of CSCR in both eyes with a chronic serous PED in the OS. BCVA of 20/25 at previous visits. Vital parameters were within normal limits, but the BCVA in OS dropped to 20/400.	41.4 (9.3) yrs (range: 30–55 yrs)	Can be associated with anemia, hypertension or hypotension, hypoxia, and other systemic morbidities, which can contribute to nerve fiber layer infarcts, haemorrhages, or microaneurysms. Vasculitis and thromboembolism also can contribute to retinal ischemia.	Patient was closely observed, and at 2-month follow-up, the tomographic picture had resolved and BCVA was back to 20/30.	(Pichi et al., 2021) [43]

Table 3. Cont.

Vitreo-Retina:

	Manifestation	Vaccine	Time of Onset (Days)	Symptoms	Case/Case Series Age/Age Range	Mechanism	Visual Prognosis	Article Reference No.
2.	Paracentral acute middle maculopathy (PAMM)	AZD1222 2nd dose	30 days	Reduced brightness sensitivity in both eyes progressed further, black spots in his central field. OCT macula revealed a significant reduction in the number and size of the hyperreflective lesions noted in the nerve fibre and ganglion cell layers. There was also a reduction in the thickness of the outer nuclear layer in both eyes.	35 yrs	Possible microvascular pathology affecting the deep capillary plexus. It is possible that small vessel vasculitis induced by vaccination resulted in these findings. It is hypothesized that the vasculitis changes may have led to the ischemia of the deep capillary plexus presenting as PAMM and AMN in the patient.	On re-examining the patient after 3 weeks he reported slight improvement of brightness sensitivity but still complained of black spots in his central field of vision. On examination, his vision was 6/6 in both eyes. His Amsler's grid charting was also normal. The OCT macula revealed a significant reduction in the number and size of the hyperreflective lesions noted in the NFL and GCL. There was also a reduction in the thickness of the outer nuclear layer in OU.	(Vinzamuri et al., 2021) [49]
		BBIBP-CorV Sinopharm	5.2 days (1–10 days)	20 min after receiving Sinopharm, they developed persistent tachycardia and raised blood pressure. Noticed inferior scotoma in OS. BCVA at presentation was 20/30 OS, with a dot hemorrhage superior to the fovea.	41.4 (9.3) yrs (30–55 yrs)	Molecular mimicry and antigen-specific cell and antibody-mediated hypersensitivity reactions may be involved.	BP was nonresponsive to treatment for 3 weeks	(Pichi et al., 2021) [43]

Table 3. Cont.

	Manifestation	Vaccine	Time of Onset (Days)	Symptoms	Case/Case Series Age/Age Range	Mechanism	Visual Prognosis	Article Reference No.
					Vitreo-Retina:			
3.	Multifocal choroiditis	AZD1222	7 days	Patient had a large unilateral serous macular detachment and severe choroidal thickening bilaterally. BCVA was 6/36, N60, and 6/6, N6 in OD and OS, respectively.	34 yrs	Autoimmunity triggered by the vaccines. Mechanisms include cytokine production, expression of human histocompatibility leukocyte antigens, modification of surface antigens, induction of novel antigens, molecular mimicry, bystander activation, epitope spreading, polyclonal activation of B cells, and an immune reaction to vaccination adjuvants known collectively as Shoenfeld syndrome are often associated with constitutional symptoms such as arthralgia, myalgia, and fatigue.	On oral prednisolone 100 mg daily (1 mg/kg body weight) tapering by 10 mg/week after 11 days the patient reported significant improvement in vision. UCVA improved to 6/6, N6. Significant resolution of choroiditis with trace residual subretinal fluid. B-scan showed significant reduction in CT.	(Goyal et al., 2021) [50]
4.	Panuveitis	BNT162b2	3 days	Patient presented with a visual acuity of 20/500 in both eyes, eye pain, eye redness, and sensitivity to light having 3-4+ anterior chamber cell with 2-3+ vitreous cell with significant choroidal thickening.	43 yrs	Direct infection of ocular structures by live strain (the COVID-19 vaccine is not a live strain * Additive-induced immune-related uveitis (which are not present in the Pfizer-Biontech vaccine) * Molecular mimicry between the vaccine and ocular structures, driving the adaptive immune system to create autoimmunity.	Within 10 days of starting oral prednisone pain resolved, her VA improved to 20/20 OU, there was no inflammation, and the choroidal thickening resolved.	(Mudie et al., 2021) [51]

Table 3. *Cont.*

	Manifestation	Vaccine	Time of Onset (Days)	Symptoms	Case/Case Series Age/Age Range	Mechanism	Visual Prognosis	Article Reference No.
					Vitreo-Retina:			
5.	Central serous chorioretinopathy (CSCR)	BNT162b2	3 days	Unilateral blurry vision. BCVA OD: 20/63; OS: 20/25 with metamorphopsia	33 yrs	Possibly due to increased serum cortisol, free extracellular mRNA, and polyethylene glycol.	At the 2-month visit, BCVA:20/40; CFT: 325 μm. At the 3-month visit, BCVA: 20/20; CFT: 211 μm. OCT showed complete resolution of subretinal fluid	(Fowler at al., 2021) [52]
6.	Acute Zonal Occult Outer Retinopathy (AZOOR)	mRNA-1273	10 days	Bilateral presentation with progressive unilateral nasal defect and bilateral flashes. At presentation, had 20/20 vision in both eyes with a yellow-white reflex in the temporal macula of her left eye.	33 yrs	Possible mechanisms include: (i) molecular mimicry, where the vaccine triggers an immune response to self-antigens; (ii) bystander activation of sequestered self-antigens from the host that can activate antigen-presenting cells and T-helper cells; (iii) cytokines secretion from macrophages that recruit additional T-helper cells; (iv) genetic polymorphisms related to the aberrant regulation of the IL-4 expression or activity, which may over-stimulate inflammatory responses	Patient was recommended a combination therapy of azathioprine and cyclosporine. Patient consulted her gynecologist prior to starting therapy as she was nursing a baby.	(Maleki et al., 2021.) [53]

Table 3. Cont.

	Manifestation	Vaccine	Time of Onset (Days)	Symptoms	Case/Case Series Age/Age Range	Mechanism	Visual Prognosis	Article Reference No.
				Vitreo-Retina:				
7.	Posterior Uveitis	BNT162b2 (4 cases) AZD1222 (4 cases) mRNA-1273 (1 case)	6.5 [1–14] after first dose 8 [2–9] after second dose	Unilateral in 8, bilateral in 1. 2 (22.2%) had history of ocular toxoplasmosis, 1 (11.1%) of AZOOR. Patients with history of ocular toxoplasmosis presented with recurrence of lesions and the patient with AZOOR had a different presentation from previous events with multifocal choroiditis. 3 (33.3%) presented with ocular toxoplasmosis, 2 (22.2%) presented with retinal vasculitis, and 1 (11.1%) presented with choroiditis for the first time.	40 yrs	Out of 3 with previous history of posterior uveitis, 2 had history of previous similar event. * Molecular mimicry secondary to resemblance between uveal peptides and vaccine peptide fragments. * Antigen-specific cell and antibody-mediated hypersensitivit. Reactions * Inflammatory damage induced by adjuvants included the vaccines stimulating innate immunity through endosolic or cytoplasmic nucleic acid receptors.	VA unaffected in 7 (77.8%) VA reduced > 3 lines in 2 (22.2%) Macular Scarring in 2 (22.2%) On being treated by topical corticosteroid in 6 and systemic corticosteroid in 3. One patient with ocular toxoplasmosis, and 1 with occlusive retinal vasculitis had persistent vision loss on the last follow-up due to macular scarring.	(Testi et al., 2021) [54]

(BCVA: Best-corrected visual acuity; CSCR: central serous chorioretinopathy; GCL: ganglion cell layer; mRNA: messenger ribonucleic acid; NFL: nerve fiber layer; OS: oculus sinistrum; PED: pigment epithelial detachment).

4. Discussion

A new variant of CoV emerged in Wuhan, China in December 2019 that caused severe respiratory illness. The World Health Organization named this virus SARS-CoV-2 and the pandemic COVID-19. According to Li, Y.-D. [55], to address the global morbidity and mortality caused by COVID-19, the development process of COVID-19 vaccines was expedited by undertaking clinical trials in parallel rather than in a linear fashion. Multiple COVID-19 vaccines directly entered clinical trials on humans without preclinical testing in animal models. The COVID-19 vaccination drive has been carried out worldwide and the evidence is overwhelming that irrespective of the type(s) of vaccine taken, the vaccines offered safety and protection against becoming seriously ill or dying due to the different variants of CoV-2.

The Vaccine Adverse Event Reporting System (VAERS) was developed by the U.S. Food and Drug Administration (FDA) in 1990 as a national early monitoring system for vaccine safety. The commonly reported adverse effects of COVID-19 vaccinations consist of the injection site's local reaction followed by several non-specific flu-like symptoms. However, several systemic and organ-specific (e.g., eye, heart) adverse effects have also been reported from across the globe. Therefore, it is imperative for ophthalmic health care providers to be familiar with the clinical presentations, pathophysiology, diagnostic criteria, and management of ocular adverse effects following COVID-19 vaccination. Early diagnosis and quick initiation of the treatment may help to provide patients with a more favorable outcome and rule out masquerading entities. With an increasing amount of literature in the form of isolated case-study reports, case series, and analysis of the VAERS database, an epidemiological montage has started to emerge [56].

A recent Lancet article questioned the effectiveness of COVID-19 vaccines and the waning of immunity over time, more pronounced in individuals with pre-existing conditions and elderly adults. According to Nordström, P. [57], in addition to the risk of infections owing to lowered immune function, the authors cited a possible risk of some organ damage caused by the vaccine that has remained somewhat sequestered in the circulatory system, without apparent clinical presentations. This can explain the slightly delayed presentation of some of the adverse effects.

Vaccines have added adjuvants within them to boost their efficacy; these adjuvants potentiate the innate and adaptive immune responses further, possibly leading to autoimmune or inflammatory conditions in some individuals. Although truncated and modified RNA traces may be present in BNT162b2 and mRNA-1273 vaccines, these aberrant proteins have a minuscule chance of eliciting allergic reactions. The active constituent of the vaccine is not always the culprit for causing adverse reactions. Excipients such as polyethylene glycol (PEG) used in the BNT162b2 and mRNA-1273 vaccines have been reported to have induced IgE-mediated allergic reactions [3].

Despite reports suggesting an association between ocular adverse effects and the vaccines due to a maladaptive immune response in susceptible individuals, the adverse issues are still considered 'rare' given the millions of people who have received either one or more vaccines or boosters.

The COVID-19 vaccines interact with the platelets or the platelet factor 4 (PF4) and this interaction results in vaccine-induced immune thrombotic thrombocytopenia (VITT). The proposed mechanisms suggest the formation of autoantibodies against PF4, antibodies induced by the free deoxyribonucleic acid (DNA) in the vaccine that cross-reacts with PF4, platelets, and adenovirus binds to the platelets causing platelet activation. VITT may explain vascular occlusions [58].

Endothelial graft rejection, herpes simplex virus (HSV) keratitis, herpes zoster ophthalmicus (HZO), anterior uveitis, eyelid edema, purpuric rashes, ischemic optic neuropathy, and cranial nerve palsies were the most reported with the BNT163b2 vaccine. Although both BNT162b2 and mRNA 1273 are mRNA vaccines, the ocular adverse effects have been relatively lesser with mRNA 1273 than those with BNT162b2.

Retinal hemorrhages (subretinal, subhyaloid, or intraretinal), vascular occlusions, and angle closure glaucoma have been the most reported with the AZD 1222 vaccine. No COVID-19 vaccine-associated adverse events have been reported in patients with age-related macular degeneration in the peer-reviewed literature to date.

The pathophysiological mechanisms underlying vaccine–corneal graft rejection are still poorly understood. However, cases of acute graft rejection have also been reported following influenza, hepatitis B, yellow fever, and tetanus toxoid vaccinations. Steinemann, T.L. and Wertheim, M.S. [59,60] proposed mechanisms for acute corneal allograft rejection include the reduction in the corneal immune privilege due to systemic immune dysregulation and activation of toll-like receptors on the ocular surface and CD4+ T helper-1 cell (Th1) immunity. Corneal edema was the leading clinical manifestation, followed by keratic precipitates in patients with corneal graft rejection. Most of the ocular adverse effects reported in the literature had a good to fair prognosis with appropriate management. Therefore, corneal graft recipients should not be discouraged from receiving COVID-19 vaccines or boosters. Additionally, the evidence is insufficient to suggest delaying keratoplasties or uptitrating topical steroid administration after a routine keratoplasty, following primary COVID vaccine or booster administration. In high-risk cases, increasing immunosuppressants in the peri-vaccination period may decrease the risk of immune reactions [9].

Studies suggest a link between COVID-19 vaccines and the reactivation of the varicella-zoster virus (VZV), resulting in vaccine-acquired immunodeficiency syndrome. Data from the works of Barda, N., Desai, H.D. and Seneff, S. [61–63] have shown that the population prevalence rates of post-vaccination ophthalmic HSV were $\leq$0.05 cases per million doses and for HZO were $\leq$0.5 cases per million doses. According to Wang, M.T.M. [64], there is no conclusive evidence to suggest the need for prophylactic antiviral treatment for patients with prior herpetic eye disease considering COVID-19 vaccination.

Regarding vaccine-associated uveitis (VAU), a recent VAERS review by Singh R B et al. reported a total of 1094 cases from 40 countries with an estimated crude reporting rate (per million doses) of 0.57, 0.44, and 0.35 for BNT162b2, mRNA-1273, and Ad26.COV2.S, respectively. More than two-thirds of cases were reported in patients who received BNT162b2. Additionally, the post hoc analysis showed a significantly shorter interval of onset for the first dose compared with the second dose and BNT162b2 compared with the mRNA 1273 vaccine. According to [65], other vaccines that have also triggered uveitis flare-ups include hepatitis A and B, influenza, Bacillus Calmette–Guérin, human papillomavirus, measles–mumps–rubella (MMR), and varicella zoster vaccines. According to Wang [64], De novo VKH cases can be the result of molecular mimicry between vaccine peptide fragments and uveal self-peptides, whereas, for cases with VKH reactivation, specific HLA haplotypes may account for the individual susceptibility of the autoimmune activation. Many patients who developed ocular adverse effects lacked medical comorbidities that may have predisposed them to the adverse effects, although a few patients were on hormone-based birth control [49,66].

Although clinical trials for all vaccines undergo rigorous safety monitoring prior to authorization for human use, some serious adverse events may not be identified in trials, especially if uncommon, because of the relatively small sample size, the selection of trial participants who may not represent the general population, restrictive eligibility criteria, and limited duration follow-up [67].

The data regarding ocular adverse effects with other approved vaccines, such as ZyCoV-D, Sputnik, Covidecia, Sputnik, Abdala, Zifivax, and Novavax are sparse. Despite the mandatory requirement by all nations to report any vaccine-associated adverse events, unreliable reporting, under-reporting, and/or delayed reporting are common. Additionally, the possibility of anti-vaccination fringe groups attempting to malign vaccines using VAERS data by adding misinformation about the safety of COVID-19 vaccinations must also be remembered.

To conclude, the scientific evidence regarding the ocular adverse effects does not outweigh the benefits of COVID immunization in patients with pre-existing systemic or ophthalmic conditions. However, patients must be counseled to seek prompt medical review for symptoms of post-vaccination deterioration of vision or primary ocular disease relapse.

Author Contributions: Conceptualization, P.I. and U.P.S.P.; methodology, S.D.; formal analysis, P.I., S.D. and U.P.S.P.; data curation, P.I., S.D. and U.P.S.P.; writing—original draft preparation, P.I., S.K. and U.P.S.P.; writing—review and editing, P.I. and S.K.; supervision, P.I.; project administration, U.P.S.P. and P.I. All authors have read and agreed to the published version of the manuscript.

Funding: This research received no external funding.

Institutional Review Board Statement: Because the study includes publicly available deidentified anonymous data from, the Institute Research Ethics Committee exempted it from ethical review.

Informed Consent Statement: Not applicable.

Data Availability Statement: Not applicable.

Conflicts of Interest: The authors declare no conflict of interest.

References

1. Marian, A.J. Current State of Vaccine Development and Targeted Therapies for COVID-19: Impact of Basic Science Discoveries. *Cardiovasc. Pathol.* **2020**, *50*, 107278. [CrossRef] [PubMed]
2. WHO Coronavirus (COVID-19) Dashboard | WHO Coronavirus (COVID-19) Dashboard with Vaccination Data. Available online: https://covid19.who.int/ (accessed on 24 September 2022).
3. Forchette, L.; Sebastian, W.; Liu, T. A Comprehensive Review of COVID-19 Virology, Vaccines, Variants, and Therapeutics. *Curr. Med. Sci.* **2021**, *41*, 1037–1051. [CrossRef] [PubMed]
4. Le Ng, X.; Betzler, B.K.; Testi, I.; Ho, S.L.; Tien, M.; Ngo, W.K.; Zierhut, M.; Chee, S.P.; Gupta, V.; Pavesio, C.E.; et al. Ocular Adverse Events After COVID-19 Vaccination. *Ocul. Immunol. Inflamm.* **2021**, *29*, 1216–1224. [CrossRef]
5. Eleiwa, T.K.; Gaier, E.D.; Haseeb, A.; ElSheikh, R.H.; Sallam, A.B.; Elhusseiny, A.M. Adverse Ocular Events Following COVID-19 Vaccination. *Inflamm. Res.* **2021**, *70*, 1005–1009. [CrossRef]
6. Phylactou, M.; Li, J.-P.O.; Larkin, D.F.P. Characteristics of Endothelial Corneal Transplant Rejection Following Immunisation with SARS-CoV-2 Messenger RNA Vaccine. *Br. J. Ophthalmol.* **2021**, *105*, 893–896. [CrossRef] [PubMed]
7. Crnej, A.; Khoueir, Z.; Cherfan, G.; Saad, A. Acute Corneal Endothelial Graft Rejection Following COVID-19 Vaccination. *J. Fr. Ophtalmol.* **2021**, *44*, e445–e447. [CrossRef] [PubMed]
8. Forshaw, T.R.J.; Jørgensen, C.; Kyhn, M.C.; Cabrerizo, J. Acute Bilateral Descemet Membrane Endothelial Keratoplasty Graft Rejection After the BNT162b2 MRNA COVID-19 Vaccine. *Int. Med. Case Rep. J.* **2022**, *15*, 201–204. [CrossRef]
9. Fujio, K.; Sung, J.; Nakatani, S.; Yamamoto, K.; Iwagami, M.; Fujimoto, K.; Shokirova, H.; Okumura, Y.; Akasaki, Y.; Nagino, K.; et al. Characteristics and Clinical Ocular Manifestations in Patients with Acute Corneal Graft Rejection after Receiving the COVID-19 Vaccine: A Systematic Review. *J. Clin. Med.* **2022**, *11*, 4500. [CrossRef]
10. Molero-Senosiain, M.; Houben, I.; Savant, S.; Savant, V. Five Cases of Corneal Graft Rejection After Recent COVID-19 Vaccinations and a Review of the Literature. *Cornea* **2022**, *41*, 669–672. [CrossRef]
11. Abousy, M.; Bohm, K.; Prescott, C.; Bonsack, J.M.; Rowhani-Farid, A.; Eghrari, A.O. Bilateral EK Rejection After COVID-19 Vaccine. *Eye Contact Lens* **2021**, *47*, 625–628. [CrossRef]
12. Simão, M.F.; Kwitko, S. Corneal Graft Rejection After Inactivated SARS-CoV-2 Vaccine: Case Report. *Cornea* **2022**, *41*, 502–504. [CrossRef] [PubMed]
13. Nahata, H.; Nagaraja, H.; Shetty, R. A Case of Acute Endothelial Corneal Transplant Rejection Following Immunization with ChAdOx1 NCoV-19 Coronavirus Vaccine. *Indian J. Ophthalmol.* **2022**, *70*, 1817–1818. [CrossRef] [PubMed]
14. Shah, A.P.; Dzhaber, D.; Kenyon, K.R.; Riaz, K.M.; Ouano, D.P.; Koo, E.H. Acute Corneal Transplant Rejection After COVID-19 Vaccination. *Cornea* **2022**, *41*, 121–124. [CrossRef]
15. Eid, E.; Abdullah, L.; Kurban, M.; Abbas, O. Herpes Zoster Emergence Following MRNA COVID-19 Vaccine. *J. Med. Virol.* **2021**, *93*, 5231–5232. [CrossRef] [PubMed]
16. van Dam, C.S.; Lede, I.; Schaar, J.; Al-Dulaimy, M.; Rösken, R.; Smits, M. Herpes Zoster after COVID Vaccination. *Int. J. Infect. Dis.* **2021**, *111*, 169–171. [CrossRef]
17. Arora, P.; Sardana, K.; Mathachan, S.R.; Malhotra, P. Herpes Zoster after Inactivated COVID-19 Vaccine: A Cutaneous Adverse Effect of the Vaccine. *J. Cosmet. Dermatol.* **2021**, *20*, 3389–3390. [CrossRef]
18. Lee, C.; Cotter, D.; Basa, J.; Greenberg, H.L. 20 Post-COVID-19 Vaccine-Related Shingles Cases Seen at the Las Vegas Dermatology Clinic and Sent to Us via Social Media. *J. Cosmet. Dermatol.* **2021**, *20*, 1960–1964. [CrossRef]
19. Rodríguez-Jiménez, P.; Chicharro, P.; Cabrera, L.-M.; Seguí, M.; Morales-Caballero, Á.; Llamas-Velasco, M.; Sánchez-Pérez, J. Varicella-Zoster Virus Reactivation after SARS-CoV-2 BNT162b2 MRNA Vaccination: Report of 5 Cases. *JAAD Case Rep.* **2021**, *12*, 58–59. [CrossRef]

20. Bostan, E.; Yalici-Armagan, B. Herpes Zoster Following Inactivated COVID-19 Vaccine: A Coexistence or Coincidence? *J. Cosmet. Dermatol.* **2021**, *20*, 1566–1567. [CrossRef]
21. Aksu, S.B.; Öztürk, G.Z. A Rare Case of Shingles after COVID-19 Vaccine: Is It a Possible Adverse Effect? *Clin. Exp. Vaccine Res.* **2021**, *10*, 198–201. [CrossRef]
22. Psichogiou, M.; Samarkos, M.; Mikos, N.; Hatzakis, A. Reactivation of Varicella Zoster Virus after Vaccination for SARS-CoV-2. *Vaccines* **2021**, *9*, 572. [CrossRef] [PubMed]
23. Richardson-May, J.; Rothwell, A.; Rashid, M. Reactivation of Herpes Simplex Keratitis Following Vaccination for COVID-19. *BMJ Case Rep.* **2021**, *14*, e245792. [CrossRef] [PubMed]
24. Rallis, K.I.; Fausto, R.; Ting, D.S.J.; Al-Aqaba, M.A.; Said, D.G.; Dua, H.S. Manifestation of Herpetic Eye Disease after COVID-19 Vaccine: A UK Case Series. *Ocul. Immunol. Inflamm.* **2022**, *30*, 1–6. [CrossRef] [PubMed]
25. Fard, A.M.; Desilets, J.; Patel, S. Recurrence of Herpetic Keratitis after COVID-19 Vaccination: A Report of Two Cases. *Case Rep. Ophthalmol. Med.* **2022**, *2022*, 7094893. [CrossRef]
26. Alkwikbi, H.; Alenazi, M.; Alanazi, W.; Alruwaili, S. Herpetic Keratitis and Corneal Endothelitis Following COVID-19 Vaccination: A Case Series. *Cureus* **2022**, *14*, e20967. [CrossRef]
27. Alkhalifah, M.I.; Alsobki, H.E.; Alwael, H.M.; al Fawaz, A.M.; Al-Mezaine, H.S. Herpes Simplex Virus Keratitis Reactivation after SARS-CoV-2 BNT162b2 MRNA Vaccination: A Report of Two Cases. *Ocul. Immunol. Inflamm.* **2021**, *29*, 1238–1240. [CrossRef]
28. You, I.-C.; Ahn, M.; Cho, N.-C. A Case Report of Herpes Zoster Ophthalmicus and Meningitis After COVID-19 Vaccination. *J. Korean Med. Sci.* **2022**, *37*, e165. [CrossRef]
29. Al-Dwairi, R.A.; Aleshawi, A.; Adi, S.; Abu-Zreig, L. Reactivation of Herpes Simplex Keratitis on a Corneal Graft Following SARS-CoV-2 MRNA Vaccination. *Med. Arch.* **2022**, *76*, 146–148. [CrossRef]
30. Murgova, S.; Balchev, G. Ophthalmic Manifestation after SARS-CoV-2 Vaccination: A Case Series. *J. Ophthalmic Inflamm. Infect.* **2022**, *12*, 20. [CrossRef]
31. Ryu, K.J.; Kim, D.H. Recurrence of Varicella-Zoster Virus Keratitis After SARS-CoV-2 Vaccination. *Cornea* **2022**, *41*, 649–650. [CrossRef]
32. Song, M.Y.; Koh, K.M.; Hwang, K.Y.; Kwon, Y.A.; Kim, K.Y. Relapsed Disciform Stromal Herpetic Keratitis Following MRNA COVID-19 Vaccination: A Case Report. *Korean J. Ophthalmol.* **2022**, *36*, 80–82. [CrossRef] [PubMed]
33. Bolletta, E.; Iannetta, D.; Mastrofilippo, V.; de Simone, L.; Gozzi, F.; Croci, S.; Bonacini, M.; Belloni, L.; Zerbini, A.; Adani, C.; et al. Uveitis and Other Ocular Complications Following COVID-19 Vaccination. *J. Clin. Med.* **2021**, *10*, 5960. [CrossRef] [PubMed]
34. Renisi, G.; Lombardi, A.; Stanzione, M.; Invernizzi, A.; Bandera, A.; Gori, A. Anterior Uveitis Onset after Bnt162b2 Vaccination: Is This Just a Coincidence? *Int. J. Infect. Dis.* **2021**, *110*, 95–97. [CrossRef] [PubMed]
35. ElSheikh, R.H.; Haseeb, A.; Eleiwa, T.K.; Elhusseiny, A.M. Acute Uveitis Following COVID-19 Vaccination. *Ocul. Immunol. Inflamm.* **2021**, *29*, 1207–1209. [CrossRef]
36. Al-Allaf, A.-W.; Razok, A.; Al-Allaf, Y.; Aker, L. Post-COVID-19 Vaccine Medium-Vessel Vasculitis and Acute Anterior Uveitis, Causation vs. Temporal Relation; Case Report and Literature Review. *Ann. Med. Surg.* **2022**, *75*, 103407. [CrossRef]
37. Duran, M. Bilateral Anterior Uveitis after BNT162b2 MRNA Vaccine: Case Report. *J. Fr. Ophtalmol.* **2022**, *45*, e311–e313. [CrossRef]
38. Alhamazani, M.A.; Alruwaili, W.S.; Alshammri, B.; Alrashidi, S.; Almasaud, J. A Case of Recurrent Acute Anterior Uveitis After the Administration of COVID-19 Vaccine. *Cureus* **2022**, *14*, e22911. [CrossRef]
39. Ortiz-Egea, J.M.; Sánchez, C.G.; López-Jiménez, A.; Navarro, O.D. Herpetic Anterior Uveitis Following Pfizer-BioNTech Coronavirus Disease 2019 Vaccine: Two Case Reports. *J. Med. Case Rep.* **2022**, *16*, 127. [CrossRef]
40. Hwang, J.H. Uveitis after COVID-19 Vaccination. *Case Rep. Ophthalmol.* **2022**, *13*, 124–127. [CrossRef]
41. Choi, M.; Seo, M.-H.; Choi, K.-E.; Lee, S.; Choi, B.; Yun, C.; Kim, S.-W.; Kim, Y.Y. Vision-Threatening Ocular Adverse Events after Vaccination against Coronavirus Disease 2019. *J. Clin. Med.* **2022**, *11*, 3318. [CrossRef]
42. Hernanz, I.; Arconada, C.; López Corral, A.; Sánchez-Pernaute, O.; Carreño, E. Recurrent Anterior Non-Necrotizing Scleritis as an Adverse Event of ChAdOx1 NCoV-19 (Vaxzevria) Vaccine. *Ocul. Immunol. Inflamm.* **2022**, *30*, 1–3. [CrossRef] [PubMed]
43. Pichi, F.; Aljneibi, S.; Neri, P.; Hay, S.; Dackiw, C.; Ghazi, N.G. Association of Ocular Adverse Events With Inactivated COVID-19 Vaccination in Patients in Abu Dhabi. *JAMA Ophthalmol.* **2021**, *139*, 1131. [CrossRef] [PubMed]
44. Austria, Q.M.; Lelli, G.J.; Segal, K.L.; Godfrey, K.J. Transient Eyelid Edema Following COVID-19 Vaccination. *Ophthalmic Plast. Reconstr. Surg.* **2021**, *37*, 501–502. [CrossRef] [PubMed]
45. Mazzatenta, C.; Piccolo, V.; Pace, G.; Romano, I.; Argenziano, G.; Bassi, A. Purpuric Lesions on the Eyelids Developed after BNT162b2 MRNA COVID-19 Vaccine: Another Piece of SARS-CoV-2 Skin Puzzle? *J. Eur. Acad. Dermatol. Venereol.* **2021**, *35*, e543–e545. [CrossRef]
46. Colella, G.; Orlandi, M.; Cirillo, N. Bell's Palsy Following COVID-19 Vaccination. *J. Neurol.* **2021**, *268*, 3589–3591. [CrossRef]
47. Book, B.A.J.; Schmidt, B.; Foerster, A.M.H. Bilateral Acute Macular Neuroretinopathy After Vaccination Against SARS-CoV-2. *JAMA Ophthalmol.* **2021**, *139*, e212471. [CrossRef]
48. Mambretti, M.; Huemer, J.; Torregrossa, G.; Ullrich, M.; Findl, O.; Casalino, G. Acute Macular Neuroretinopathy Following Coronavirus Disease 2019 Vaccination. *Ocul. Immunol. Inflamm.* **2021**, *29*, 730–733. [CrossRef]
49. Vinzamuri, S.; Pradeep, T.G.; Kotian, R. Bilateral Paracentral Acute Middle Maculopathy and Acute Macular Neuroretinopathy Following COVID-19 Vaccination. *Indian J. Ophthalmol.* **2021**, *69*, 2862–2864. [CrossRef]

50. Goyal, M.; Murthy, S.I.; Annum, S. Bilateral Multifocal Choroiditis Following COVID-19 Vaccination. *Ocul. Immunol. Inflamm.* **2021**, *29*, 753–757. [CrossRef]
51. Mudie, L.I.; Zick, J.D.; Dacey, M.S.; Palestine, A.G. Panuveitis Following Vaccination for COVID-19. *Ocul. Immunol. Inflamm.* **2021**, *29*, 741–742. [CrossRef]
52. Fowler, N.; Mendez Martinez, N.R.; Pallares, B.V.; Maldonado, R.S. Acute-Onset Central Serous Retinopathy after Immunization with COVID-19 MRNA Vaccine. *Am. J. Ophthalmol. Case Rep.* **2021**, *23*, 101136. [CrossRef] [PubMed]
53. Maleki, A.; Look-Why, S.; Manhapra, A.; Foster, C.S. COVID-19 Recombinant MRNA Vaccines and Serious Ocular Inflammatory Side Effects: Real or Coincidence? *J. Ophthalmic Vis. Res.* **2021**, *16*, 490–501. [CrossRef] [PubMed]
54. Testi, I.; Brandão-de-Resende, C.; Agrawal, R.; Pavesio, C. COVID-19 Vaccination Ocular Inflammatory Events Study Group Ocular Inflammatory Events Following COVID-19 Vaccination: A Multinational Case Series. *J. Ophthalmic Inflamm. Infect.* **2022**, *12*, 4. [CrossRef] [PubMed]
55. Li, Y.-D.; Chi, W.-Y.; Su, J.-H.; Ferrall, L.; Hung, C.-F.; Wu, T.-C. Coronavirus Vaccine Development: From SARS and MERS to COVID-19. *J. Biomed. Sci.* **2020**, *27*, 104. [CrossRef] [PubMed]
56. Nyankerh, C.N.A.; Boateng, A.K.; Appah, M. Ocular Complications after COVID-19 Vaccination, Vaccine Adverse Event Reporting System. *Vaccines* **2022**, *10*, 941. [CrossRef] [PubMed]
57. Nordström, P.; Ballin, M.; Nordström, A. Risk of Infection, Hospitalisation, and Death up to 9 Months after a Second Dose of COVID-19 Vaccine: A Retrospective, Total Population Cohort Study in Sweden. *Lancet* **2022**, *399*, 814–823. [CrossRef]
58. Lee, E.-J.; Cines, D.B.; Gernsheimer, T.; Kessler, C.; Michel, M.; Tarantino, M.D.; Semple, J.W.; Arnold, D.M.; Godeau, B.; Lambert, M.P.; et al. Thrombocytopenia Following Pfizer and Moderna SARS-CoV-2 Vaccination. *Am. J. Hematol.* **2021**, *96*, 534–537. [CrossRef]
59. Steinemann, T.L.; Koffler, B.H.; Jennings, C.D. Corneal Allograft Rejection Following Immunization. *Am. J. Ophthalmol.* **1988**, *106*, 575–578. [CrossRef]
60. Wertheim, M.S.; Keel, M.; Cook, S.D.; Tole, D.M. Corneal Transplant Rejection Following Influenza Vaccination. *Br. J. Ophthalmol.* **2006**, *90*, 925. [CrossRef]
61. Barda, N.; Dagan, N.; Ben-Shlomo, Y.; Kepten, E.; Waxman, J.; Ohana, R.; Hernán, M.A.; Lipsitch, M.; Kohane, I.; Netzer, D.; et al. Safety of the BNT162b2 MRNA COVID-19 Vaccine in a Nationwide Setting. *N. Engl. J. Med.* **2021**, *385*, 1078–1090. [CrossRef]
62. Desai, H.D.; Sharma, K.; Shah, A.; Patoliya, J.; Patil, A.; Hooshanginezhad, Z.; Grabbe, S.; Goldust, M. Can SARS-CoV-2 Vaccine Increase the Risk of Reactivation of Varicella Zoster? A Systematic Review. *J. Cosmet. Dermatol.* **2021**, *20*, 3350–3361. [CrossRef] [PubMed]
63. Seneff, S.; Nigh, G.; Kyriakopoulos, A.M.; McCullough, P.A. Innate Immune Suppression by SARS-CoV-2 MRNA Vaccinations: The Role of G-Quadruplexes, Exosomes, and MicroRNAs. *Food Chem. Toxicol.* **2022**, *164*, 113008. [CrossRef] [PubMed]
64. Wang, M.T.M.; Niederer, R.L.; McGhee, C.N.J.; Danesh-Meyer, H.V. COVID-19 Vaccination and The Eye. *Am. J. Ophthalmol.* **2022**, *240*, 79–98. [CrossRef] [PubMed]
65. Singh, R.B.; Singh Parmar, U.P.; Kahale, F.; Agarwal, A.; Tsui, E. Vaccine-Associated Uveitis Following SARS-CoV-2 Vaccination: A CDC-VAERS Database Analysis. *Ophthalmology* **2022**. [CrossRef] [PubMed]
66. Valenzuela, D.A.; Groth, S.; Taubenslag, K.J.; Gangaputra, S. Acute Macular Neuroretinopathy Following Pfizer-BioNTech COVID-19 Vaccination. *Am. J. Ophthalmol. Case Rep.* **2021**, *24*, 101200. [CrossRef] [PubMed]
67. Haseeb, A.A.; Solyman, O.; Abushanab, M.M.; Abo Obaia, A.S.; Elhusseiny, A.M. Ocular Complications Following Vaccination for COVID-19: A One-Year Retrospective. *Vaccines* **2022**, *10*, 342. [CrossRef]

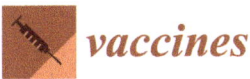

Case Report

Recurrent Multiple Evanescent White Dot Syndrome (MEWDS) Following First Dose and Booster of the mRNA-1273 COVID-19 Vaccine: Case Report and Review of Literature

Matias Soifer [1], Nam V. Nguyen [1,2], Ryan Leite [1,3], Josh Fernandes [4] and Shilpa Kodati [1,*]

[1] National Eye Institute, National Institutes of Health, Bethesda, MD 20892, USA
[2] College of Medicine, University of Nebraska Medical Center, Omaha, NE 68198, USA
[3] School of Medicine, Georgetown University, Washington, DC 20007, USA
[4] DC Retina, Silver Spring, MD 20902, USA
* Correspondence: shilpa.kodati@nih.gov; Tel.: +301-435-5139; Fax: +301-480-1122

Abstract: Abstract: Purpose To report a rare case of a patient with two recurrent episodes of Multiple Evanescent White Dot Syndrome (MEWDS) associated with the second dose and second booster of the mRNA-1273 COVID-19 vaccine (Moderna), and to perform a literature review on COVID-19-vaccine-associated MEWDS. **Case Report:** A 31-year-old female was evaluated for a temporal scotoma and photopsias that started two weeks after the second dose of the Moderna COVID-19 vaccine. Dilated fundus findings were remarkable for unilateral, small whitish-yellow dots scattered around posterior pole of the left eye, consistent with a diagnosis of MEWDS. The symptoms resolved three months later without treatment. Approximately one year after the first vaccine, the patient received the second Moderna COVID-19 vaccine booster and experienced a recurrence of symptoms with an enlarged scotoma and similar examination findings. The patient was treated with a course of systemic corticosteroids with subsequent clinical improvement. **Conclusion:** Although uveitis following COVID-19 vaccines is rare, our case highlights a need for increased awareness amongst practitioners regarding COVID-19-vaccine-associated onset or recurrence of ocular inflammatory diseases.

Keywords: white dot syndromes; MEWDS; COVID-19 vaccine; mRNA vaccine

Citation: Soifer, M.; Nguyen, N.V.; Leite, R.; Fernandes, J.; Kodati, S. Recurrent Multiple Evanescent White Dot Syndrome (MEWDS) Following First Dose and Booster of the mRNA-1273 COVID-19 Vaccine: Case Report and Review of Literature. *Vaccines* 2022, 10, 1776. https://doi.org/10.3390/vaccines10111776

Academic Editor: Antonella Caputo

Received: 14 August 2022
Accepted: 19 October 2022
Published: 22 October 2022

Publisher's Note: MDPI stays neutral with regard to jurisdictional claims in published maps and institutional affiliations.

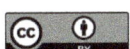

Copyright: © 2022 by the authors. Licensee MDPI, Basel, Switzerland. This article is an open access article distributed under the terms and conditions of the Creative Commons Attribution (CC BY) license (https://creativecommons.org/licenses/by/4.0/).

1. Introduction

The white dot syndromes (WDS) refer to a group of ocular diseases that characteristically involve the outer retina and/or choroid and present with white-yellow lesions of varying morphologies on fundus examination. Amongst them, multiple evanescent white dot syndrome (MEWDS) has distinctive features, characterized by small spots at the level of the outer retina or RPE and is more commonly unilateral. This disease is usually self-limiting and occurs largely in healthy young adult females [1,2].

Although the pathogenesis of MEWDS remains poorly understood, different theories implicate a genetic and autoimmune predisposition contributing to the development of this disease. Interestingly, its onset has been associated with different viral vaccines including hepatitis A and B, human papillomavirus, influenza, measles-mumps-rubella, varicella virus, yellow fever, and most recently COVID-19 vaccines [3].

The Food and Drug Administration (FDA) authorized the messenger RNA (mRNA) vaccines from Moderna and Pfizer-BioNTech for SARS-CoV-2 virus (COVID-19) disease for emergency use in December 2020 [3]. Since then, other vaccines with different compositions have been widely utilized around the world, and the efforts have reduced the morbidity and mortality effectively caused by the COVID-19 virus [4,5]. There have been approximately 600 million COVID-19 infections with 6.5 million associated deaths to date worldwide. The number of vaccinations has now exceeded 12.5 billion, and the incidences of infections and death have decreased significantly since January 2022 [6]. The positive global effect that these vaccines have had is unquestionable. Nevertheless, reports of very rare side effects including ophthalmic findings have been noted with their use [3,7].

Herein, we report a case of recurrent MEWDS associated with the mRNA-1273 COVID-19 vaccine. Furthermore, we performed a literature review on COVID-19-vaccine-associated cases of MEWDS reported until 20 July 2022, using PubMed and Google scholar search engines for terms "multiple evanescent white dot syndrome, MEWDS, uveitis, and COVID-19 vaccine".

2. Case Report

A 31-year-old white female was evaluated for a new onset temporal scotoma and photopsias, 14 days after the second dose of the mRNA-1273 COVID-19 vaccine (Moderna). She was seen by an outside ophthalmologist, and her fundus examination was remarkable for multifocal, outer retinal dots scattered around the posterior pole in the left eye consistent with a diagnosis of MEWDS. The patient was observed without any intervention, and her symptoms resolved within 3 months. Approximately 12 months after the second dose, the patient received the second booster dose and experienced a recurrence of symptoms, which prompted referral to our clinic.

On our evaluation, the patient reported an enlarged scotoma in her left eye with increased photopsias. Past medical history was unremarkable, except for a remote episode of Lyme disease, which was successfully treated with doxycycline. Past ocular history was significant for myopia, and she was status-post myopic LASIK surgery in both eyes in 2019. On examination, best-corrected visual acuity (BCVA) was 20/16 on the right eye (OD) and 20/50 on the left eye (OS), and intraocular pressure (IOP) was 13 mm Hg in both eyes (OU). Slit-lamp examination revealed a quiet anterior chamber in both eyes and trace pigmented anterior vitreous cells in the left eye. On dilated fundus examination, a few scattered faint hypopigmented round dots of differing sizes, especially nasal to the optic nerve (Figure 1B) were noted. Optical Coherence Tomography (OCT) of the left eye revealed multifocal areas of ellipsoid zone (EZ) loss with associated areas of outer retinal hyperreflectivity (Figure 2A–C). Fundus autofluorescence (FAF) of the left eye revealed a confluent area of hyperautofluorescence in the posterior pole with scattered hyperautofluorescent dots (Figure 3B). Fluorescein angiography (FA) of the left eye demonstrated hyperfluorescent staining of the corresponding areas. Late-phase indocyanine green (ICG) imaging showed diffuse hypocyanescent spots in the posterior pole (Figure 1D). The clinical examination and imaging studies of the right eye were unremarkable. A uveitic laboratory work-up was performed, which was unrevealing for QuantiFERON, syphilis IgG antibody and angiotensin converting enzyme. The clinical presentation, examination, and imaging findings were thought to be consistent with MEWDS. After a discussion with the patient, a course of 60 mg of oral prednisone tapered over 8 weeks was started. The patient returned for follow-up two weeks later with improvement in symptoms and BCVA OS had improved to 20/25 OS. Four-weeks after the initiation of prednisone, BCVA OS remained stable at 20/25. OCT revealed reconstitution of the EZ and a decrease in outer retinal hyperreflectivity (Figure 2C,D), and FAF demonstrated a reduction in hyperautofluoresence (Figure 3D).

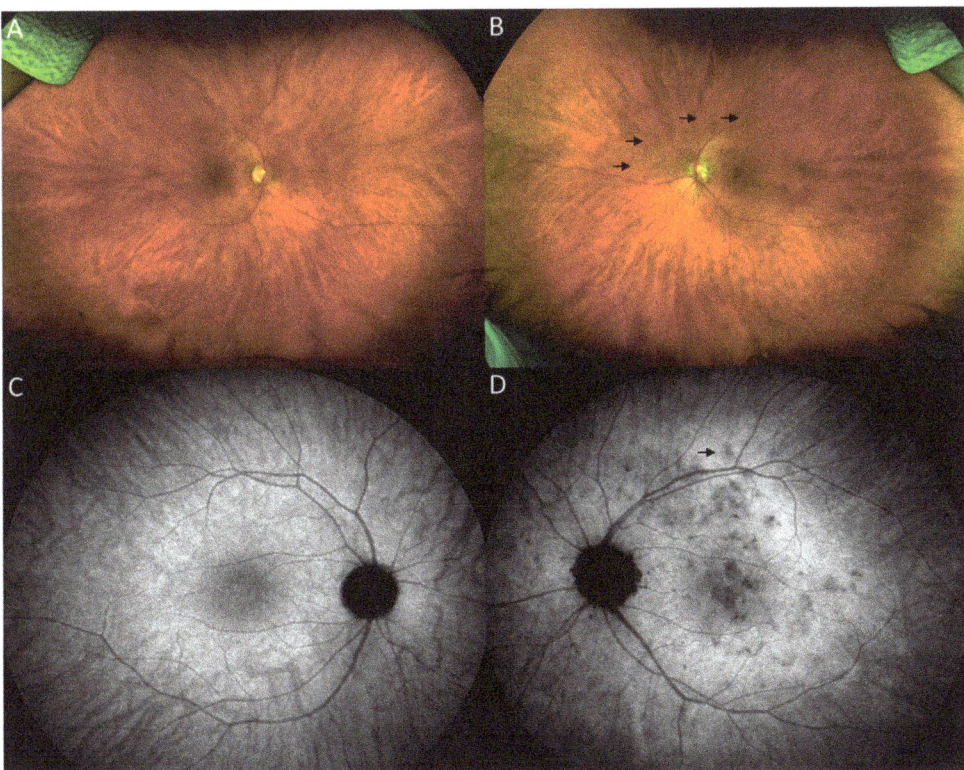

Figure 1. Optos ultrawide-field fundus images of the right eye showing normal fundus (**A**). The left eye demonstrates a mottled appearance of the macula and areas of multiple scattered hypopigmented spots in the posterior pole (dark arrows) (**B**). Late-phase indocyanine green angiography (ICG) of the left eye shows multiple spots of hypocyanescence in the posterior pole, some of which correspond to the spots on color fundus photos (**D**). Late-phase ICG of the right eye (**C**) was unremarkable.

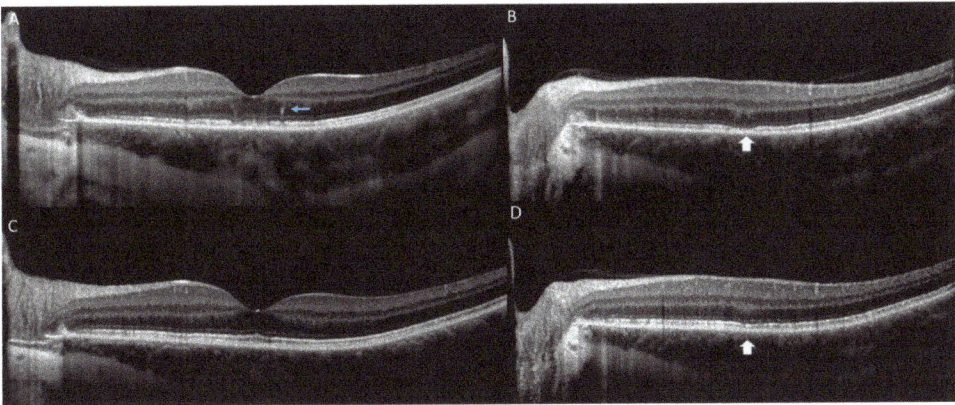

Figure 2. Optical coherence tomography (OCT) of the left eye at the initial presentation is notable for presence of hyperreflective dots in outer retina (blue arrow) and multifocal loss of the ellipsoid zone (EZ) (white arrow) (**A**,**B**). At 1 month follow up, reconstitution of the EZ (white arrow) is observed and improvement in outer retinal hyperreflectivity (**C**,**D**).

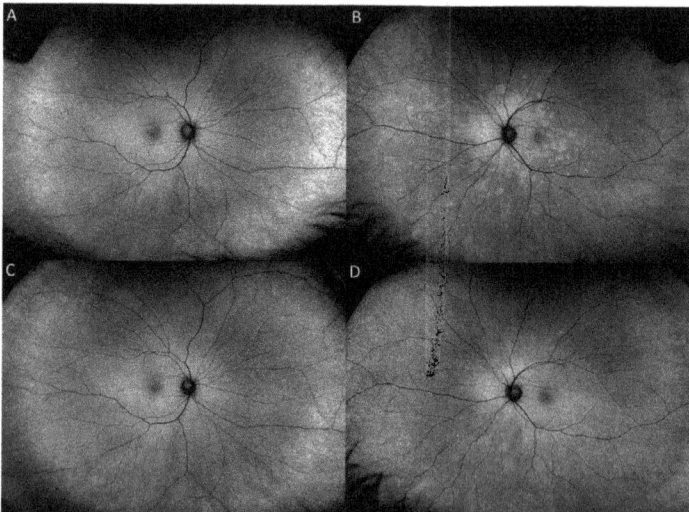

Figure 3. Fundus autofluorescence (FAF) at presentation of the left eye at presentation demonstrates a confluent area of hyperautofluorescence surrounding the optic nerve and posterior pole with hyperautofluorescent dots extending to the temporal macula and mid nasal periphery (**B**) FAF at 1 month follow-up demonstrates decreased hyperautofluoresence and ill-defined borders. (**D**). FAF of the right eye at presentation and final visit are unremarkable (**A**,**C**).

3. Discussion

We report a de novo case of MEWDS following the second dose of COVID-19 mRNA-vaccination and a subsequent recurrence after the second booster. To the best of our knowledge, this is the second case of COVID-19-vaccine-associated MEWDS which developed a recurrent course, with both episodes temporally associated with vaccine doses. Recurrences are uncommonly reported in MEWDS. A large retrospective cohort of 111 patients with MEWDS, observed recurrent disease in only 14% of cases [8] Although our patient had improved symptoms after the initiation of corticosteroids, the efficacy of treatment with systemic corticosteroids for MEWDS remains unclear. In a study of 51 patients with MEWDS, those who received systemic prednisone did not achieve a better final BCVA than those who did not; however, lower baseline BCVA at presentation and younger age were predictive of worse outcomes [9]. Although the use of corticosteroids with this subpopulation is reasonable, further studies are needed to determine the efficacy of corticosteroids in MEWDS.

The association between COVID-19 vaccines and MEWDS is yet to be elucidated. The causality assessment of an adverse event following immunization (AEFI) provides criteria to assess causality between a vaccine and an adverse event [10]. In our case, factors supporting a causal association are that this presentation occurred in an otherwise healthy patient, without a previous history of uveitis, and was temporally associated, as the doses of the vaccine preceded the onset of disease within the "plausible" time window on both occasions. Notably, the patient denied a viral prodrome, which is commonly associated with MEWDS. Finally, MEWDS has been reported in association with different vaccines [11], as well as more recently, COVID-19 immunizations (Table 1).

To date, 13 cases of COVID-19-vaccine-associated MEWDS have been reported to date in the literature (Table 1). The average patient age was 39.5 years (ranging from 15 to 71 years old) with a female predominance (9:4), and the only reported races (5/13) were Asian (3) or White (2). Notably, these demographics and clinical features are similar to non-vaccine related MEWDS [2]. The most common vaccine manufacturer was Pfizer-BioNTech (9/13) followed by CoronaVac (2/13), Medigen (1/13), and Moderna (1/13). Of note, approximately 360 million Pfizer doses have been administered worldwide compared to Moderna's 229 million [12], which may bias the data towards a greater association between the Pfizer vaccine and MEWDS than with the Moderna vaccine or others. From our review, six cases developed symptoms after the first dose, seven patients after the second dose, and one after the first booster. Interestingly, the large majority of cases (12/13) had their first onset of MEWDS following the vaccine. One case had a previous episode of MEWDS nine years prior and experienced recurrence with the vaccine [13]. Of note, one case developed a new episode following the first dose, then a recurrence of MEWDS in the same eye following the second vaccine [13]. Nine patients received no treatment, and four patients received a short course of systemic corticosteroids. Nearly all patients had complete resolution of visual symptoms, with majority having 20/20 as their final visual acuity [13].

These findings are highly comparable with those of other reported vaccine-associated MEWDS presentations. Ng et al. reviewed eight cases of vaccine-associated MEWDS, which included immunizations against rabies, HPV, hepatitis A and B, meningococcal, yellow fever, and influenza [11]. Patients had an average age of 31.7 years (ranging from 16 to 53) with female predominance (2:1), and the disclosed racial data indicated that only White (44.4%) and Asian (22.2%) races were affected; however, this association should not be restricted to these ethnic populations. Overall, patients had significant visual recovery, although one reported a gradual loss of peripheral vision for 2 years following MEWDS [11]. Altogether, MEWDS associated with the COVID-19 vaccines and others, typically occurs in young to middle age healthy females, has a good prognosis and mostly monophasic course of disease.

The Pfizer BNT and Moderna COVID-19 vaccines are both mRNA vaccines and received their authorizations almost simultaneously in December 2020 (FDA and UK). This vaccine encapsulates the mRNA in lipid nanoparticles (LNP) that encode for the S protein of SARS-CoV-2 [14]. Unlike most vaccines, the mRNA molecules function as both the antigen and the adjuvant; thus, it can avoid the need for added molecules that may induce toxicity. Although the exact mechanisms by which the mRNA COVID-19 vaccines cause uveitis is still unclear, it has been proposed that these vaccines can activate type I interferon (IFN) proinflammatory cascades which can stimulate autoimmunity in predisposed individuals [15,16]. The inoculated mRNA may activate intracellular RNA-sensors, namely endosomal Toll-like receptors, with a subsequent increase in IFN production which may stimulate autoimmunity [17]. However, although we are reporting an association of MEWDS with the mRNA COVID-19 Moderna vaccine, the underlying pathogenesis is likely due to a shared etiological mechanism across different vaccines, given the reports of MEWDS following COVID-19 non-mRNA vaccines as well as non-COVID-19 vaccines. Many theories have been proposed to explain this phenomenon which include molecular mimicry [18], hypersensitivity reactions [19], and autoimmunity induced by adjuvants (ASIA) [20]. Future work is needed to better understand the multifactorial risk factors including genetic and environmental associations that predispose certain individuals to the development of MEWDS.

COVID-19 vaccines have been associated with multiple ocular inflammatory diseases including anterior uveitis [21], acute macular neuroretinopathy, bilateral acute zonal occult outer retinopathy (AZOOR) [15], Vogt–Koyanagi–Harada [22], optic neuropathies [23] and corneal graft rejection [24,25]. It is important to note that the uveitis following COVID-19 vaccine have a good prognosis as shown by multinational case series of 70 patients with onset of ocular inflammatory diseases associated with different COVID-19 vaccines [3]. In this series, the majority of patients presented with anterior uveitis (58.6%), followed by posterior uveitis and scleritis. Most of these were not severe and their course was notable for unchanged final visual acuity in 93% of cases. The majority were either observed without treatment or received topical corticosteroids (70%) [3]. In our case and literature review, all patients improved with visual acuity greater than 20/40, and the majority improved to 20/20 (73%).

Table 1. Summary of cases of COVID-19-vaccine-associated MEWDS.

Authors	Age	Sex	Race	Vaccine	Dose	Time from Vaccine to Symptoms (Days)	Ocular Symptoms	Past History	Course	Initial VA	Final VA	Treatment	Resolution
Bolletta et al. [26]	53	M	–	Pfizer BNT162b2	2nd	28	Decreased VA, scotoma,	None	Acute	20/25	20/20	Observation	Complete resolution
	18	F	–	Pfizer BNT162b2	1st	4	Blurred vision, visual field defect	None	Acute	20/66	20/20	Observation	Complete resolution
	48	M	–	Pfizer BNT162b2	1st	7	Decreased VA	None	Acute	20/400	20/20	Observation	Complete resolution
Xu et al. [13]	49	F	–	Sinovac-CoronaVac vaccine (Inactivated)	1st	2	Blurred vision	MEWDS	Recurrent	20/100	20/20	Tapered prednisone, starting with 20 mg	Complete resolution
Lin et al. [27]	36	F	Taiwanese	Medigen Vaccine Biologics Corporation (MVC) COVID-19 Vaccine	1st	2	Photopsia	High myopia (−9.75D/−7.5D)	Acute	20/25	20/20	observation	Complete resolution in 4 weeks
Smith et al. [28]	15	M	–	Pfizer BNT162b2	2nd	14	Blurred vision, myodesopsia, photopsia	None	Acute	20/100	20/20	Tapered oral prednisone, starting at 40 mg	Complete resolution in 2 weeks
	21	F	–	Pfizer BNT162b2	2nd	21	Blurred vision	None	Acute	20/60	20/20	Tapered oral prednisone, starting at 40 mg	Complete resolution in 2 weeks
Yasuda et al. [29]	67	F	Japanese	Pfizer BNT162b2	2nd	1	Scotoma, photopsia, blurred vision	None	Acute	20/100	20/25	–	Patient also developed moderate vitritis, almost complete resolution at 2 weeks.
Inagawa et al. [30]	30	F	Japanese	Pfizer BNT162b2	1st, 2nd	7 and 3, respectively	Blurred vision	None	Recurrent	20/20 OU	20/30	Topical 0.1% fluorometholone for 21 days	Both eyes had fundus abnormalities L>R
Tomishige et al. [31]	38	F	White	Sinovac-CoronaVac vaccine (Inactivated)	1st	7	Photopsia, decreased VA	None	Acute	20/400	20/20	Tapered oral prednisone, starting at 80 mg oral prednisone	Complete resolution in 4 weeks
Rabinovitch et al. [32]	28	F	–	Pfizer BNT162b2	2nd	0	Blurred vision, scotoma, photopsia	None	Acute	–	–	–	Significant improvement on FU
	39	M	–	Pfizer BNT162b2	2nd	–	Blurred vision, scotoma, photopsia	None	Acute	–	–	–	Significant improvement on FU
Alhabshan et al. [33]	71	F	White	Moderna mRNA-1273	1st booster	3	Blurred vision and scotoma	Myopic and retinal tear	Acute	20/30	–	–	Spontaneous improvement

4. Conclusions

In conclusion, we have reported a case of recurrent episodes of MEWDS following COVID-19 mRNA-1273 vaccines. The majority of vaccine-associated MEWDS episodes were previously in healthy, young females and resembled those of non-COVID-19-vaccine-associated MEWDS. Although the prognosis for this disease is favorable, physicians should be aware of this association so that these patients can be rapidly identified and offered prompt management and counseling.

Author Contributions: M.S. and S.K.: Conceptualization; M.S., S.K. and J.F.: Investigation; M.S., N.V.N. and R.L.: Original Draft Preparation; M.S. and N.V.N.: Visualization; M.S., N.V.N., R.L., J.F. and S.K.: Writing—Review and Editing. All authors have read and agreed to the published version of the manuscript.

Funding: National Eye Institute Intramural Research Program.

Institutional Review Board Statement: Not applicable.

Informed Consent Statement: Not applicable.

Data Availability Statement: Not applicable.

Conflicts of Interest: The authors declare no conflict of interest.

References

1. Jampol, L.M.; Sieving, P.A.; Pugh, D.; Fishman, G.A.; Gilbert, H. Multiple evanescent white dot syndrome. I. Clinical findings. *Arch. Ophthalmol.* **1984**, *102*, 671–674. [CrossRef] [PubMed]
2. Papasavvas, I.; Mantovani, A.; Tugal-Tutkun, I.; Herbort, C.P. Multiple evanescent white dot syndrome (MEWDS): Update on practical appraisal, diagnosis and clinicopathology; a review and an alternative comprehensive perspective. *J. Ophthalmic Inflamm. Infect.* **2021**, *11*, 45. [CrossRef] [PubMed]
3. Testi, I.; Brandão-de-Resende, C.; Agrawal, R.; Pavesio, C. Ocular inflammatory events following COVID-19 vaccination: A multinational case series. *J. Ophthalmic Inflamm. Infect.* **2022**, *12*, 4. [CrossRef]
4. Watson, O.J.; Barnsley, G.; Toor, J.; Hogan, A.B.; Winskill, P.; Ghani, A.C. Global impact of the first year of COVID-19 vaccination: A mathematical modelling study. *Lancet Infect. Dis.* **2022**, *22*, 1293–1302. [CrossRef]
5. Sharif, N.; Alzahrani, K.J.; Ahmed, S.N.; Dey, S.K. Efficacy, Immunogenicity and Safety of COVID-19 Vaccines: A Systematic Review and Meta-Analysis. *Front. Immunol.* **2021**, *12*, 714170. [CrossRef]
6. WHO Coronavirus (COVID-19) Dashboard. Available online: https://covid19.who.int (accessed on 10 September 2022).
7. Rosenblum, H.G.; Hadler, S.C.; Moulia, D.; Shimabukuro, T.T.; Su, J.R.; Tepper, N.K.; Ess, K.C.; Woo, E.J.; Mba-Jonas, A.; Alimchandani, M.; et al. Use of COVID-19 Vaccines After Reports of Adverse Events Among Adult Recipients of Janssen (Johnson & Johnson) and mRNA COVID-19 Vaccines (Pfizer-BioNTech and Moderna): Update from the Advisory Committee on Immunization Practices—United States, July 2021. *MMWR Morb. Mortal. Wkly. Rep.* **2021**, *70*, 1094–1099. [CrossRef]
8. Ramakrishnan, M.S.; Patel, A.P.; Melles, R.; Vora, R.A. Multiple Evanescent White Dot Syndrome: Findings from a Large Northern California Cohort. *Ophthalmol. Retina.* **2021**, *5*, 850–854. [CrossRef] [PubMed]
9. Bosello, F.; Westcott, M.; Casalino, G.; Agorogiannis, G.; Micciolo, R.; Rees, A.; Pavesio, C. Multiple evanescent white dot syndrome: Clinical course and factors influencing visual acuity recovery. *Br. J. Ophthalmol.* **2022**, *106*, 121–127. [CrossRef]
10. WHO. *Causality Assessment of an Adverse Event Following Immunization (AEFI): User Manual for the Revised WHO Classification*, 2nd ed.; 2019 Update; WHO: Geneva, Switzerland, 2019. Available online: https://www.who.int/publications-detail-redirect/9789241516990 (accessed on 25 September 2022).
11. Ng, C.C.; Jumper, J.M.; Cunningham, E.T. Multiple evanescent white dot syndrome following influenza immunization—A multimodal imaging study. *Am. J. Ophthalmol. Case Rep.* **2020**, *19*, 100845. [CrossRef]
12. COVID Vaccinations Administered Number by Manufacturer U.S. 2022. Statista. Available online: https://www.statista.com/statistics/1198516/covid-19-vaccinations-administered-us-by-company/ (accessed on 10 September 2022).
13. Chen, Y.; Xu, Z.; Wang, P.; Li, X.M.; Shuai, Z.W.; Ye, D.Q.; Pan, H.F. New-onset autoimmune phenomena post-COVID-19 vaccination. *Immunology* **2022**, *165*, 386–401. [CrossRef]
14. Yadav, T.; Srivastava, N.; Mishra, G.; Dhama, K.; Kumar, S.; Puri, B.; Saxena, S.K. Recombinant vaccines for COVID-19. *Hum. Vaccines Immunother.* **2020**, *16*, 2905–2912. [CrossRef]
15. Maleki, A.; Look-Why, S.; Manhapra, A.; Foster, C.S. COVID-19 Recombinant mRNA Vaccines and Serious Ocular Inflammatory Side Effects: Real or Coincidence? *J. Ophthalmic Vis. Res.* **2021**, *16*, 490–501. [CrossRef] [PubMed]
16. Ngo, S.T.; Steyn, F.J.; McCombe, P.A. Gender differences in autoimmune disease. *Front. Neuroendocrinol.* **2014**, *35*, 347–369. [CrossRef] [PubMed]

17. Choubey, D.; Moudgil, K.D. Interferons in Autoimmune and Inflammatory Diseases: Regulation and Roles. *J. Interferon Cytokine Res.* **2011**, *31*, 857–865. [CrossRef] [PubMed]
18. Vojdani, A.; Kharrazian, D. Potential antigenic cross-reactivity between SARS-CoV-2 and human tissue with a possible link to an increase in autoimmune diseases. *Clin. Immunol. Orlando Fla.* **2020**, *217*, 108480. [CrossRef]
19. Sawant, O.B.; Wright, S.S.E.; Jones, K.M.; Titus, M.S.; Dennis, E.; Hicks, E.; Majmudar, P.A.; Kumar, A.; Mian, S.I. Prevalence of SARS-CoV-2 in human post-mortem ocular tissues. *Ocul. Surf.* **2021**, *19*, 322–329. [CrossRef]
20. Bragazzi, N.L.; Hejly, A.; Watad, A.; Adawi, M.; Amital, H.; Shoenfeld, Y. ASIA syndrome and endocrine autoimmune disorders. *Best Pract. Res. Clin. Endocrinol. Metab.* **2020**, *34*, 101412. [CrossRef]
21. Rabinovitch, T.; Ben-Arie-Weintrob, Y.; Hareuveni-Blum, T.; Shaer, B.; Vishnevskia-Dai, V.; Shulman, S.; Newman, H.; Biadsy, M.; Masarwa, D.; Fischer, N.; et al. Uveitis after the BNT162b2 mRNA vaccination against SARS-CoV-2 Infection: A Possible Association. *Retina Phila Pa* **2021**, *41*, 2462–2471. [CrossRef]
22. Haseeb, A.A.; Solyman, O.; Abushanab, M.M.; Abo Obaia, A.S.; Elhusseiny, A.M. Ocular Complications Following Vaccination for COVID-19: A One-Year Retrospective. *Vaccines* **2022**, *10*, 342. [CrossRef]
23. Elnahry, A.G.; Asal, Z.B.; Shaikh, N.; Dennett, K.; Elmohsen, M.N.A.; Elnahry, G.A.; Shehab, A.; Vytopil, M.; Ghaffari, L.; Athappilly, G.K.; et al. Optic neuropathy after COVID-19 vaccination: A report of two cases. *Int. J. Neurosci.* **2021**, 1–7. [CrossRef]
24. Nioi, M.; d'Aloja, E.; Fossarello, M.; Napoli, P.E. Dual Corneal-Graft Rejection after mRNA Vaccine (BNT162b2) for COVID-19 during the First Six Months of Follow-Up: Case Report, State of the Art and Ethical Concerns. *Vaccines* **2021**, *9*, 1274. [CrossRef] [PubMed]
25. Jin, S.X.; Juthani, V.V. Acute Corneal Endothelial Graft Rejection With Coinciding COVID-19 Infection. *Cornea* **2021**, *40*, 123–124. [CrossRef] [PubMed]
26. Bolletta, E.; Iannetta, D.; Mastrofilippo, V.; Simone, L.D.; Gozzi, F.; Croci, S.; Bonacini, M.; Belloni, L.; Zerbini, A.; Adani, C.; et al. Uveitis and Other Ocular Complications Following COVID-19 Vaccination. *J. Clin. Med.* **2021**, *10*, 5960. [CrossRef] [PubMed]
27. Multiple Evanescent White Dot Syndrome Following Medigen Vaccine Biologics Corporation COVID-19 Vaccination—PubMed. Available online: https://pubmed.ncbi.nlm.nih.gov/35442848/ (accessed on 19 July 2022).
28. Multiple Evanescent White Dot Syndrome following COVID-19 mRNA Vaccination in Two Patients—PubMed. Available online: https://pubmed.ncbi.nlm.nih.gov/35201960/ (accessed on 19 July 2022).
29. Yasuda, E.; Matsumiya, W.; Maeda, Y.; Kusuhara, S.; Nguyen, Q.D.; Nakamura, M.; Hara, R. Multiple evanescent white dot syndrome following BNT162b2 mRNA COVID-19 vaccination. *Am. J. Ophthalmol. Case Rep.* **2022**, *26*, 101532. [CrossRef] [PubMed]
30. Inagawa, S.; Onda, M.; Miyase, T.; Murase, S.; Murase, H.; Mochizuki, K.; Sakaguchi, H. Multiple evanescent white dot syndrome following vaccination for COVID-19: A case report. *Medicine* **2022**, *101*, e28582. [CrossRef]
31. Tomishige, K.S.; Novais, E.A.; Finamor, L.P.D.S.; Nascimento, H.M.d.; Belfort, R. Multiple evanescent white dot syndrome (MEWDS) following inactivated COVID-19 vaccination (Sinovac-CoronaVac). *Arq. Bras. Oftalmol.* **2022**, *85*, 186–189. [CrossRef]
32. Uveitis after the BNT162b2 mRNA Vaccination against SARS-CoV-2 Infection: A Possible Association—PubMed. Available online: https://pubmed.ncbi.nlm.nih.gov/34369440/ (accessed on 19 July 2022).
33. Alhabshan, R.; Scales, D. Multiple Evanescent White Dot Syndrome Developing Three Days following Administration of mRNA-1273 Booster Vaccine: Case Report. *Case Rep. Ophthalmol.* **2022**, *13*, 570–577. [CrossRef]

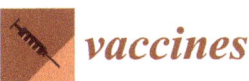

Review

COVID-19 Vaccine-Associated Optic Neuropathy: A Systematic Review of 45 Patients

Ayman G. Elnahry [1,2,*], Mutaz Y. Al-Nawaflh [2,3], Aisha A. Gamal Eldin [4], Omar Solyman [5,6], Ahmed B. Sallam [7], Paul H. Phillips [7] and Abdelrahman M. Elhusseiny [7]

1. Department of Ophthalmology, Faculty of Medicine, Cairo University, Cairo 11956, Egypt
2. Division of Epidemiology and Clinical Applications, National Eye Institute, National Institutes of Health, Bethesda, MD 20892, USA
3. Division of Ophthalmology, King Hussein Hospital, Jordanian Royal Medical Services, Amman 11855, Jordan
4. Maryland Eye Care Center, Silver Spring, MD 20910, USA
5. Department of Ophthalmology, Research Institute of Ophthalmology, Giza 11261, Egypt
6. Department of Ophthalmology, Qassim University Medical City, Al-Qassim 52571, Saudi Arabia
7. Department of Ophthalmology, Harvey and Bernice Jones Eye Institute, University of Arkansas for Medical Sciences, Little Rock, AR 72205, USA
* Correspondence: ayman.elnahry@nih.gov; Tel.: +1-2159667024

Citation: Elnahry, A.G.; Al-Nawaflh, M.Y.; Gamal Eldin, A.A.; Solyman, O.; Sallam, A.B.; Phillips, P.H.; Elhusseiny, A.M. COVID-19 Vaccine-Associated Optic Neuropathy: A Systematic Review of 45 Patients. *Vaccines* 2022, 10, 1758. https://doi.org/10.3390/vaccines10101758

Academic Editor: Rohan Bir Singh

Received: 25 September 2022
Accepted: 19 October 2022
Published: 20 October 2022

Publisher's Note: MDPI stays neutral with regard to jurisdictional claims in published maps and institutional affiliations.

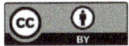

Copyright: © 2022 by the authors. Licensee MDPI, Basel, Switzerland. This article is an open access article distributed under the terms and conditions of the Creative Commons Attribution (CC BY) license (https://creativecommons.org/licenses/by/4.0/).

Abstract: We provide a systematic review of published cases of optic neuropathy following COVID-19 vaccination. We used Ovid MEDLINE, PubMed, and Google Scholar. Search terms included: "COVID-19 vaccination", "optic neuropathy", "optic neuritis", and "ischemic optic neuropathy". The titles and abstracts were screened, then the full texts were reviewed. Sixty eyes from forty-five patients (28 females) were included. Eighteen eyes from fourteen patients (31.1%) were diagnosed with anterior ischemic optic neuropathy (AION), while 34 eyes from 26 patients (57.8%) were diagnosed with optic neuritis (ON). Other conditions included autoimmune optic neuropathy and Leber hereditary optic neuropathy. Fifteen patients (33.3%) had bilateral involvement. The mean age of all patients was 47.4 ± 17.1 years. The mean age of AION patients was 62.9 ± 12.2 years and of ON patients was 39.7 ± 12.8 years ($p < 0.001$). The mean time from vaccination to ophthalmic symptoms was 9.6 ± 8.7 days. The mean presenting visual acuity (VA) was logMAR 0.990 ± 0.924. For 41 eyes with available follow-up, the mean presenting VA was logMAR 0.842 ± 0.885, which improved to logMAR 0.523 ± 0.860 at final follow-up ($p < 0.001$). COVID-19 vaccination may be associated with different forms of optic neuropathy. Patients diagnosed with ON were more likely to be younger and to experience visual improvement. More studies are needed to further characterize optic neuropathies associated with COVID-19 vaccination.

Keywords: CNS inflammation; COVID-19; ischemic optic neuropathy; ocular inflammation; optic neuritis; optic neuropathy; vaccination

1. Introduction

In 2021, vaccination against severe acute respiratory syndrome coronavirus 2 (SARS-CoV-2) became a primary focus of public health efforts to control the COVID-19 pandemic. Even though they were generally found to be safe and effective in multiple large controlled clinical trials, the relatively fast and wide deployment of COVID-19 vaccines has made them a subject of considerable scrutiny and analysis since the time of their introduction to the public.

The COVID-19 disease itself has affected the eye in many ways. Previous research demonstrated a link between COVID-19 infection and ophthalmic manifestations, both directly and indirectly. For example, it was reported that inflammatory conditions such as conjunctivitis, scleritis, orbital inflammation, keratitis, and retinal affection may be directly linked to COVID-19 infection [1–9]. Regarding indirect impact, several studies have addressed the relationship between eye strain and dry eye symptoms and the increased screen time in both pediatric and adult populations during the pandemic [7,10].

Since their deployment, COVID-19 vaccines have been linked to various ophthalmic manifestations [11,12]. These manifestations have involved the orbit [13], cornea [14,15], uvea [16,17], optic nerve [18,19], retina [20,21], and retinal vessels [22]. Regarding neuro-ophthalmic manifestations, several cranial nerve palsies were reported following COVID-19 vaccines that involved the oculomotor [23], abducens [24], and facial nerves [25–28]. Recently, multiple reports were published on the development of optic neuropathy following COVID-19 vaccination [19,29–34]. In this study, we provide a systematic review of all cases of optic neuropathy following COVID-19 vaccination published to date.

2. Materials and Methods

We performed a systematic literature search using Ovid MEDLINE, PubMed, and Google Scholar for published cases of optic neuropathy that followed COVID-19 vaccination up to 10 September 2022. We used a combination of the following terms: "COVID-19 vaccination", "optic neuropathy", "optic neuritis", "papillitis", "retrobulbar optic neuritis", "ischemic optic neuropathy", "NAION", and "AION". We initially screened titles and abstracts for the identification of studies, then the full texts were retrieved for eligible studies for a complete review and inclusion in the final analysis. We only included cases that were published in the English language, peer-reviewed, and that included details on optic nerve involvement. There were no restrictions on study type, and all studies, including case reports and case series, were eligible for inclusion. Exclusion criteria included insufficient evidence or details of optic nerve involvement.

Data Extraction and Statistical Analysis

The following data were extracted from the included studies: type of study, age of patients, gender of patients, type of vaccine, the dose of vaccination, the duration between administration of the vaccine and the onset of ocular symptoms, the presenting, and the final visual acuity, presenting symptoms and signs, results of systemic and ocular investigations, diagnoses, and mode of treatment. For continuous variables, we reported the mean as mean ± standard deviation. We made comparisons of populations, when appropriate, using a two-tailed two-sample t-test for means. A p-value of <0.05 was considered statistically significant.

3. Results

3.1. Studies and Patients

We identified 29 studies (21 case reports and 8 case series) that reported on patients that developed optic neuropathy following COVID-19 vaccination. From those, a total of 60 eyes from 45 patients that developed optic neuropathy following COVID-19 vaccination met the inclusion criteria (Table 1). Eighteen eyes from fourteen patients (31.1%) were diagnosed with anterior ischemic optic neuropathy (AION), while 34 eyes from 26 patients (57.8%) were diagnosed with optic neuritis. One patient was diagnosed with papillitis in one eye and neuroretinitis in the other, while four eyes from three patients were diagnosed with autoimmune optic neuropathy (AON). In addition, one patient was diagnosed with Leber hereditary optic neuropathy (LHON), which was genetically confirmed (m.14568A > G mutation in MT-ND6). Fifteen patients (33.3% of the total), therefore, had bilateral optic nerve involvement. Regarding AION, five eyes from three patients were diagnosed with arteritic anterior ischemic optic neuropathy (AAION), all confirmed by temporal artery biopsy, while the remaining eyes (13 eyes from 11 patients) were diagnosed as non-arteritic anterior ischemic optic neuropathy (NAION). In addition to optic neuropathy, one patient was diagnosed with central nervous system (CNS) inflammatory syndrome, one with acute disseminated encephalomyelitis (ADEM), three with giant cell arteritis (GCA), three with neuromyelitis optica spectrum disorder (NMOSD), and five with myelin-oligodendrocyte-glycoprotein (MOG) antibody-associated disease.

3.2. Demographic Data

Twenty-eight patients (62.2%) were females, while 17 (37.8%) were males. The mean age of all patients was 47.4 ± 17.1 years (Range: 15–87 years). The mean age of AION patients was 62.9 ± 12.2 years (Range: 40–87 years), while the mean age of optic neuritis patients was 39.7 ± 12.8 years (Range: 19–65 years) ($p < 0.001$). The mean time from vaccination to onset of ophthalmic symptoms was 9.6 ± 8.7 days (Range: 0–42 days).

3.3. Visual Acuity Outcomes

The mean presenting visual acuity of all patients was logMAR 0.990 ± 0.924 (20/200 in Snellen notation). Of the 41 eyes (32 patients) that had both presenting and final follow-up visual acuity, 21 eyes (52.5%) from 18 patients (56.3%) experienced an improvement in visual acuity, with 16 eyes (76.2%) due to optic neuritis, 3 (14.3%) due to AION, and 2 (9.5%) due to AON. For those 41 eyes, the mean presenting visual acuity was logMAR 0.842 ± 0.885 (20/140 in Snellen notation), while at final follow-up, it significantly improved to logMAR 0.523 ± 0.860 (20/70 in Snellen notation; $p < 0.001$). For the 18 eyes (14 patients) with AION, the mean presenting visual acuity was logMAR 0.987 ± 0.929 (20/200 in Snellen notation), comparable to the 32 eyes (25 patients) with optic neuritis (2 eyes from one patient had no reported visual acuity), who had mean presenting visual acuity of logMAR 1.068 ± 0.980 (20/230 in Snellen notation) ($p = 0.772$). However, for cases with available follow-up visual acuity, the final visual acuity for 14 eyes (11 patients) with AION was logMAR 0.970 ± 1.012 (20/185 in Snellen notation), which was significantly worse than that for 21 eyes (17 patients) with optic neuritis with available follow-up (final visual acuity of logMAR 0.227 ± 0.659 (20/35 in Snellen notation), $p = 0.025$).

Table 1. Summary of cases of optic neuropathy following COVID-19 vaccination.

Author	Article Type	Age	Sex	Vaccine, Dose	Time from Vaccine to Symptoms (Days)	Baseline VA	Eye	Systemic Conditions (Pre-Vaccination)	Manifestations	Outcome	Final VA
Elnahry et al., 2021 [19]	CS	69	F	BNT162b2, #2	16	CF	OD	Hypertension, DM, cutaneous T-cell lymphoma	Blurry vision OU with immediate OS clearing but persistent blurring OD. The exam showed optic nerve head edema (OD > OS) and RAPD OD. OCT imaging and CSF confirmed a diagnosis of CNS inflammatory syndrome with neuroretinitis OD and papillitis OS.	Significant improvement of optic disc edema with stable vision after 5 days of IV methylprednisolone.	CF
						20/20	OS				20/20
Garcia-Estrada et al., 2021 [29]	CR	32	F	COVISHIELD, #1	4	20/30	OS	None	Blurred vision with superior field defect OS. Examination revealed optic disc swelling and RAPD with decreased RNFL thickness. MRI was consistent with optic neuritis	Significant improvement of optic nerve head swelling and improved VF defect and VA after 3 days of IV methylprednisolone followed by PO prednisone.	20/20
Girbardt et al., 2021 [30]	CR	19	F	Ad26.COV2.S, #1	7	20/20	OS	None	Ocular pain and vision loss OS, with exam revealing amaurosis, RAPD, and papillitis.	Resolution of symptoms and papillitis after 5 days of IV methylprednisolone followed by a PO prednisolone.	20/20
Leber et al., 2021 [31]	CR	67	M	Vaxveria, #1	2	20/200	OD	DM, hypercholesterolemia	Decreased vision and scotomas OD with exam revealing an elevated, congested optic nerve head with surrounding intraretinal hemorrhages and cotton-wool spots. NAION was diagnosed	NR	NR
	CR	32	F	Corona Vac, #2	0	20/200	OS	NR	Rapidly progressive worsening vision and pain with EOM OS. Exam revealed RAPD OS and disc swelling OD and OS. MRI revealed optic neuritis OU.	Improvement in symptoms and vision after 5 days of IV methylprednisolone.	20/20
						20/20	OD				20/25
Nachbor et al., 2021 [32]	CR	64	F	BNT162b2, #1	6	20/80	OS	DM	Acute, painless, unilateral vision loss with superior sectoral optic disc edema OS after 1st dose. After 2nd dose, VA was CF with persistent APD OS. RNFL OCT showed diffuse thickening OS. NAION was diagnosed OS.	Improvement of symptoms with PO prednisone over 1 week. Resolution of optic disc edema followed by optic nerve pallor.	20/100
Pawar et al., 2021 [33]	CR	28	F	AstraZeneca, #1	21	20/120	OS	None	Sudden vision loss OS, with exam revealing mild blurring of the optic disc margin. MRI was consistent with optic neuritis OS.	Resolution of symptoms after IV methylprednisolone followed by PO steroid.	20/20
Maleki et al., 2021 [34]	CR	79	F	BNT162b2, #2	2	20/1250	OD	None	Bilateral sudden loss of vision, OD>OS, with 3+ RAPD OD. OCT, FA, ICG, and temporal artery biopsy consistent with bilateral AAION.	Initiated on subcutaneous tocilizumab. Prognosis was NR.	NR
						20/40	OS				NR

Table 1. Cont.

Author	Article Type	Age	Sex	Vaccine, Dose	Time from Vaccine to Symptoms (Days)	Baseline VA	Eye	Systemic Conditions (Pre-Vaccination)	Manifestations	Outcome	Final VA
Tsukii et al., 2021 [35]	CR	55	F	BNT162b2, #1	3	20/20	OD	None	Visual disturbance with RAPD OD. Fundoscopy revealed diffuse optic disc swelling OD. An inferior VF defect suggesting AION.	vision remained normal and there was diffuse pallor OD, although no treatment was initiated	20/20
Lin et al., 2022 [36]	CR	61	F	ChAdOx1nCoV-19 #1	7	20/50	OS	Hypertension, hyperlipidemia	Scotoma in inferior field with hazy vision OS and headache. Fundus exam: optic disc edema OS. VF: inferior altitudinal field defect. OCT: peripapillary RNFL edema and GCL thinning in the superior macula. FA: filling delay, decreased choroidal perfusion, and optic disc leakage consistent with NAION OS.	PO prednisolone with gradual tapering. After 6 weeks, VA became 20/80 OS, and disc edema resolved	20/80
Chung et al., 2022 [37]	CR	65	F	AstraZeneca #2	15	CF	OD	None	RAPD OD. Fundus exam: a swollen disc with several splinter hemorrhages OD. VF: inferior arcuate and cecocentral visual field defects. OCT: thickened peripapillary RNFL and thinning of RNFL. MRI: no increased signal intensity or abnormal enhancement. NAION OD diagnosed	IV methylprednisolone followed by PO steroid taper. VA improved to 20/200 with optic disc pallor and no improvement in VF defect.	20/200
Sanjay et al., 2022 [38]	CR	52	F	COVISHIELD #2	4	20/20	OS	DM	Blurring of temporal disc margin with hyperemia OS. RAPD OS. Color vision was abnormal OU. NAION OS diagnosed.	PO aspirin for 1 month. BCVA OS was 20/20 at 1 month with resolved disc edema.	20/20
Roy et al., 2022 [39]	CS	27	F	COVISHIELD #1	4	20/200	OS	None	Progressive blurring of vision OS. RAPD and color desaturation OS. Fundus exam: diffuse swelling of the optic nerve head. VF: an enlarged blind spot. MRI brain and orbit: enhancement of left optic nerve just behind the disc. VEP: flat wave OS compared to OD. Diagnosed as optic neuritis OS.	IV methylprednisolone followed by PO steroid taper. BCVA improved to 20/40 OS with decreased disc swelling.	20/40
		48	F	COVISHIELD #2	2	20/80	OS	NR	RAPD OS. Fundus: swollen optic disc with blurred margins. OCT: peripapillary swelling of the retina. VF: an inferior arcuate defect. VEP: delayed latency and decreased amplitude OS. Optic neuritis OS was diagnosed	IV methylprednisolone. BCVA improved to 20/30 OS with improved VF.	20/30
		40	M	COVISHIELD #1	5	20/200	OD	NR	Sluggishly reacting pupils OU. Fundus: bilaterally blurred and swollen optic disc margin. VF: generalized depression OU. VEP: flat waves. Diagnosis of bilateral optic neuritis was made.	BCVA and VF improved OU after steroid therapy.	20/30
						20/200	OS				20/40

115

Table 1. Cont.

Author	Article Type	Age	Sex	Vaccine, Dose	Time from Vaccine to Symptoms (Days)	Baseline VA	Eye	Systemic Conditions (Pre-Vaccination)	Manifestations	Outcome	Final VA
Elhusseiny et al., 2022 [40]	CR	51	M	BNT162b2 #2	1	CF 3 ft	OS	DM	Fundus exam: optic disc edema, peripapillary hemorrhages, and blunted foveal reflex OS. FA: optic disc leakage OS. OCT: marked thickening of the peripapillary retina, intraretinal fluid and hyperreflective foci consistent with exudates, and subretinal fluid under the fovea. NAION OS diagnosed.	PO prednisone over 1 month. Disc swelling and subretinal fluid resolved with BCVA of 20/400 OS.	20/400
Madina et al., 2022 [41]	CS	65	F	BNT162b2 #1	5	PL	OD	Medullary thyroid cancer, hypothyroidism, prediabetic, hyperlipidemia	Had vision loss and pain with eye movements OD. RAPD OD, optic disc swelling associated with cotton-wool spots and flame hemorrhages. MRI orbits: evidence of right optic neuritis. Optic neuritis OD diagnosed.	IV methylprednisolone and IVIG BCVA improved to 20/100 OD.	20/100
		67	M	Moderna #2	1	20/40	OD	Prediabetic, hyperlipidemia	bilateral eye redness, chemosis, and blurring of vision. Had RAPD OS. MRI orbits: evidence of left optic neuritis. Optic neuritis OU diagnosed.	IV methylprednisolone. BCVA improved to 20/20 OD with a normal visual field, but he continued to have NPL OS.	20/20
						NPL	OS				NPL
Franco et al., 2022 [42]	CS	53	M	BNT162b2/Comirnaty vaccine #2	10	20/20	OD	None	RAPD OS and fundus exam showed optic disc swelling with peripapillary hemorrhages OU. Disc edema confirmed by OCT OU. VF: constriction of peripheral visual field OS and an incomplete lower nasal scotoma OD. NAION OU diagnosed.	Stable BCVA with sluggish pupils. Fundus exam: pale discs OU without any hemorrhages. VF did not change OD, but OS was slightly better.	20/20
						20/40	OS				20/40
		65	M	BNT162b2/Comirnaty vaccine #1	12	20/200	OD	Hypertension	RAPD with optic disc swelling and peripapillary hemorrhages OD. NAION diagnosed.	No specific treatment was given. No vision improvement with dyschromatopsia (Ishihara test: 1/17), temporal optic disc pallor, and blind spot enlargement with centrocecal scotoma on VF.	20/200

Table 1. Cont.

Author	Article Type	Age	Sex	Vaccine, Dose	Time from Vaccine to Symptoms (Days)	Baseline VA	Eye	Systemic Conditions (Pre-Vaccination)	Manifestations	Outcome	Final VA
Norman et al., 2022 [43]	CS	62	M	BNT162b2 #1	6	20/20	OS	None	RAPD OS. Inferior optic nerve swelling OS. VF: superior altitudinal defect. Diagnosed as presumed AON OS.	Stable BCVA and color vision, while VF continued to show superior altitudinal defect. Had complete resolution of disc edema, with some pallor and loss of the RNFL inferiorly.	20/20
		48	F	BNT162b2 #1	5	20/70	OD	Hypertension, migraine, asthma, trigeminal neuralgia	Trace RAPD OS. VF: paracentral scotoma OD with full field and no scotomas OS. Optic nerve head: temporal pallor and trace edema OD and temporal pallor OS. Labs: elevated ESR and CRP. Diagnosed as papillitis OU due to AON.	Started on steroids. VA improved OU, RAPD disappeared, with resolved disc swelling.	20/50
						20/200	OS				20/80
		38	M	BNT162b2 #1	3	20/25	OS	Hypertension, hyperlipidemia	Color Plates showed 12/14 OS with 2+ RAPD. VF: superior and inferior arcuate defects OS. Optic nerve head had a 0.1 cup-to-disc ratio with severe pallid edema, enlarged capillaries, and small disc hemorrhages. Diagnosed as presumed AON OS	IV methylprednisolone followed by PO steroid taper. Stable VA, persistent 2+ RAPD OS, with improved disc swelling and VF defects.	20/25
Rizk et al., 2022 [44]	CR	15	M	BNT162b2 #2	7	20/200	OD	None	No RAPD. Color vision: 8/17 OD and 6/17 OS. Hyperemic telangiectatic vessels on optic disc OU. VF: cecocentral scotoma OU. Diagnosis of LHON OU was confirmed genetically.	Started on idebenone 300 mg 3 times daily and counselled about lifestyle changes and triggers.	NR
						20/200	OS				NR
Kumar et al., 2022 [45]	CR	73	M	COVISHEILD #1	5	20/1200	OD	None	Bilateral sluggish and poorly sustained pupillary reactions. Exam: edematous disks and chorioretinal changes inferonasal to the disk OS. NAION diagnosed OU	Patient did not report any appreciable visual gain.	20/1200
						20/120	OS				20/120
Che et al., 2022 [46]	CR	87	F	BNT162b2 #1	1	HM	OD	Hypertension	Bilateral optic disc edema with focal disc hemorrhage. FFA: peripapillary choroidal filling delay in the vertical watershed zone OD. MRI: circumferential enhancement of the intraorbital portion of the optic nerve sheath bilaterally. Biopsy of the right temporal artery confirmed the diagnosis of GCA and AAION OU.	IV methylprednisolone followed by PO steroid taper. BCVA improved to 0.1 logMAR OS but worsened to NPL OD at 4 months after treatment.	NPL
					4	20/30	OS				20/25
Raxwal et al., 2022 [47]	CR	47	F	Moderna #1	8	20/50	OS	Hypertension	Blurring and RAPD OS. There was no pallor of the optic nerve and no evidence of papilledema OU. Optic neuritis diagnosed OS	IV methylprednisolone followed by PO steroid taper. Follow-up revealed normal eye exam and normal VA.	20/20

Table 1. Cont.

Author	Article Type	Age	Sex	Vaccine, Dose	Time from Vaccine to Symptoms (Days)	Baseline VA	Eye	Systemic Conditions (Pre-Vaccination)	Manifestations	Outcome	Final VA
Wang et al., 2022 [48]	CS	21	F	Sinopharm #1 and #2	42 and 21	20/30	OD	None	RAPD OD. Fundus exam: blurred optic disc margin with congestion and edema OD. FA: early hyperfluorescence and late enhancement of the right optic papilla. OCT: significant thickening of the RNFL. VF: central scotoma. VEP: decreased amplitude. MRI brain: a small ischemic focus in the left frontal lobe. orbital MRI: no significant abnormalities. Optic neuritis diagnosed OD.	IV methylprednisolone followed by PO steroid taper. Papillary congestion and edema OD gradually resolved. BCVA recovered to 1.0 after 1 month.	20/20
		38	F	Sinopharm #1	21	CF 1 m	OD	None	RAPD OD. Fundus exam: blurred borders of the optic disc with congestion and edema OD. FA: early hyperfluorescence of the optic papilla OD with late staining. OCT: significant thickening of RNFL. VEP: prolonged P100 wave latency and decreased amplitude. VF: centripetal narrowing. Orbital CT: hypointense thickening of optic nerve. Optic neuritis diagnosed OD.	IV methylprednisolone followed by PO steroid taper. Papillary congestion and edema gradually resolved OD. BCVA recovered to 1.0 after 1 month.	20/20
Haseeb et al., 2022 [49]	CR	40	M	BNT162b2 #1	4	20/40	OS	DM	Vision loss OS. Exam: RAPD OS and an edematous pale optic disc with blurred edges and splinter hemorrhages. FA: early leakage OS with late staining. NAION diagnosed OS	NR	NR
Helmchen et al., 2022 [50]	CR	40	F	AstraZeneca #1	14	NR	OD	Multiple sclerosis	Progressive diminution of vision over 48 h. CSF: severe pleocytosis, increased lactate and strongly elevated protein. Cranial MRI: numerous old white matter lesions compatible with MS and increased signal intensity in the chiasm, optic nerves and tracts. Mild optic chiasm enhancement was observed. VEP: unrecordable OU. Spinal MRI: increased longitudinal centrally located signal intensities throughout the thoracic myelon. Diagnosed with NMOSD and optic neuritis OU.	Two days after receiving IV methylprednisolone, there was no contrast enhancement visible. she was also treated with plasmapheresis and immunoadsorption with slight recovery of visual functions but paraplegia, loss of sensory function below T5, and incontinence persisted. Two months after subacute onset, with even more improved BCVA but unchanged paraplegia follow-up spinal	NR
						NR	OS				NR

Table 1. Cont.

Author	Article Type	Age	Sex	Vaccine, Dose	Time from Vaccine to Symptoms (Days)	Baseline VA	Eye	Systemic Conditions (Pre-Vaccination)	Manifestations	Outcome	Final VA
Nagaratnam et al., 2022 [51]	CR	36	F	ChAdOx1nCoV-19 #1	12	20/50	OD	None	CSF analysis on day 2 of admission showed a normal protein with pleocytosis. CSF oligoclonal IgG bands were present, suggestive of intrathecal IgG synthesis. VEP: unrecordable OS and delayed OD, consistent with demyelinating pathology of anterior visual pathways OU but OS>OD. MRI brain: multiple T2/FLAIR hyperintense lesions in subcortical white matter, posterior limb of bilateral internal capsules, pons and left middle cerebellar peduncle. No definite abnormal signal or enhancement of optic nerves. Patient diagnosed with ADEM and optic neuritis OU.	IV methylprednisolone followed by PO steroid taper. VA improved to near baseline with full color vision OU. Both optic nerves were pale.	20/16
						20/100	OS				20/20
Shirah et al., 2022 [52]	CR	31	F	BNT162b2 #1	14	20/20	OS	Systemic lupus erythematosus	Diagnosed with SLE 10 years earlier. Fundus exam: normal OU without optic disc swelling. VF: paracentral VF contraction OU. Aquaporin-4 IgG antibody titer was positive at 1:1000. OCT: mild paracentral optic nerve thickening OS. VEP: mild to moderate prechiasmatic optic pathway dysfunction OS with secondary axonal loss. MRI: abnormal signal intensity and enhancement within the intraocular and intraorbital optic nerve OS. Optic neuritis diagnosed OS.	IV methylprednisolone followed by plasmapheresis, however, there was: no improvement. Rituximab was also started. Blurred vision OS remained unchanged, but ocular pain subsided.	20/20
Pirani et al., 2022 [53]	CS	31	F	BNT162b2 #1	6	20/200	OD	Ankylosing spondylitis	Fundus exam): mildly blurred margins of optic disc OD. VF showed scotoma OD. MRI brain, orbits and spine: no demyelination. T1-weighted MRI brain and orbits: enhancement of retrobulbar optic nerve OD; diagnosed with retrobulbar optic neuritis OD.	IV methylprednisolone followed by PO prednisone taper. On the third day BCVA improved to 20/20 OD.	20/20
		46	F	BNT162b2 #1	8	20/40	OD	Hashimoto thyroiditis	Slit-lamp exam OU was unremarkable. VF testing and MRI confirmed the diagnosis of retrobulbar optic neuritis OD.	IV methylprednisolone followed by PO steroid taper. BCVA improved to 20/25 OD and VF deficit resolved.	20/25
Singu et al., 2022 [54]	CR	39	F	BNT162b2 #1	12	20/20	OS	None	Ocular pain OS and headache without any other neurologic deficits. MRI: slight left optic neural swelling and perineuritis OS. Anti- MOG antibody: positive Diagnosed with optic neuritis and perineuritis OS.	Visual disturbance never recurred, and her ocular pain and headache subsided only with anti-inflammatory agents.	20/20

Table 1. Cont.

Author	Article Type	Age	Sex	Vaccine, Dose	Time from Vaccine to Symptoms (Days)	Baseline VA	Eye	Systemic Conditions (Pre-Vaccination)	Manifestations	Outcome	Final VA
Xia et al., 2022 [55]	CR	68	M	ChAdOx1nCoV-19 #2	29	NPL	OS	Chronic obstructive pulmonary disease	Bilateral jaw claudication and profound lethargy, but no scalp tenderness, fever, weight loss, and no shoulder, neck, or hip pain. Labs: normal ESR with mildly elevated CRP. Bilateral temporal artery biopsy confirmed GCA. AAION diagnosed OS.	Treated with oral and IV steroids. Had episodes of blurred vision OD on day 3 so a fourth dose of methylprednisolone was given.	NPL
Netravathi et al., 2022 [56]	CS	29	F	ChAdOx1nCoV-19 #1	11	HM	OD	NR	RAPD OD. Anti-MOG- positive VEP: absent waveform OD, normal OS. MRI brain: T2/FLAIR hyperintensity of long intraorbital segment of optic nerve OD with contrast enhancement. MOG-antibody-associated optic neuritis OD diagnosed.	IV methylprednisolone followed by PO steroid taper and plasmapheresis.	NR
		39	M	ChAdOx1nCoV-19 #1	14	CF	OD	NR	RAPD OD. VF: right inferonasal quadrant involvement. MOG-antibody-associated optic neuritis OD diagnosed.	IV methylprednisolone followed by PO steroid taper	NR
		54	M	ChAdOx1nCoV-19 #1	14	20/40	OS	NR	RAPD OS. VEP: normal OD, absent waveform OS. Anti-MOG: positive. MRI brain and spine: hyperintensity in Rt pons. MOG-associated optic neuritis diagnosed OS.	IV methylprednisolone followed by PO steroid taper	NR
		34	M	ChAdOx1nCoV-19 #1	1	PL	OD	NR	Non-reactive pupil OD. VEP: absent waveform OD. MRI: optic nerve tortuosity with prominent perioptic sheath and fat stranding OD. Optic neuritis diagnosed OD.	IV methylprednisolone followed by PO steroid taper	NR
		45	F	ChAdOx1nCoV-19 #1	21	20/40	OD	NR	RAPD OS. Normal pupillary reaction OD. MOG-associated optic neuritis diagnosed OU.	IV methylprednisolone followed by PO steroid taper and plasmapheresis.	NR
						HM	OS				NR
		30	M	ChAdOx1nCoV-19 #1	14	NPL	OD	NR	Optic disc edema OU. VEP: non-recordable OU. CSF lymphocytosis. MRI brain: subcortical hyperintense foci in both cerebral hemispheres. MRI Optic nerves: OD>OS intraneural hyperintensities Optic neuritis diagnosed OU.	IV methylprednisolone followed by plasmapheresis and Rituximab.	NR
						20/600	OS				NR
		40	M	ChAdOx1nCoV-19 #1	10	20/60	OD	NR	Serum MOG positive. MRI brain: T2 Hyperintensities in pons, bilateral thalami, right frontal cortex. MRI spine: longitudinally extensive myelitis. MOG-associated opticomyelopathy with optic neuritis OU diagnosed.	IV methylprednisolone followed by PO steroid taper and mycophenolate mofetil.	NR
						20/60	OS				NR

120

Table 1. Cont.

Author	Article Type	Age	Sex	Vaccine, Dose	Time from Vaccine to Symptoms (Days)	Baseline VA	Eye	Systemic Conditions (Pre-Vaccination)	Manifestations	Outcome	Final VA
		65	F	ChAdOx1nCoV-19 #1	42	HM	OD	NR	VEP OD non-recordable. CSF cells. Elevated ESR. NMO antibodies: positive. MRI brain: few hyperintensities in frontal subcortex. MRI Spine: hyperintensity with patchy contrast enhancement and bright spotty areas. NMO with optic neuritis OD diagnosed.	Received 3 cycles plasmapheresis followed by IV methylprednisolone then PO prednisolone 40 mg PO and mycophenolate mofetil.	NR

Abbreviations. #1 indicates that the event occurred following the first dose of vaccination, while #2 indicates that it occurred following the second dose. AAION = arteritic anterior ischemic optic neuropathy, AION = anterior ischemic optic neuropathy, ADEM = acute disseminated encephalomyelitis, ANA = anti-nuclear antibodies, AON = autoimmune optic neuropathy, BCVA = best corrected visual acuity, CF = counting fingers, CR = case report, CS = case series, CNS = central nervous system, CSF = cerebrospinal fluid, GCA = giant cell arteritis, DM = diabetes mellitus, ESR = erythrocyte sedimentation rate, GCL = ganglion cell layer, FA = fluorescein angiography, HM = hand movement, ICG = indocyanine green, IV = intravenous, LHON= Leber hereditary optic neuropathy, MOG = myelin-oligodendrocyte-glycoprotein, MRI = magnetic resonance imaging, MS = multiple sclerosis, NAION = non-arteritic anterior ischemic optic neuropathy, NMOSD = neuromyelitis optica spectrum disorder, NPL = no perception of light, NR = not reported, OCT = ocular coherence tomography, OD = right eye, OS = left eye, OU = both eyes, PL = perception of light, PO = oral, RAPD = relative afferent pupillary defect, RNFL = retinal nerve fiber layer, SLE = systemic lupus erythematosus, VA = visual acuity, VDRL = venereal disease research laboratory, VEP = visual evoked potential, VF = visual field.

4. Discussion

In this systematic review of published cases of optic neuropathy following COVID-19 vaccination, we found that COVID-19 vaccination was associated with several forms of optic neuropathy, most commonly AION and optic neuritis. All subtypes of COVID-19 vaccines, including mRNA, viral vector, and inactivated viral vaccines were associated with optic neuropathy. However, protein subunit vaccines, such as the Novavax vaccine, were not reported as a cause of optic neuropathy in the current review. The temporal association between vaccine administration and the development of optic neuropathies in these cases makes a causal link plausible, with a mean time from vaccination to the development of ocular symptoms of 9.6 ± 8.7 days. Cases with a late onset of optic neuropathy, however, are less likely to be related to vaccination and could be coincidental. Vaccines and their adjuvants are meant to robustly activate the innate immune system, and adaptive immunity then follows. Overactivation of this response, however, may occur in some patients and lead to rare immune-mediated complications.

AION is an important cause of loss of vision in adults and is classically divided into AAION and NAION. Previously, the incidences per 100,000 individuals for NAION and AAION, respectively, were reported as 2.30 and 0.36 [57]. Regarding pathogenesis, AAION results from inflammation and thrombosis of the short posterior ciliary arteries, which causes optic nerve head infarction [58,59]. It occurs mainly in the setting of GCA. It is an ophthalmic emergency and requires immediate treatment with systemic steroids [58]. NAION is classically idiopathic [58], though there is an association with various conditions including sleep apnea [60–62], certain drugs such as sildenafil and interferon [63–65], and ocular conditions such as optic disc drusen and crowded discs [66–68]. It commonly manifests as an altitudinal field defect. Post-vaccination NAION was also reported following the administration of the influenza vaccine [69,70].

Most of the post-vaccination inflammatory syndromes affecting the CNS were related to influenza vaccines, and optic neuritis is the most common clinical presentation of these syndromes [71]. The number of people receiving COVID-19 vaccines annually is even larger than those who receive influenza vaccines. This possibly makes the appearance of complications following COVID-19 vaccination seem more common. Certain individuals may also be at a higher risk of developing complications such as patients with diabetes, hypertension, or patients with autoimmune diseases, as suggested in the current review. The development of cerebral venous sinus thrombosis in women under 50 years of age was associated with the AstraZeneca-Oxford COVID-19 vaccine owing to a vaccine-induced immune thrombotic thrombocytopenia [72]. This complication was excluded by magnetic resonance venography in most of the reported cases of post-COVID-19 vaccination optic neuropathy included in this review.

Historically, gender type seems to influence the incidence and type of optic neuropathy. Previous studies have demonstrated a female predominance of incident optic neuritis, with one large study from the UK demonstrating that almost 70% of new cases over 22 years involved females [73]. Lee et al., however, previously showed in a cohort of patients with diabetes that the male gender increases the risk of developing AION by around 32% [74]. In the current review, we found that 62.2% of cases of optic neuropathy following COVID-19 vaccination occurred in females. This percentage was even higher (73.1%) when looking at only patients who developed optic neuritis, indicating a possible higher risk of optic neuropathy, especially optic neuritis, in females following COVID-19 vaccination. This could be due to hormonal or genetic differences and requires further analysis in larger prospective studies.

Ocular side effects including ocular inflammation, were reported following COVID-19 vaccination but are thought to be rare. In a relatively large multinational study of ocular inflammatory events following COVID-19 vaccination, 70 patients were reported to develop ocular inflammation within 14 days of COVID-19 vaccination, but only 2 (2.9%) patients were diagnosed with optic neuritis [75]. This indicates that the incidence of optic neuropathy following COVID-19 vaccination could be low. The latter study, however, did not provide specific details on cases with optic nerve involvement and so were not included in this review.

We have previously described that an autoimmune mechanism underlies the development of optic neuropathies following vaccination [11]. Previously, Stübgen et al. reported that there is no long-term risk of developing optic neuropathy following vaccination, but that the presence of adjuvants contributes to the process [76]. However, in the absence of adjuvants in several of the COVID-19 vaccines, this explanation is insufficient [19]. Clinically, it is challenging to differentiate between AION and optic neuritis, and the diagnosis is usually based on both clinical impression and multimodal imaging findings including neuroimaging [77–79]. Some differentiating features include older age of onset, altitudinal field defect, and worse visual outcomes in patients with AION, which was also found in our study; however, these features cannot confidently distinguish between both conditions [77]. Furthermore, the pathophysiology (and treatment) of both types of optic neuropathies is suggested to be different and it is not currently clear why some patients develop AION while others develop optic neuritis following vaccination. Documented risk factors for NAION include small cup-to-disc ratio, diabetes, hyperlipidemia, and hypertension, and it is likely that the development of NAION is a multifactorial process that includes the pre-existing structural compromise of the optic nerve [36,80,81].

Tsukii et al. have proposed that neutralizing antibodies directed against SARS-CoV-2 spike proteins after vaccination may cross-react with proteins in the retinal vasculature and retinal pigment epithelial cells, a mechanism also endorsed by Maleki et al. [34,35]. It is possible that these antibodies also cross-react with elements of the CNS including the optic nerve, a phenomenon suggested by the co-occurrence of CNS disease in several patients reported in this review. It is, therefore, conceivable that both processes may have played a role in the development of optic neuropathy in the cases reported herein. This is also supported by reports on cases of optic neuritis that developed following COVID-19 infection and was suggested to be due to molecular mimicry between viral antigens, which are also partly present in the vaccines, and CNS proteins [82–84]. Another possible explanation for the development of post-vaccination optic neuropathy that could link inflammation and ischemia was recently elucidated by Francis and colleagues in patients that developed optic neuropathy with immune checkpoint inhibitors used for the treatment of cancer [85]. These immunotherapy agents, such as vaccines, enhance the adaptive immune response resulting in a range of adverse inflammatory events including both ophthalmic and neurologic phenomena [85]. Francis and colleagues also indicated that this class of drugs could result in optic papillitis, a specific type of optic neuritis that involves the optic nerve head, leading to ischemia of the optic nerve head and an AION-like picture [85,86].

This review has limitations, including that it relies on a cohort of a relatively small number of case reports. Larger case-control studies would have provided a more optimal analysis of the association and the temporal relationship between COVID-19 vaccines and optic nerve disease, but unfortunately, no studies exist to date. Optic neuritis and AION are among the most common optic neuropathies even among the unvaccinated, with predisposing risk factors similar to those seen in patients in the current report. Therefore, the association of optic neuropathy with vaccination in many patients could be coincidental and unrelated to vaccination. Furthermore, the number of cases of optic neuropathy reported to date is very small, despite billions of individuals having already received COVID-19 vaccines, suggesting that the incidence of this complication is very low. The frequency of optic neuropathy following COVID-19 vaccination, however, is currently unknown and cannot be determined based on the available data.

5. Conclusions

In conclusion, several cases of optic neuropathy were reported following the administration of COVID-19 vaccines, suggesting an association and perhaps a cause–effect relationship, with at least one case reporting a positive rechallenge phenomenon following the second dose of vaccination [48]. Nevertheless, the benefits of vaccination against SARS-CoV-2 are substantial and outweigh the associated risks. Many reported cases were self-limiting and had a good prognosis with available treatments. Future studies should further evaluate the risk factors, both ocular and systemic, that may contribute to the development of optic neuropathy following COVID-19 vaccination within larger and more diverse populations and elucidate the mechanisms that underly the development of these conditions. This could further assist in the causality assessment of optic neuropathy as an adverse event following COVID-19 vaccination and help optimize the follow-up and treatment of this rare but sight-threatening complication [87].

Author Contributions: Conceptualization, A.G.E. and A.M.E.; methodology, A.G.E., A.A.G.E. and M.Y.A.-N.; validation, O.S., A.B.S. and P.H.P.; formal analysis, A.G.E., A.B.S., P.H.P. and A.M.E.; investigation, A.A.G.E. and M.Y.A.-N.; resources, A.G.E. and A.M.E.; data curation, M.Y.A.-N. and A.A.G.E.; writing—original draft preparation, A.G.E.; writing—review and editing, A.B.S., P.H.P., O.S. and A.M.E.; visualization, A.G.E. and A.M.E.; supervision, P.H.P. and A.M.E.; project administration, A.M.E. All authors have read and agreed to the published version of the manuscript.

Funding: This research received no external funding.

Institutional Review Board Statement: The study was conducted in accordance with the Declaration of Helsinki. Ethical review and approval were waived for this study since it was a review article. The authors declare that they adhered to the PRISMA guidelines/methodology.

Informed Consent Statement: Not applicable.

Data Availability Statement: Not applicable.

Conflicts of Interest: The authors declare no conflict of interest.

References

1. Singh, S.; Garcia, G., Jr.; Shah, R.; Kramerov, A.A.; Wright, R.E., 3rd; Spektor, T.M.; Ljubimov, A.V.; Arumugaswami, V.; Kumar, A. SARS-CoV-2 and its beta variant of concern infect human conjunctival epithelial cells and induce differential antiviral innate immune response. *Ocul. Surf.* **2022**, *23*, 184–194. [CrossRef] [PubMed]
2. Barros, A.; Queiruga-Piñeiro, J.; Lozano-Sanroma, J.; Alcalde, I.; Gallar, J.; Fernández-Vega Cueto, L.; Alfonso, J.F.; Quirós, L.M.; Merayo-Lloves, J. Small fiber neuropathy in the cornea of COVID-19 patients associated with the generation of ocular surface disease. *Ocul. Surf.* **2022**, *23*, 40–48. [CrossRef] [PubMed]
3. Wang, J.; Li, Y.; Musch, D.C.; Wei, N.; Qi, X.; Ding, G.; Li, X.; Li, J.; Song, L.; Zhang, Y.; et al. Progression of Myopia in School-Aged Children After COVID-19 Home Confinement. *JAMA Ophthalmol.* **2021**, *139*, 293–300. [CrossRef] [PubMed]
4. Rokohl, A.C.; Grajewski, R.S.; Matos, P.; Kopecky, A.; Heindl, L.M.; Cursiefen, C. Ocular Involvement in COVID-19: Conjunctivitis and More. *Klin Monbl Augenheilkd.* **2021**, *238*, 555–560. [CrossRef] [PubMed]
5. Loffredo, L.; Pacella, F.; Pacella, E.; Tiscione, G.; Oliva, A.; Violi, F. Conjunctivitis and COVID-19: A meta-analysis. *J. Med. Virol.* **2020**, *92*, 1413–1414. [CrossRef]
6. Ahuja, A.S.; Farford, B.A.; Forouhi, M.; Abdin, R.; Salinas, M. The Ocular Manifestations of COVID-19 Through Conjunctivitis. *Cureus* **2020**, *12*, e12218. [CrossRef]
7. Elhusseiny, A.M.; Eleiwa, T.K.; Yacoub, M.S.; George, J.; ElSheikh, R.H.; Haseeb, A.; Kwan, J.; Elsaadani, I.A.; Abo Shanab, S.M.; Solyman, O.; et al. Relationship between screen time and dry eye symptoms in pediatric population during the COVID-19 pandemic. *Ocul. Surf.* **2021**, *22*, 117–119. [CrossRef]
8. Eleiwa, T.K.; Elmaghrabi, A.; Helal, H.G.; Abdelrahman, S.N.; ElSheikh, R.H.; Elhusseiny, A.M. Phlyctenular Keratoconjunctivitis in a Patient With COVID-19 Infection. *Cornea* **2021**, *40*, 1502–1504. [CrossRef]
9. Eleiwa, T.; Abdelrahman, S.N.; ElSheikh, R.H.; Elhusseiny, A.M. Orbital inflammatory disease associated with COVID-19 infection. *J. Am. Assoc. Pediatr. Ophthalmol. Strabismus* **2021**, *25*, 232–234. [CrossRef]
10. Sawalha, K.; Adeodokun, S.; Kamoga, G.R. COVID-19-Induced Acute Bilateral Optic Neuritis. *J. Investig. Med. High Impact Case Rep.* **2020**, *8*, 6018. [CrossRef]
11. Eleiwa, T.K.; Gaier, E.D.; Haseeb, A.; ElSheikh, R.H.; Sallam, A.B.; Elhusseiny, A.M. Adverse Ocular Events following COVID-19 Vaccination. *Inflamm. Res.* **2021**, *70*, 1005–1009. [CrossRef] [PubMed]
12. Ng, X.L.; Betzler, B.K.; Testi, I.; Ho, S.L.; Tien, M.; Ngo, W.K.; Zierhut, M.; Chee, S.P.; Gupta, V.; Pavesio, C.E.; et al. Ocular Adverse Events After COVID-19 Vaccination. *Ocul. Immunol. Inflamm.* **2021**, *29*, 1216–1224. [CrossRef] [PubMed]
13. Bayas, A.; Menacher, M.; Christ, M.; Behrens, L.; Rank, A.; Naumann, M. Bilateral superior ophthalmic vein thrombosis, ischaemic stroke, and immune thrombocytopenia after ChAdOx1 nCoV-19 vaccination. *Lancet* **2021**, *397*, e11. [CrossRef]

14. Crnej, A.; Khoueir, Z.; Cherfan, G.; Saad, A. Acute corneal endothelial graft rejection following COVID-19 vaccination. *J. Fr. Ophtalmol.* **2021**, *44*, e445–e447. [CrossRef]
15. Phylactou, M.; Li, J.O.; Larkin, D. Characteristics of endothelial corneal transplant rejection following immunisation with SARS-CoV-2 messenger RNA vaccine. *Br. J. Ophthalmol.* **2021**, *105*, 893–896. [CrossRef]
16. Rabinovitch, T.; Ben-Arie-Weintrob, Y.; Hareuveni-Blum, T.; Shaer, B.; Vishnevskia-Dai, V.; Shulman, S.; Newman, H.; Biadsy, M.; Masarwa, D.; Fischer, N.; et al. Uveitis after the bnt162b2 mrna vaccination against sars-cov-2 infection: A Possible Association. *Retina* **2021**, *41*, 2462–2471. [CrossRef]
17. ElSheikh, R.H.; Haseeb, A.; Eleiwa, T.K.; Elhusseiny, A.M. Acute Uveitis following COVID-19 Vaccination. *Ocul. Immunol. Inflamm.* **2021**, *29*, 1207–1209. [CrossRef]
18. Lee, C.; Park, K.A.; Ham, D.I.; Seong, M.; Kim, H.J.; Lee, G.I.; Oh, S.Y. Neuroretinitis after the second injection of a SARS-CoV-2-vaccine: A case report. *Am. J. Ophthalmol. Case Rep.* **2022**, *27*, 101592. [CrossRef]
19. Elnahry, A.G.; Asal, Z.B.; Shaikh, N.; Dennett, K.; Abd Elmohsen, M.N.; Elnahry, G.A.; Shehab, A.; Vytopil, M.; Ghaffari, L.; Athappilly, G.K.; et al. Optic neuropathy after COVID-19 vaccination: A report of two cases. *Int. J. Neurosci.* **2021**, 1–7. [CrossRef]
20. Bøhler, A.D.; Strøm, M.E.; Sandvig, K.U.; Moe, M.C.; Jørstad, Ø.K. Acute macular neuroretinopathy following COVID-19 vaccination. *Eye* **2022**, *36*, 644–645. [CrossRef]
21. Book, B.; Schmidt, B.; Foerster, A. Bilateral Acute Macular Neuroretinopathy After Vaccination Against SARS-CoV-2. *JAMA Ophthalmol.* **2021**, *139*, e212471. [CrossRef] [PubMed]
22. Endo, B.; Bahamon, S.; Martínez-Pulgarín, D.F. Central retinal vein occlusion after mRNA SARS-CoV-2 vaccination: A case report. *Indian J. Ophthalmol.* **2021**, *69*, 2865–2866. [CrossRef] [PubMed]
23. Pappaterra, M.C.; Rivera, E.J.; Oliver, A.L. Transient Oculomotor Palsy Following the Administration of the Messenger RNA-1273 Vaccine for SARS-CoV-2 Diplopia Following the COVID-19 Vaccine. *J. Neuroophthalmol.* **2021**, 1369. [CrossRef]
24. Reyes-Capo, D.P.; Stevens, S.M.; Cavuoto, K.M. Acute abducens nerve palsy following COVID-19 vaccination. *J. Am. Assoc. Pediatr. Ophthalmol. Strabismus* **2021**, *25*, 302–303. [CrossRef] [PubMed]
25. Khouri, C.; Roustit, M.; Cracowski, J.L. Adverse event reporting and Bell's palsy risk after COVID-19 vaccination. *Lancet Infect. Dis.* **2021**, *21*, 1490–1491. [CrossRef]
26. Ozonoff, A.; Nanishi, E.; Levy, O. Bell's palsy and SARS-CoV-2 vaccines. *Lancet Infect. Dis.* **2021**, *21*, 450–452. [CrossRef]
27. Shibli, R.; Barnett, O.; Abu-Full, Z.; Gronich, N.; Najjar-Debbiny, R.; Doweck, I.; Rennert, G.; Saliba, W. Association between vaccination with the BNT162b2 mRNA COVID-19 vaccine and Bell's palsy: A population-based study. *Lancet Reg. Health Eur.* **2021**, *11*, 100236. [CrossRef]
28. Wong, I.; Wan, E.; Chui, C.; Li, X.; Chan, E. Adverse event reporting and Bell's palsy risk after COVID-19 vaccination—Authors' reply. *Lancet Infect. Dis.* **2021**, *21*, 1492–1493. [CrossRef]
29. García-Estrada, C.; Gómez-Figueroa, E.; Alban, L.; Arias-Cárdenas, A. Optic neuritis after COVID-19 vaccine application. *Clin. Exp. Neuroimmunol.* **2022**, *13*, 72–74. [CrossRef]
30. Girbardt, C.; Busch, C.; Al-Sheikh, M.; Gunzinger, J.M.; Invernizzi, A.; Xhepa, A.; Unterlauft, J.D.; Rehak, M. Retinal Vascular Events after mRNA and Adenoviral-Vectored COVID-19 Vaccines-A Case Series. *Vaccines* **2021**, *9*, 1349. [CrossRef]
31. Leber, H.M.; Sant'Ana, L.; Konichi da Silva, N.R.; Raio, M.C.; Mazzeo, T.; Endo, C.M.; Nascimento, H.; de Souza, C.E. Acute Thyroiditis and Bilateral Optic Neuritis following SARS-CoV-2 Vaccination with CoronaVac: A Case Report. *Ocul. Immunol. Inflamm.* **2021**, *29*, 1200–1206. [CrossRef] [PubMed]
32. Nachbor, K.M.; Naravane, A.V.; Adams, O.E.; Abel, A.S. Nonarteritic Anterior Ischemic Optic Neuropathy Associated With COVID-19 Vaccination. *J. Neuroophthalmol.* **2021**, *2021*, 1423. [CrossRef] [PubMed]
33. Pawar, N.; Maheshwari, D.; Ravindran, M.; Padmavathy, S. Ophthalmic complications of COVID-19 vaccination. *Indian J. Ophthalmol.* **2021**, *69*, 2900–2902. [CrossRef] [PubMed]
34. Maleki, A.; Look-Why, S.; Manhapra, A.; Foster, C.S. COVID-19 Recombinant mRNA Vaccines and Serious Ocular Inflammatory Side Effects: Real or Coincidence? *J. Ophthalmic. Vis. Res.* **2021**, *16*, 490–501. [CrossRef] [PubMed]
35. Tsukii, R.; Kasuya, Y.; Makino, S. Nonarteritic Anterior Ischemic Optic Neuropathy following COVID-19 Vaccination: Consequence or Coincidence. *Case Rep. Ophthalmol. Med.* **2021**, *2021*, 5126254. [CrossRef]
36. Lin, W.Y.; Wang, J.J.; Lai, C.H. Non-Arteritic Anterior Ischemic Optic Neuropathy Following COVID-19 Vaccination. *Vaccines* **2022**, *10*, 931. [CrossRef]
37. Chung, S.A.; Yeo, S.; Sohn, S.Y. Nonarteritic Anterior Ischemic Optic Neuropathy Following COVID-19 Vaccination: A Case Report. *Korean J. Ophthalmol.* **2022**, *36*, 168–170. [CrossRef]
38. Sanjay, S.; Acharya, I.; Rawoof, A.; Shetty, R. Non-arteritic anterior ischaemic optic neuropathy (NA-AION) and COVID-19 vaccination. *BMJ Case Rep.* **2022**, *15*, e248415. [CrossRef]
39. Roy, M.; Chandra, A.; Roy, S.; Shrotriya, C. Optic neuritis following COVID-19 vaccination: Coincidence or side-effect?—A case series. *Indian J. Ophthalmol.* **2022**, *70*, 679–683. [CrossRef]
40. Elhusseiny, A.M.; Sanders, R.N.; Siddiqui, M.Z.; Sallam, A.B. Non-arteritic Anterior Ischemic Optic Neuropathy with Macular Star following COVID-19 Vaccination. *Ocul. Immunol. Inflamm.* **2022**, *30*, 1274–1277. [CrossRef]
41. Sookaromdee, P.; Wiwanitkit, V. Atypical Optic Neuritis After COVID-19 Vaccination. *J. Neuroophthalmol.* **2022**, 1595. [CrossRef] [PubMed]

42. Valsero Franco, S.; Fonollosa, A. Ischemic Optic Neuropathy After Administration of a SARS-CoV-2 Vaccine: A Report of 2 Cases. *Am. J. Case Rep.* **2022**, *23*, e935095. [CrossRef] [PubMed]
43. Saffra, N.A.; Emborgo, T.S.; Kelman, S.E.; Kirsch, D.S. Presumed Autoimmune Optic Neuropathy After Pfizer-BioNTech (BNT162b2) COVID-19 Vaccine. *J. Neuroophthalmol.* **2022**, 1620. [CrossRef]
44. Rizk, M.; Dunya, I.; Seif, R.; Megarbane, A.; Sadaka, A. A Case of Leber Hereditary Optic Neuropathy Triggered by Pfizer-BioNTech Vaccine: Evidence of Pathogenesis of a Novel Mutation. *J. Neuroophthalmol.* **2022**, 1665. [CrossRef]
45. Kumar, K.; Kohli, P.; Babu, N.; Rajan, R.P.; Ramasamy, K. Bilateral Optic Neuropathy After First Dose of COVID-19 Vaccine. *J. Neuroophthalmol.* **2022**, 1636. [CrossRef]
46. Che, S.A.; Lee, K.Y.; Yoo, Y.J. Bilateral Ischemic Optic Neuropathy From Giant Cell Arteritis Following COVID-19 Vaccination. *J. Neuroophthalmol.* **2022**, 1570. [CrossRef] [PubMed]
47. Raxwal, T.; Akel, Z.; Naidu, J.; Sundaresh, K. Neuro-Ophthalmologic Symptoms Associated with the Moderna mRNA COVID-19 Vaccine: A Case Report. *Cureus* **2022**, *14*, e28523. [CrossRef] [PubMed]
48. Wang, J.; Huang, S.; Yu, Z.; Zhang, S.; Hou, G.; Xu, S. Unilateral optic neuritis after vaccination against the coronavirus disease: Two case reports. *Doc. Ophthalmol.* **2022**, *145*, 65–70. [CrossRef]
49. Haseeb, A.; Elhusseiny, A.M.; Chauhan, M.Z.; Elnahry, A.G. Optic neuropathy after COVID-19 vaccination: Case report and systematic review. *Neuroimmunol. Rep.* **2022**, *2*, 100121. [CrossRef]
50. Helmchen, C.; Buttler, G.M.; Markewitz, R.; Hummel, K.; Wiendl, H.; Boppel, T. Acute bilateral optic/chiasm neuritis with longitudinal extensive transverse myelitis in longstanding stable multiple sclerosis following vector-based vaccination against the SARS-CoV-2. *J. Neurol.* **2022**, *269*, 49–54. [CrossRef]
51. Nagaratnam, S.A.; Ferdi, A.C.; Leaney, J.; Lee, R.L.K.; Hwang, Y.T.; Heard, R. Acute disseminated encephalomyelitis with bilateral optic neuritis following ChAdOx1 COVID-19 vaccination. *BMC Neurol.* **2022**, *22*, 54. [CrossRef] [PubMed]
52. Shirah, B.; Mulla, I.; Aladdin, Y. Optic Neuritis Following the BNT162b2 mRNA COVID-19 Vaccine in a Patient with Systemic Lupus Erythematosus Uncovering the Diagnosis of Neuromyelitis Optica Spectrum Disorders. *Ocul. Immunol. Inflamm.* **2022**, 1–3. [CrossRef] [PubMed]
53. Pirani, V.; Pelliccioni, P.; Carpenè, M.J.; Nicolai, M.; Barbotti, F.; Franceschi, A.; Mariotti, C. Optic neuritis following COVID-19 vaccination: Do autoimmune diseases play a role? *Eur. J. Ophthalmol.* **2022**. [CrossRef] [PubMed]
54. Singu, T.; Nakajima, M.; Ueda, A.; Nakahara, K.; Nomura, T.; Kojima, S.; Inoue, T.; Ueda, M. Transient optic neuritis and perineuritis associated with anti-MOG antibody after SARS-CoV-2 mRNA vaccination. *Neuroimmunol. Rep.* **2022**, *2*, 100077. [CrossRef]
55. Xia, C.; Edwards, R.; Omidvar, B. A Case of Giant Cell Arteritis with a Normal Erythrocyte Sedimentation Rate (ESR) Post ChAdOx1 nCoV-19 Vaccination. *Cureus* **2022**, *14*, e25388. [CrossRef]
56. Netravathi, M.; Dhamija, K.; Gupta, M.; Tamborska, A.; Nalini, A.; Holla, V.V.; Nitish, L.K.; Menon, D.; Pal, P.K.; Seena, V.; et al. COVID-19 vaccine associated demyelination & its association with MOG antibody. *Mult. Scler. Relat. Disord.* **2022**, *60*, 103739. [CrossRef]
57. Hattenhauer, M.G.; Leavitt, J.A.; Hodge, D.O.; Grill, R.; Gray, D.T. Incidence of nonarteritic anterior ischemic optic neuropathy. *Am. J. Ophthalmol.* **1997**, *123*, 103–107. [CrossRef]
58. Hayreh, S.S. Ischemic optic neuropathy. *Prog. Retin. Eye Res.* **2009**, *28*, 34–62. [CrossRef]
59. Hayreh, S.S. Anterior ischemic optic neuropathy. *Clin. Neurosci.* **1997**, *4*, 251–263.
60. Wu, Y.; Zhou, L.M.; Lou, H.; Cheng, J.W.; Wei, R.L. The Association Between Obstructive Sleep Apnea and Nonarteritic Anterior Ischemic Optic Neuropathy: A Systematic Review and Meta-Analysis. *Curr. Eye Res.* **2016**, *41*, 987–992. [CrossRef]
61. Aptel, F.; Khayi, H.; Pépin, J.L.; Tamisier, R.; Levy, P.; Romanet, J.P.; Chiquet, C. Association of Nonarteritic Ischemic Optic Neuropathy with Obstructive Sleep Apnea Syndrome: Consequences for Obstructive Sleep Apnea Screening and Treatment. *JAMA Ophthalmol.* **2015**, *133*, 797–804. [CrossRef] [PubMed]
62. Mojon, D.S.; Hedges, T.R., 3rd; Ehrenberg, B.; Karam, E.Z.; Goldblum, D.; Abou-Chebl, A.; Gugger, M.; Mathis, J. Association between sleep apnea syndrome and nonarteritic anterior ischemic optic neuropathy. *Arch. Ophthalmol.* **2002**, *120*, 601–605. [CrossRef] [PubMed]
63. Sharif, W.; Sheikh, K.; De Silva, I.; Elsherbiny, S. Nonarteritic anterior ischemic optic neuropathy associated with interferon and ribavirin in a patient with hepatitis C. *Am. J. Ophthalmol. Case Rep.* **2017**, *5*, 52–55. [CrossRef] [PubMed]
64. Purvin, V.A. Anterior ischemic optic neuropathy secondary to interferon alfa. *Arch Ophthalmol.* **1995**, *113*, 1041–1044. [CrossRef]
65. Gupta, R.; Singh, S.; Tang, R.; Blackwell, T.A.; Schiffman, J.S. Anterior ischemic optic neuropathy caused by interferon alpha therapy. *Am. J. Med.* **2002**, *112*, 683–684. [CrossRef]
66. Purvin, V.; King, R.; Kawasaki, A.; Yee, R. Anterior ischemic optic neuropathy in eyes with optic disc drusen. *Arch. Ophthalmol.* **2004**, *122*, 48–53. [CrossRef]
67. Newman, W.D.; Dorrell, E.D. Anterior ischemic optic neuropathy associated with disc drusen. *J. Neuroophthalmol.* **1996**, *16*, 7–8. [CrossRef]
68. Elnahry, A.G. Anterior ischemic optic neuropathy in a patient with optic disc Drusen while on FOLFOX Chemotherapy for colon cancer: The value of Occam's Razor and Hickam's dictum. *Rom. J. Ophthalmol.* **2019**, *63*, 174–177.
69. Kawasaki, A.; Purvin, V.A.; Tang, R. Bilateral anterior ischemic optic neuropathy following influenza vaccination. *J. Neuroophthalmol.* **1998**, *18*, 56–59. [CrossRef]

70. Manasseh, G.; Donovan, D.; Shao, E.H.; Taylor, S.R. Bilateral sequential non-arteritic anterior ischaemic optic neuropathy following repeat influenza vaccination. *Case. Rep. Ophthalmol.* **2014**, *5*, 267–269. [CrossRef]
71. Karussis, D.; Petrou, P. The spectrum of post-vaccination inflammatory CNS demyelinating syndromes. *Autoimmun. Rev.* **2014**, *13*, 215–224. [CrossRef] [PubMed]
72. Cines, D.B.; Bussel, J.B. SARS-CoV-2 vaccine-induced immune thrombotic thrombocytopenia. *N. Engl. J. Med.* **2021**, *384*, 2254–2256. [CrossRef] [PubMed]
73. Braithwaite, T.; Subramanian, A.; Petzold, A.; Galloway, J.; Adderley, N.J.; Mollan, S.P.; Plant, G.T.; Nirantharakumar, K.; Denniston, A.K. Trends in Optic Neuritis Incidence and Prevalence in the UK and Association with Systemic and Neurologic Disease. *JAMA Neurol.* **2020**, *77*, 1514–1523. [CrossRef]
74. Lee, M.S.; Grossman, D.; Arnold, A.C.; Sloan, F.A. Incidence of nonarteritic anterior ischemic optic neuropathy: Increased risk among diabetic patients. *Ophthalmology* **2011**, *118*, 959–963. [CrossRef]
75. Testi, I.; Brandão-de-Resende, C.; Agrawal, R.; Pavesio, C. COVID-19 Vaccination Ocular Inflammatory Events Study Group. Ocular inflammatory events following COVID-19 vaccination: A multinational case series. *J. Ophthalmic. Inflamm. Infect.* **2022**, *12*, 4. [CrossRef] [PubMed]
76. Stubgen, J.P. A literature review on optic neuritis following vaccination against virus infections. *Autoimmun. Rev.* **2013**, *12*, 990–997. [CrossRef]
77. Levin, L.A.; Rizzo, J.F., 3rd; Lessell, S. Neural network differentiation of optic neuritis and anterior ischaemic optic neuropathy. *Br. J. Ophthalmol.* **1996**, *80*, 835–839. [CrossRef]
78. Elnahry, A.G.; Elnahry, G.A. Response to: Optic neuritis induced by 5-fluorouracil chemotherapy: Case report and review of the literature. *J. Oncol. Pharm. Pract.* **2020**, *26*, 775. [CrossRef]
79. Raina, A.J.; Gilbar, P.J.; Grewal, G.D.; Holcombe, D.J. Optic neuritis induced by 5-fluorouracil chemotherapy: Case report and review of the literature. *J. Oncol. Pharm. Pract.* **2020**, *26*, 511–516. [CrossRef]
80. Behbehani, R.; Ali, A.; Al-Moosa, A. Risk factors and visual outcome of Non-Arteritic Ischemic Optic Neuropathy (NAION): Experience of a tertiary center in Kuwait. *PLoS ONE* **2021**, *16*, e0247126. [CrossRef]
81. Tsai, R.K.; Liu, Y.T.; Su, M.Y. Risk factors of non-arteritic anterior ischemic optic neuropathy (NAION): Ocular or systemic. *Kaohsiung J. Med. Sci.* **1998**, *14*, 221–225. [PubMed]
82. Jossy, A.; Jacob, N.; Sarkar, S.; Gokhale, T.; Kaliaperumal, S.; Deb, A.K. COVID-19-associated optic neuritis—A case series and review of literature. *Indian J. Ophthalmol.* **2022**, *70*, 310–316. [CrossRef] [PubMed]
83. Assavapongpaiboon, B.; Apinyawasisuk, S.; Jariyakosol, S. Myelin oligodendrocyte glycoprotein antibody-associated optic neuritis with COVID-19 infection: A case report and literature review. *Am. J. Ophthalmol. Case Rep.* **2022**, *26*, 101491. [CrossRef]
84. Rojas-Correa, D.X.; Reche-Sainz, J.A.; Insausti-García, A.; Calleja-García, C.; Ferro-Osuna, M. Post COVID-19 Myelin Oligodendrocyte Glycoprotein Antibody-Associated Optic Neuritis. *Neuroophthalmology* **2021**, *46*, 115–121. [CrossRef] [PubMed]
85. Francis, J.H.; Jaben, K.; Santomasso, B.D.; Canestraro, J.; Abramson, D.H.; Chapman, P.B.; Berkenstock, M.; Aronow, M.E. Immune Checkpoint Inhibitor-Associated Optic Neuritis. *Ophthalmology* **2020**, *127*, 1585–1589. [CrossRef] [PubMed]
86. Francis, J.H.; Jaben, K.; Santomasso, B.D.; Canestraro, J.; Abramson, D.H.; Berkenstock, M.; Aronow, M.E. Reply. *Ophthalmology* **2020**, *127*, e106–e107. [CrossRef]
87. *Causality Assessment of an Adverse Event Following Immunization (AEFI): User Manual for the Revised WHO Classification*, 2nd ed.; 2019 update; World Health Organization: Geneva, Switzerland, 2019.

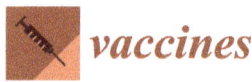

Article

Recurrent and De Novo Toxoplasmosis Retinochoroiditis following Coronavirus Disease 2019 Infection or Vaccination

Mélanie Hébert [1], Soumaya Bouhout [2], Julie Vadboncoeur [2,3] and Marie-Josée Aubin [2,3,4,*]

1. Department of Ophthalmology, Université Laval, Quebec, QC G1V 0A6, Canada
2. Department of Ophthalmology, Université de Montréal, Montreal, QC H3T 1J4, Canada
3. Ophthalmology Department, Centre Universitaire d'Opthalmologie (CUO), Centre Intégré Universitaire de Santé et de Services Sociaux de l'Est-de-l'Île-de-Montréal—Hôpital Maisonneuve-Rosemont, Montreal, QC H1T 2M4, Canada
4. Department of Social and Preventive Medicine, School of Public Health, Université de Montréal, Montreal, QC H3T 1J4, Canada
* Correspondence: marie-josee.aubin@umontreal.ca; Tel.: +1-514-252-3400

Abstract: This study reports three cases of toxoplasmosis retinochoroiditis following coronavirus disease 2019 (COVID-19) infection or vaccination from the national Canadian COVID-19 Eye Registry between December 2020 and September 2021. A 56-year-old male presented 15 days after a positive COVID-19 test with toxoplasmosis retinochoroiditis. He later relapsed 8 days following a first Pfizer-BioNTech vaccine dose. Two patients presented with toxoplasmosis retinochoroiditis following COVID-19 vaccination: A 58-year-old female presenting 4 days following a first Pfizer-BioNTech vaccine dose with anterior uveitis and a posterior pole lesion discovered 3 months later and a 39-year-old female presenting 17 days after a first Moderna vaccine dose. Resolution was achieved with oral clindamycin, oral trimethoprim/sulfamethoxazole, and topical prednisolone acetate 1%. Patients were offered prophylactic trimethoprim/sulfamethoxazole for subsequent doses without relapse. Following COVID-19 infection or vaccination, patients may be at risk for toxoplasmosis retinochoroiditis. Prophylactic antibiotics for future doses may be offered to patients with known ocular toxoplasmosis to prevent recurrence.

Keywords: coronavirus disease 2019; vaccination; mRNA vaccine; SARS-CoV-2; toxoplasmosis retinochoroiditis; inflammation; antibiotic prophylaxis; ophthalmic adverse events; COVID-19 vaccination

Citation: Hébert, M.; Bouhout, S.; Vadboncoeur, J.; Aubin, M.-J. Recurrent and De Novo Toxoplasmosis Retinochoroiditis following Coronavirus Disease 2019 Infection or Vaccination. *Vaccines* **2022**, *10*, 1692. https://doi.org/10.3390/vaccines10101692

Academic Editor: Rohan Bir Singh

Received: 11 August 2022
Accepted: 30 September 2022
Published: 10 October 2022

Publisher's Note: MDPI stays neutral with regard to jurisdictional claims in published maps and institutional affiliations.

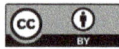

Copyright: © 2022 by the authors. Licensee MDPI, Basel, Switzerland. This article is an open access article distributed under the terms and conditions of the Creative Commons Attribution (CC BY) license (https://creativecommons.org/licenses/by/4.0/).

1. Introduction

Toxoplasmosis, caused by the protozoan parasite *Toxoplasma gondii*, is an opportunistic infection which can affect healthy adults but targets immunosuppressed people, causing more severe disease [1]. When this affects the eye, ocular toxoplasmosis can cause severe vision loss especially with macular involvement [1,2]. Many causes of relative immune suppression have reportedly caused reactivations of ocular toxoplasmosis, such as dexamethasone intravitreal implants [3] and azathioprine treatment for inflammatory bowel disease [4].

Another emerging cause of relative immunosuppression is the coronavirus disease 2019 (COVID-19). It triggers dysfunction and reduced numbers of T cells, natural killer cells, monocytes, and dendritic cells [5]. This may explain reports of de novo infections or reactivations following COVID-19 disease, including herpes simplex keratitis [6] and herpes zoster ophthalmicus even in children [7].

Another possible immune modulator is COVID-19 vaccination. These were shown to be safe and effective [8–10], allowing for the reduction in virus transmission [11,12]. However, these have also been associated with autoimmune and infectious diseases, such as graft rejections [13] and herpes zoster ophthalmicus [14].

Changes in immunity related to both COVID-19 infection and vaccination may increase the risk of ocular toxoplasmosis relapse. Three cases following COVID-19 vaccination have recently been reported [15]. This case series aims to report three cases of new or recurrent toxoplasmosis retinochoroiditis following COVID-19 infection or vaccination.

2. Methods

This study reports results from the COVID-19 Eye Registry (COVER). COVER is a national Canadian registry recording ocular manifestations following COVID-19 infection or vaccination [16]. Patients who were reported between December 2020 and September 2021 with new or recurrent toxoplasmosis retinochoroiditis were presented. Basic demographic data, type of vaccine (i.e., Moderna Spikevax® (ModernaTX, Inc., Cambridge, MA, USA), Pfizer-BioNTech Comirnaty® (BioNTech Manufacturing GmbH, Mainz, Germany), or AstraZeneca Vaxzevria® (AstraZeneca BioPharmaceuticals, Cambridge, England)), timing of presentation relative to COVID-19 infection or vaccination, clinical presentation, management, and final visual acuity (VA) are reported.

3. Results

Three eyes of three patients were reported. Of these, a patient presented with de novo toxoplasmosis retinochoroiditis following COVID-19 infection followed by reactivation after a first dose of COVID-19 vaccine. Two other patients presented with unilateral panuveitis and active chorioretinal lesions following COVID-19 vaccination.

3.1. Case 1

A 56-year-old male known for high blood pressure and oral herpes simplex virus, with no history of toxoplasmosis, presented with hypertensive anterior uveitis in his right eye (OD). Initial VA was 20/40-2 and dilated fundus examination (DFE) at the time did not show any chorioretinal lesion. He was found to be COVID-19 positive 10 days later. At follow-up 15 days after his positive COVID-19 test, his VA had decreased to 20/70 and repeat DFE showed a unilateral white chorioretinal lesion in the posterior pole without pigmentary or atrophic scarring (Figure 1) associated with vitritis, consistent with ocular toxoplasmosis. Anti-toxoplasmosis immunoglobulin (Ig) G was positive (97.80 g/L), while anti-toxoplasmosis IgM was negative when requested at the follow-up visit. Moreover, the patient tested negative for syphilis but positive for HLA-B27. Resolution was achieved with a course of topical prednisolone acetate 1% with oral clindamycin 450 mg three times daily and trimethoprim/sulfamethoxazole 800/160 mg twice daily over 2 months. One month following the end of treatment, VA was 20/20, no inflammation was observed, and the chorioretinal lesions were cicatricial and inactive. He later presented a retinochoroiditis relapse 8 days following a first dose of Pfizer-BioNTech vaccine, which resolved with the same therapeutic regimen.

A prophylactic course of trimethoprim/sulfamethoxazole 800/160 mg three times per week was started 2 days before his second dose and continued over 2 weeks. No recurrence was observed. He was not seen in clinic prior to his third booster dose to receive a prophylactic prescription. Nevertheless, no recurrence was detected when assessed 1 week later. His final VA was 20/25-1.

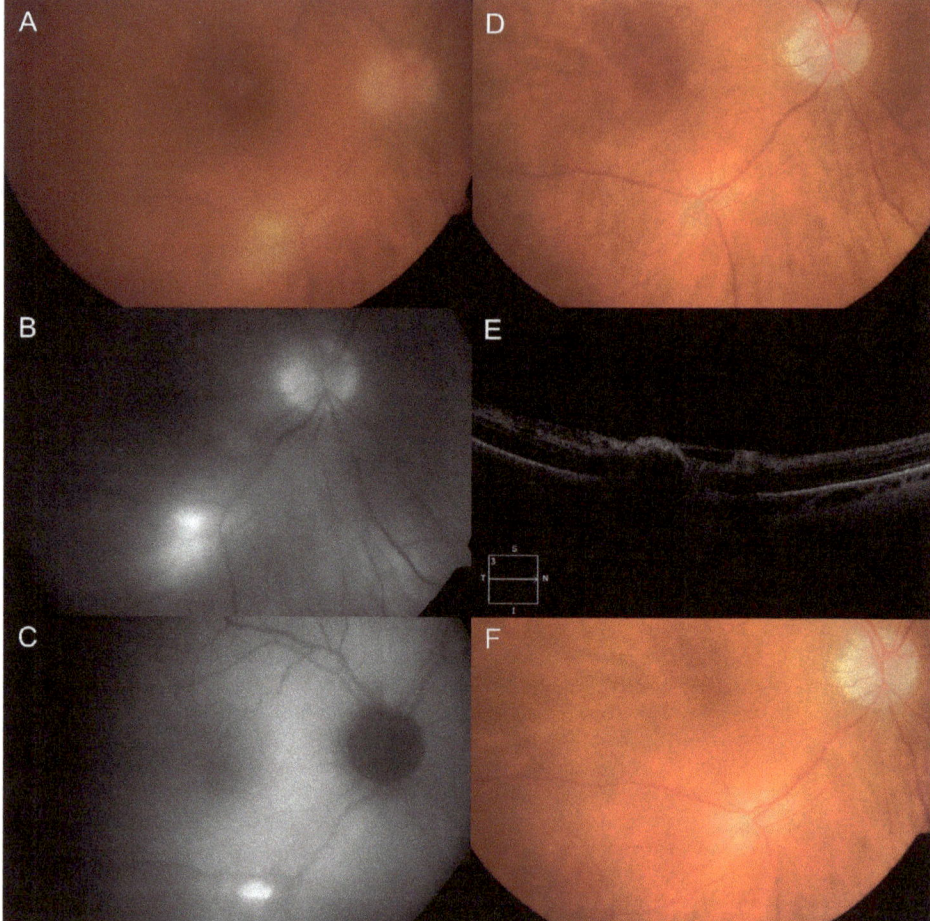

Figure 1. Case 1 with active toxoplasmosis retinochoroiditis following a diagnosis of coronavirus disease 2019 (COVID-19) and recurrence after COVID-19 vaccination. (**A**) Color fundus photography showing a single, white, deep chorioretinal lesion along the inferior arcade with vitritis at initial presentation. (**B**) Initial red-free monochromatic fundus photograph showing the same lesion which becomes more apparent. (**C**) Initial fundus autofluorescence showing a hyperautofluorescent lesion with distinct borders corresponding to the retinochoroiditis. (**D**) Four months after presentation, the lesion is now cicatricial without vitritis with (**E**) a horizontal optical coherence tomography scan through the lesion. (**F**) The patient had a recurrence 1 month later, 8 days after his first COVID-19 vaccine dose.

3.2. Case 2

A 58-year-old female known for high blood pressure, dyslipidemia, type II diabetes mellitus, and fibromyalgia was previously treated for anterior uveitis in her left eye (OS) by an optometrist 4 days following her first dose of Pfizer-BioNTech vaccine with topical prednisolone acetate 1% over 1 month. It is unknown whether DFE was performed initially and whether signs of vitritis or chorioretinal lesions were already present. Three months post-vaccination, she was referred to our service for increasing floaters, discomfort, and VA of 20/50. Examination revealed panuveitis with posterior hyaloid precipitates and a slightly elevated, yellow whitish lesion with surrounding pigmentary changes

(Figure 2A). Serological testing revealed positive anti-toxoplasmosis IgG (18.80 g/L) and negative anti-toxoplasmosis IgM. Other uveitis testing was negative, including HLA-B27, antinuclear antibodies, anti-double stranded DNA, extractable nuclear antigen antibodies, antineutrophil cytoplasmic antibodies, Lyme, syphilis, and QuantiFERON-TB Gold. She was treated with topical prednisolone acetate 1% four times daily tapered over a month, 6 weeks of trimethoprim/sulfamethoxazole 800/160 mg twice daily, and a short course of oral prednisone starting at 40 mg daily tapered over 5 weeks. Six weeks after the treatment started, there was no intraocular inflammation, the chorioretinal lesion was cicatricial (Figure 2B), and final VA was 20/20. The patient received the same prophylactic trimethoprim/sulfamethoxazole regimen as Case 1 for her second vaccine doses, but not for her third dose, and she did not relapse in both instances.

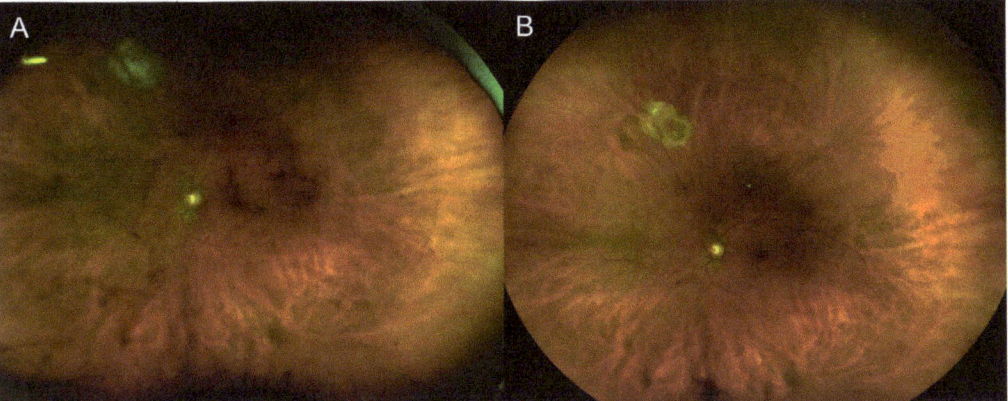

Figure 2. Case 2 with active toxoplasmosis retinochoroiditis 3 months after a first dose of COVID-19 vaccination. (**A**) Fundus photography showing the initial elevated, yellow whitish lesion with surrounding pigmentary changes. (**B**) Six weeks later, the main lesion became cicatricial.

The patient was not known to have had a previous COVID-19 infection prior to their vaccination or during follow-up. At follow-up, she later received a dose of pneumococcal polysaccharide vaccine (Pneumovax® 23, Merck & Co., Inc., Kenilworth, NJ, USA) and had a recurrence of retinochoroiditis that responded to the same treatment of prednisolone.

3.3. Case 3

A 39-year-old female presented 17 days after a first dose of Moderna vaccine with floaters and VA of 20/100. This patient was known to the center's uveitis service for toxoplasmosis retinochoroiditis since 2011 with no relapse since 2016 without prophylaxis and was otherwise healthy. Her initial exam showed panuveitis with an active fundus lesion around the known chorioretinal scar (Figure 3). She was treated with topical prednisolone acetate 1%, oral clindamycin 600 mg three times daily and trimethoprim/sulfamethoxazole 800/160 mg twice daily over 6 weeks, and a short course of oral prednisone starting at 10 mg with a taper over 4 weeks. She received her second dose of Moderna 12 weeks after presentation while still under trimethoprim/sulfamethoxazole 800/160 mg twice daily without recurrence. At her last follow-up 2 months later, the final VA was 20/20 and the lesion was cicatricial 4 months after the initial presentation. She was offered the same prophylactic trimethoprim/sulfamethoxazole regimen as Case 1 in the event of a third booster dose. The patient was not known to have had a previous COVID-19 infection prior to their vaccination or during follow-up.

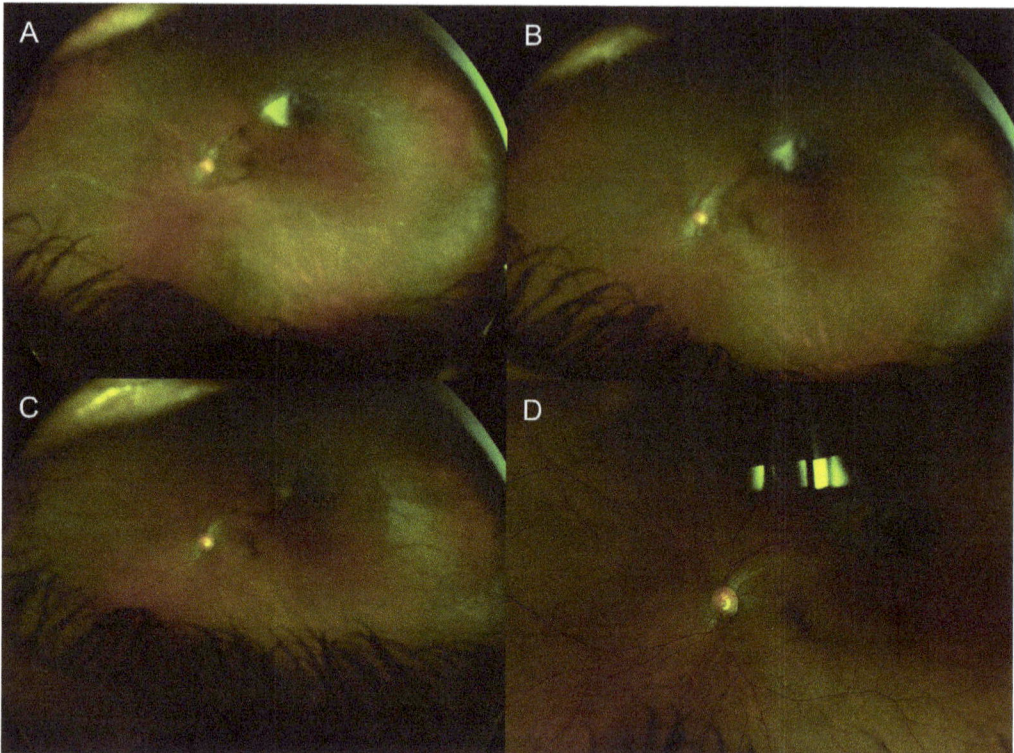

Figure 3. Case 3 with a previous, cicatricial toxoplasmosis scar with recurrence of active toxoplasmosis retinochoroiditis 17 days after COVID-19 vaccination. (**A**) Fundus photography showcasing the old toxoplasmosis scar with an area of active retinochoroiditis adjacent to it. There is diffuse sheathing consistent with vasculitis. (**B**) Three weeks later, the new area of retinochoroiditis has decreased in size and activity as did the vasculitis. (**C**) At seven weeks, there was still an area of activity within the chorioretinal scar, thus the treatment was further extended. (**D**) At final follow-up 4 months later, the area had scarred, and no inflammation was observed.

4. Discussion

We report one case of toxoplasmosis retinochoroiditis following COVID-19 infection with recurrence after COVID-19 vaccination, as well as two cases of toxoplasmosis retinochoroiditis following COVID-19 vaccination. Both Cases 1 and 3 had recurrences of ocular toxoplasmosis within 2–3 weeks following COVID-19 vaccination. Both had previous episodes of toxoplasmosis retinochoroiditis (after COVID-19 infection in Case 1), which may explain the rapid reactivation following vaccination. In Case 2, anterior uveitis was initially diagnosed 4 days after vaccination. As an outside optometrist assessed her, it is unknown whether DFE may have revealed vitritis and retinochoroidal involvement. This patient also recurred following pneumococcal polysaccharide vaccine.

COVID-19 infection disrupts the function and number of T cells, natural killer cells, monocytes, and dendritic cells [5]. This may increase ocular toxoplasmosis reactivation risk as the principal cytokine responsible for the response against *T. gondii* is interferon (IFN)-γ. It is produced by CD4 and CD8 positive T cells, natural killer cells, and neutrophils through a trigger by interleukin 12, produced by dendritic cells [1]. Production of IFN-γ is reduced in active COVID-19 infection [5]. In IFN-γ deficient mice, the extent of toxoplasmosis is more severe with cerebral dissemination and occasionally more severe ocular toxoplasmosis [17]. In humans, serum IFN-γ levels are lower in patients with ocular toxoplasmosis reactivations and old toxoplasmosis scars [18]. Decreased aqueous humor IFN-γ is also associated with increased risk of severe ocular complications and longer time to recovery from reactivations [18]. This is consistent with the fact that various polymorphisms of the *IFNG* gene modify chorioretinal scar severity [1].

The pathophysiology for ocular toxoplasmosis reactivation following COVID-19 vaccination is less clear. The Spike protein targeted by all currently available vaccines can produce robust CD4 and CD8 positive T cell responses [19]. This in turn should produce IFN-γ which should also be efficient against *T. gondii* as part of the innate and early adaptive immune response. This production of IFN-γ is important in protecting against COVID-19, since patients with deficient IFN-γ do not mount an appropriate defense against COVID-19 in the early phases of the disease, leading to more severe illness [19]. However, whether there may be a phenomenon of immune modulation responsible for decreased protection against toxoplasmosis in the immediate post-vaccination period remains to be studied. Moreover, this holds true for other vaccines, such as in Case 2 where the patient experienced a second reactivation after pneumococcal polysaccharide vaccination, which may suggest an underlying immune reaction to vaccinations in general, and not specifically to COVID-19, in susceptible patients. Additionally, with the breadth of the vaccination campaigns around the world, it is also possible that ocular findings after vaccination may occur coincidentally without a true association.

Whether patients known for ocular toxoplasmosis might require prophylactic antibiotics for COVID-19 vaccination is debatable. Antibiotic treatments for toxoplasmosis include combinations of pyrimethamine, sulfadiazine, and leucovorin or trimethoprim-sulfamethoxazole [20,21]. For prophylaxis, trimethoprim-sulfamethoxazole is the preferred option [20]. There is a lack of studies that provide level I evidence to support the antibiotics treatment of toxoplasmosis retinochoroiditis, as it does not seem to reduce lesion size or improve visual outcomes [21,22]. However, there does seem to be a reduced risk of reactivation with prophylactic treatment [21,22], which could be of particular interest in the setting of COVID-19 vaccination in patients with known toxoplasmosis retinochoroiditis, especially in those with posterior pole lesions. This remains to be studied but could be discussed with patients as possible management options in the absence of more evidence.

Limitations

There is no definitive causal relationship between COVID-19 infections or vaccines and toxoplasmosis retinochoroiditis. The temporal relationship makes this plausible although it could be a coincidence given the billions of vaccine doses administered worldwide. Since recurrences of ocular toxoplasmosis are treatable and preventable, it should not deter vaccination efforts. Similarly, we could not be certain of the temporality of Case 2 wherein a reliable DFE was not performed despite increasing floaters and discomfort between 4 days and 3 months post-vaccination.

5. Conclusions

In conclusion, following COVID-19 infection or vaccination, patients may be at risk for new or relapsing toxoplasmosis retinochoroiditis, possibly due to changes in immune modulation. Physicians should be aware of this and may propose prophylactic antibiotics for future vaccine doses in patients known for ocular toxoplasmosis, especially those with vision-threatening posterior pole lesions.

Author Contributions: Conceptualization, M.H., S.B., J.V. and M.-J.A.; methodology, M.H., S.B., J.V. and M.-J.A.; validation, M.H., S.B., J.V. and M.-J.A.; resources, M.-J.A.; writing—original draft preparation, M.H. and S.B.; writing—review and editing, J.V. and M.-J.A.; visualization, M.H.; supervision, J.V. and M.-J.A.; project administration, M.-J.A.; funding acquisition, M.H. and M.-J.A. All authors have read and agreed to the published version of the manuscript.

Funding: This project is partially funded by the Common Infrastructures program of the Vision Health Research Network and the philanthropic funds of the Vice-Dean of Research and Development of the Université de Montréal.

Institutional Review Board Statement: The Institutional Review Board of the CIUSSS de l'Est-de-l'Île-de-Montréal approved the COVID-19 Eye Registry (MP-12-2021-2307) and the publication of cases from the registry (2022-2935).

Informed Consent Statement: Patients provided written consent for inclusion in the registry.

Data Availability Statement: The data are available upon reasonable request made to the data access committee of the COVID-19 Eye Registry.

Acknowledgments: The authors wish to acknowledge and thank the patients for their participation in the registry.

Conflicts of Interest: The authors declare no conflict of interest.

References

1. Smith, J.R.; Ashander, L.M.; Arruda, S.L.; Cordeiro, C.A.; Lie, S.; Rochet, E.; Belfort, R., Jr.; Furtado, J.M. Pathogenesis of ocular toxoplasmosis. *Prog. Retin. Eye Res.* **2021**, *81*, 100882. [CrossRef] [PubMed]
2. Vishnevskia-Dai, V.; Achiron, A.; Buhbut, O.; Berar, O.V.; Musika, A.A.; Elyashiv, S.M.; Hecht, I. Chorio-retinal toxoplasmosis: Treatment outcomes, lesion evolution and long-term follow-up in a single tertiary center. *Int. Ophthalmol.* **2020**, *40*, 811–821. [CrossRef] [PubMed]
3. Olson, D.J.; Parhiz, A.T.; Wirthlin, R.S. Reactivation of Latent Toxoplasmosis Following Dexamethasone Implant Injection. *Ophthalmic Surg. Lasers Imaging Retin.* **2016**, *47*, 1050–1052. [CrossRef] [PubMed]
4. Puga, M.; Carpio, D.; Sampil, M.; Zamora, M.J.; Fernandez-Salgado, E. Ocular Toxoplasmosis Reactivation in a Patient With Inflammatory Bowel Disease Under Treatment With Azathioprine. *J. Clin. Gastroenterol.* **2016**, *50*, 610. [CrossRef] [PubMed]
5. Zhou, R.; To, K.K.; Wong, Y.C.; Liu, L.; Zhou, B.; Li, X.; Huang, H.; Mo, Y.; Luk, T.Y.; Lau, T.T.; et al. Acute SARS-CoV-2 Infection Impairs Dendritic Cell and T Cell Responses. *Immunity* **2020**, *53*, 864–877.e5. [CrossRef]
6. Majtanova, N.; Kriskova, P.; Keri, P.; Fellner, Z.; Majtan, J.; Kolar, P. Herpes Simplex Keratitis in Patients with SARS-CoV-2 Infection: A Series of Five Cases. *Medicina* **2021**, *57*, 412. [CrossRef]
7. Nofal, A.; Fawzy, M.M.; Sharaf ELDeen, S.M.; El-Hawary, E.E. Herpes zoster ophthalmicus in COVID-19 patients. *Int. J. Dermatol.* **2020**, *59*, 1545–1546. [CrossRef]
8. Polack, F.P.; Thomas, S.J.; Kitchin, N.; Absalon, J.; Gurtman, A.; Lockhart, S.; Perez, J.L.; Marc, G.P.; Pérez, G.; Moreira, E.D.; et al. Safety and Efficacy of the BNT162b2 mRNA Covid-19 Vaccine. *N. Engl. J. Med.* **2020**, *383*, 2603–2615. [CrossRef]
9. Baden, L.R.; El Sahly, H.M.; Essink, B.; Kotloff, K.; Frey, S.; Novak, R.; Diemert, D.; Spector, S.A.; Rouphael, N.; Creech, C.B.; et al. Efficacy and Safety of the mRNA-1273 SARS-CoV-2 Vaccine. *N. Engl. J. Med.* **2021**, *384*, 403–416. [CrossRef]
10. Voysey, M.; Clemens, S.A.; Madhi, S.A.; Weckx, L.Y.; Folegatti, P.M.; Aley, P.K.; Angus, B.; Baillie, V.L.; Barnabas, S.L.; Bhorat, Q.E.; et al. Safety and efficacy of the ChAdOx1 nCoV-19 vaccine (AZD1222) against SARS-CoV-2: An interim analysis of four randomised controlled trials in Brazil, South Africa, and the UK. *Lancet* **2021**, *397*, 99–111. [CrossRef]
11. Amit, S.; Regev-Yochay, G.; Afek, A.; Kreiss, Y.; Leshem, E. Early rate reductions of SARS-CoV-2 infection and COVID-19 in BNT162b2 vaccine recipients. *Lancet* **2021**, *397*, 875–877. [CrossRef]
12. Nordström, P.; Ballin, M.; Nordström, A. Association Between Risk of COVID-19 Infection in Nonimmune Individuals and COVID-19 Immunity in Their Family Members. *JAMA Intern. Med.* **2021**, *181*, 1–8. [CrossRef] [PubMed]
13. Abousy, M.; Bohm, K.; Prescott, C.; Bonsack, J.M.; Rowhani-Farid, A.; Eghrari, A.O. Bilateral EK Rejection After COVID-19 Vaccine. *Eye Contact Lens.* **2021**, *47*, 625–628. [CrossRef] [PubMed]
14. Papasavvas, I.; de Courten, C.; Herbort, C.P. Varicella-zoster virus reactivation causing herpes zoster ophthalmicus (HZO) after SARS-CoV-2 vaccination–report of three cases. *J. Ophthalmic Inflamm. Infect.* **2021**, *11*, 28. [CrossRef]
15. Bolletta, E.; Iannetta, D.; Mastrofilippo, V.; De Simone, L.; Gozzi, F.; Croci, S.; Bonacini, M.; Belloni, L.; Zerbini, A.; Adani, C.; et al. Uveitis and Other Ocular Complications Following COVID-19 Vaccination. *J. Clin. Med.* **2021**, *10*, 5960. [CrossRef]
16. Hébert, M.; Buys, Y.M.; Damji, K.F.; Yin, V.T.; Aubin, M.J. Data reporting in ophthalmology during COVID-19 pandemic: Need for a Canadian registry. *Can. J. Ophthalmol.* **2021**, *56*, e75–e76. [CrossRef]
17. Jones, L.A.; Alexander, J.; Roberts, C.W. Ocular toxoplasmosis: In the storm of the eye. *Parasite Immunol.* **2006**, *28*, 635–642. [CrossRef]
18. Rudzinski, M.; Argüelles, C.; Couto, C.; Oubiña, J.R.; Reina, S. Immune Mediators against Toxoplasma Gondii during Reactivation of Toxoplasmic Retinochoroiditis. *Ocul. Immunol. Inflamm.* **2019**, *27*, 949–957. [CrossRef]
19. Sette, A.; Crotty, S. Adaptive immunity to SARS-CoV-2 and COVID-19. *Cell* **2021**, *184*, 861–880. [CrossRef]
20. Gajurel, K.; Dhakal, R.; Montoya, J.G. Toxoplasma prophylaxis in haematopoietic cell transplant recipients: A review of the literature and recommendations. *Curr. Opin. Infect. Dis.* **2015**, *28*, 283–292. [CrossRef]

21. Pradhan, E.; Bhandari, S.; Gilbert, R.E.; Stanford, M. Antibiotics versus no treatment for toxoplasma retinochoroiditis. *Cochrane Database Syst Rev.* **2016**, *5*. [CrossRef] [PubMed]
22. Kim, S.J.; Scott, I.U.; Brown, G.C.; Brown, M.M.; Ho, A.C.; Ip, M.S.; Recchia, F.M. Interventions for toxoplasma retinochoroiditis: A report by the American Academy of Ophthalmology. *Ophthalmology* **2013**, *120*, 371–378. [CrossRef] [PubMed]

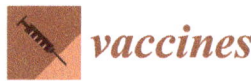

Article

Glaucoma Cases Following SARS-CoV-2 Vaccination: A VAERS Database Analysis

Rohan Bir Singh [1,2,3], Uday Pratap Singh Parmar [4], Wonkyung Cho [1] and Parul Ichhpujani [4,*]

1. Massachusetts Eye and Ear, Department of Ophthalmology, Harvard Medical School, Boston, MA 02114, USA
2. Department of Ophthalmology, Leiden University Medical Center, 2333 Leiden, The Netherlands
3. Discipline of Ophthalmology and Visual Sciences, Faculty of Health and Medical Sciences, Adelaide Medical School, University of Adelaide, Adelaide 5000, Australia
4. Glaucoma Service, Department of Ophthalmology, Government Medical College and Hospital, Chandigarh 160019, India
* Correspondence: parul77@rediffmail.com

Abstract: Background: To counter the rapidly spreading severe acute respiratory syndrome coronavirus 2 (SARS-CoV-2), global vaccination efforts were initiated in December 2020. We assess the risk of glaucoma following SARS-CoV-2 vaccination and evaluate its onset interval and clinical presentations in patients. **Methods:** We performed a retrospective analysis of the glaucoma cases reported to the Vaccine Adverse Event Reporting System (VAERS) database between 16 December 2020, and 30 April 2022. We assessed the crude reporting rate of glaucoma, clinical presentations, onset duration, and associated risk factors. **Results:** During this period, 161 glaucoma cases were reported, with crude reporting rates (per million doses) of 0.09, 0.06, and 0.07 for BNT162b2, mRNA-1273, and Ad26.COV2.S, respectively. The mean age of the patients was 60.41 ± 17.56 years, and 67.7% were women. More than half (56.6%) of the cases were reported within the first week of vaccination. The cumulative-incidence analysis showed a higher risk of glaucoma in patients who received the BNT162b2 vaccines compared with mRNA-1273 ($p = 0.05$). **Conclusions:** The incidence of glaucoma following vaccination with BNT162b2, mRNA-1273, or Ad26.COV2.S is extremely rare. Amongst the patients diagnosed with glaucoma, the onset interval of adverse events was shorter among those who received the BNT162b2 and rAd26.COV2.S vaccines compared with mRNA-1273. Most glaucoma cases were reported within the first week following vaccination in female patients and from the fifth to seventh decade. This study provides insights into the possible temporal association between reported glaucoma events and SARS-CoV-2 vaccines; however, further investigations are required to identify the potential causality link and pathological mechanisms.

Keywords: SARS-CoV-2 vaccines; glaucoma; VAERS; adverse events; COVID-19

Citation: Singh, R.B.; Parmar, U.P.S.; Cho, W.; Ichhpujani, P. Glaucoma Cases Following SARS-CoV-2 Vaccination: A VAERS Database Analysis. *Vaccines* **2022**, *10*, 1630. https://doi.org/10.3390/vaccines10101630

Academic Editor: François Meurens

Received: 1 September 2022
Accepted: 26 September 2022
Published: 28 September 2022

Publisher's Note: MDPI stays neutral with regard to jurisdictional claims in published maps and institutional affiliations.

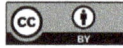

Copyright: © 2022 by the authors. Licensee MDPI, Basel, Switzerland. This article is an open access article distributed under the terms and conditions of the Creative Commons Attribution (CC BY) license (https://creativecommons.org/licenses/by/4.0/).

1. Introduction

In response to the COVID-19 pandemic, large-scale global vaccination efforts were launched in December 2020 [1]. As the COVID-19 vaccines were approved for emergency-use authorization by the United States Food and Drug Administration (FDA), the Centers for Disease Control and Prevention (CDC) expanded its passive surveillance system (known as the Vaccine Adverse Event Reporting System (VAERS)) to include a wide array of adverse events of interest, including ophthalmic disorders, such as glaucoma [2].

Glaucoma is a group of ocular disorders that cause characteristic optic neuropathy with corresponding visual-field defects that result from the progressive degeneration of the retinal ganglion cells in the optic disc and the loss of their axons in the optic nerve [3]. In 2020, an estimated 76.02 million people were reported to have glaucoma worldwide [4]. A raised intraocular pressure (IOP) has been identified as a significant risk factor. These pathological changes lead to progressive peripheral-visual-field defects and may result in blindness. Despite the clinical insights into primary and secondary glaucoma, the pathological mechanisms at the cellular and subcellular levels are poorly understood, and the factors that significantly contribute to the disease progression are yet to be delineated [5]. Although several reports highlight ocular adverse events associated with COVID-19 vaccination, the literature associating COVID-19 vaccination with glaucoma is sparse. Moreover, the COVID-19 vaccine-related information portals categorically report the absence of evidence linking vaccination with glaucoma.

We used the VAERS database to evaluate the reports of glaucoma cases for three FDA-approved COVID-19 vaccines: BNT162b2 (Pfizer Inc./BioNTech SE, Mainz, Germany), mRNA-1273 (Moderna Therapeutics Inc., Cambridge, MA, USA), and Ad26.COV2.S (Janssen Pharmaceuticals, Beerse, Belgium). We determined the crude reporting rate of glaucoma in vaccine recipients since the initiation of the vaccination program. Additionally, we assessed the clinical characteristics and association between age, sex, and duration of onset (following vaccination) in patients who received one of the three vaccines.

2. Methods

VAERS is a passive surveillance platform that functions as an early warning system for potential vaccine related adverse events [2]. The VAERS data are available through Wide-ranging Online Data for Epidemiologic Research (WONDER), a database developed and operated by the CDC, an agency of the United States federal government. The VAERS database compiles reports of all post-vaccination adverse events from patients, parents (for minor patients), clinicians, vaccine manufacturers, and regulatory bodies globally. The database includes a detailed report of the adverse events experienced by patients following vaccination. The data recorded in VAERS are verified by third-party professional coders who assign appropriate medical terminology (based on the preferred terms of the Medical Dictionary for Regulatory Activities) from the data in the submitted reports [6]. A false VAERS report violates federal law (18 U.S. Code § 1001) and is punishable by a fine and imprisonment. CDC WONDER allows access to the information freely, as well as the use, copying, distributing, or publishing of this information without additional or explicit permission [7]. This study was conducted in compliance with the tenets of the Declaration of Helsinki and the National Statement on Ethical Conduct in Human Research 2007. As the study includes publicly available, deidentified anonymous data, the University of Adelaide Human Research Ethics Committee exempted it from ethical review.

The VAERS data included in this study were accessed via CDC WONDER on April 30, 2022 [8]. The data query included all SARS-CoV-2 vaccine-adverse events for all vaccine types administered to patients of all ages and genders for glaucoma (unspecified type), angle-closure glaucoma, open-angle glaucoma, uveitic glaucoma, and uveitis-glaucoma–hyphema syndrome. The results were grouped by symptoms, age, sex, state/territory, and onset interval. The additional measures included in the results were—an adverse-event description, lab data, current illness, adverse events after prior vaccination, medications at the time of vaccination, and history/allergies. The data included in the analysis were clinical presentation, date of vaccination and adverse-event onset, ocular and systemic history, and prescribed drugs and surgeries performed on the patients before the presentation. Some of the patients' reports also included the interventions post-glaucoma diagnosis.

The unspecified glaucoma data were stratified broadly into open-angle glaucoma (OAG) and angle-closure glaucoma (ACG), as per the reported clinical presentations by a glaucoma specialist (PI). The patients presenting with elevated IOP and general ocular symptoms, such as eye pain without any associated ocular morbidity, were broadly considered open-angle glaucoma. The patients who were categorically reported with vision loss/blindness associated with colored haloes and redness were classified as angle-closure glaucoma. However, this classification may have discrepancies as the gonioscopy findings were not reported.

3. Statistical Analysis

The statistical analysis was performed using R Studio (R Foundation for Statistical Computing, Vienna, Austria). The crude reporting rates were estimated using the number of glaucoma reports (by vaccine type) per million SARS-CoV-2 vaccine doses administered. We performed a descriptive analysis of the social and demographic characteristics and vaccination data. We assessed the association between the onset interval of glaucoma and the vaccine type, age, sex, and dosage using the one-way analysis of variance (ANOVA) test. The t-test was used to evaluate the association between glaucoma diagnosis and a prior history of COVID-19. A cumulative-incidence analysis was performed for BNT162b2 and mRNA-1273 vaccines. The Ad26.COV2.S vaccine was excluded from this analysis due to few reports. As the primary outcome measure (i.e., glaucoma diagnosis) was categorical, the analysis was performed to investigate the risk factors associated with it using Pearson's chi-square test of association. The missing values in the data were indicated and Na.rm code was used to account for them during the analysis. The onset-interval data are reported as means ± standard errors of means (SEMs).

4. Results

A total of 2,061,557,270 COVID-19 vaccine doses were administered during the study period: 80.7% were BNT162b2, 16.8% were mRNA-1273, and 2.5% were Ad26.COV2.S [1]. During this period, 1,250,310 (0.06% of all doses) adverse events post-COVID-19 vaccinations were recorded in CDC VAERS, including 166 reports of glaucoma [2]. In our analysis, 161 reports were included, four were duplicated, and one report did not include any information except the type of vaccine administered. The cases were reported by drug regulatory agencies (n = 99, 61.5%), physicians (n = 18, 11.2%), directly by patients (n = 26, 16.1%), and vaccine manufacturers (n = 16, 9.9%). The estimated crude reporting rates (per million doses) for BNT162b2, mRNA-1273, and Ad26.COV2.S were 0.09, 0.06, and 0.07, respectively. All the cases in the cohort were classified as "medically significant" adverse events by the CDC VAERS. The average age of the patients included in the study was 60.41 ± 17.56 years, and 67.7% (n = 109) were female (Table 1). The cases were reported from the United States (48, 28.81%), Europe (86, 53.4%), and Asia (18, 11.2%) (Supplementary Table S1). The state-by-state crude reporting rates for the three vaccines administered in the United States are reported in Supplementary Table S2.

In the study cohort, the majority of the patients (n = 130, 80.7%) were administered the BNT162b2 vaccine, while 27 patients (16.8%) received the mRNA-1273 vaccine, and four patients (2.5%) received the rAd26.COV2.S vaccine (Table 2). Most of the cases (n = 91, 56.5%) were reported within the first week, including 18% (n = 29) of the cases on the day of vaccination (Figure 1).

A total of 77 cases (47.8%) were reported after the first dose, 59 cases (36.6%) were reported after the second dose, and 13 cases (8.1%) were reported after the third dose of the vaccine (Figure 2). Only five patients (3.1%) reported a prior history of COVID-19. On stratifying the patients based on the clinical descriptions, we found that most of the cases (n = 105, 65.2%) had OAG. The patients presented with ocular pain (n = 60, 37.3%), reduced/blurry vision (47, 29.2%), and complete vision loss/blindness (n = 35, 21.7%). An elevated IOP was reported in 48 (29.8%) cases. The other ocular signs included flashes (n = 6, 3.7%), floaters (n = 5, 3.1%), and photophobia (n = 5, 3.1%). Notably, 28 patients (17.3%) had a prior history of glaucoma and had controlled IOP at the time of vaccination. Seven patients (4.3%) had a history of uveitis. The patients also presented with severe headache (n = 48, 29.8%), general body pain (n = 17, 10.6%), and high blood pressure (n = 8, 5.0%). The patients had a prior history of cardiovascular diseases (n = 33, 20.5%) and hypertension (n = 13, 8.1%). The ocular and systemic presentation and history of the patients included in the study are summarized in Table 3.

Table 1. Demographics of patients who were diagnosed with glaucoma following SARS-CoV-2 vaccination.

	Frequency (n)	%
Mean Age (in years)	60.41 ± 17.56	
Age Range		
10–19	2	1.2
20–29	9	5.6
30–39	9	5.6
40–49	9	5.6
50–59	42	26.1
60–69	21	13.0
70–79	38	23.6
80–89	16	9.9
90+	4	2.5
Unknown	11	6.8
Sex		
Female	109	67.7
Male	51	31.7
Unknown	1	0.6
Origin		
Australia	1	0.6
Asia	18	11.2
Europe	86	53.4
United States	48	29.8
Foreign (nonspecific)	3	1.9
Unknown	5	3.1

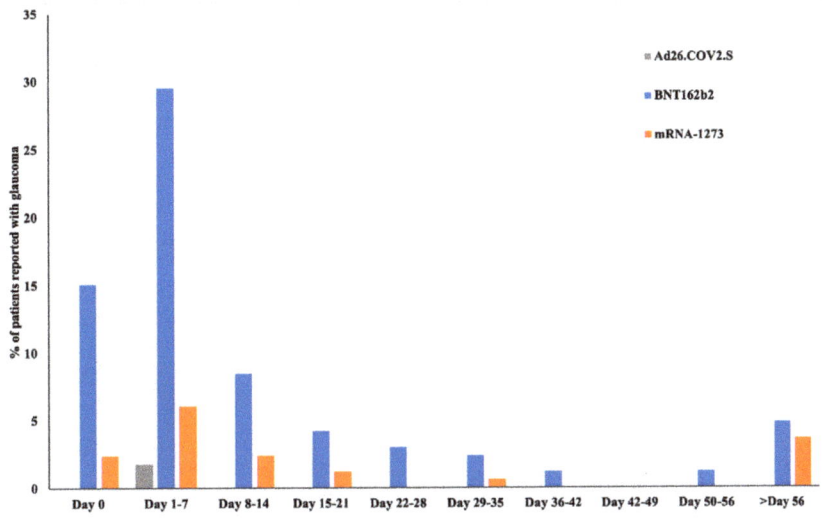

Figure 1. Cases of glaucoma following vaccination with BNT162b2, mRNA-1273, and Ad26.COV2.S on day 0 (i.e., day of vaccination) and in subsequent weeks.

Table 2. Vaccination data of patients who were diagnosed with glaucoma following vaccination.

	Frequency (*n*)	%
Type of Vaccine		
Ad26.COV2.S	4	2.5
BNT162b2	130	80.7
mRNA-1273	27	16.8
Dosage		
1	77	47.8
2	59	36.6
3	13	8.1
Unknown	12	7.5
Median Onset Interval (in days)	4	
Onset Interval Post-Vaccination		
Day 0	29	18.0
Days 1–7	62	38.5
Days 8–14	18	11.2
Days 15–21	9	5.6
Days 22–28	5	3.1
Days 29–35	5	3.1
Days 36–42	2	1.2
Days 42–49	0	0.0
Days 50–56	2	1.2
Days 56+	14	8.7
Unknown	15	9.3

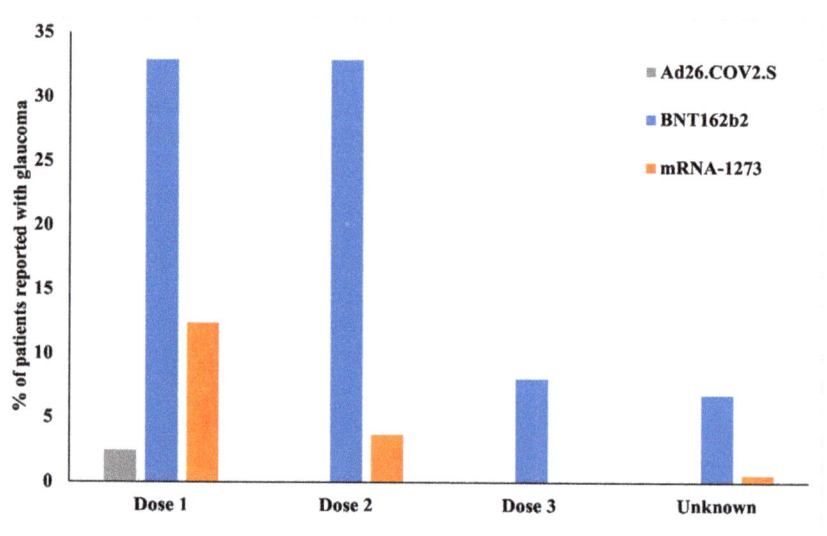

Figure 2. Cases of glaucoma post-vaccination with protocol doses (Doses 1 and 2 for BNT162b2 and mRNA-1273 and Dose 1 for Ad26.COV2.S) and boosters.

Table 3. Ocular and systemic history and presentation in patients diagnosed with glaucoma following SARS-CoV-2 vaccination.

	Frequency	%
History of COVID-19	5	3.1
Glaucoma Diagnosis		
Open-angle glaucoma	105	65.2
Angle-closure glaucoma	45	27.6
Unknown	11	6.8
Ocular Presentations		
Flashes	6	3.7
Floaters	5	3.1
High IOP	48	29.8
Ocular pain	60	37.3
Photophobia	5	3.1
Reduced/blurry vision	47	29.2
Vision loss/blindness	35	21.7
Ocular History		
Conjunctivitis	4	2.5
Glaucoma (controlled)	28	17.3
Hemorrhage	3	1.9
Herpes zoster ophthalmicus	5	3.1
Keratitis	2	1.2
Ocular ischemic syndrome	1	0.6
Optic ischemic neuropathy	1	0.6
Retinal artery occlusion	1	0.6
Retinal vein occlusion	6	3.7
Uveitis	7	4.3
Vitreous detachment	2	1.2
Systemic Presentation		
Headache	48	29.8
Pain	17	10.6
Nausea	12	7.5
Palpitations	4	2.5
High blood pressure	8	5.0
Vaccine site induration/rash	6	3.7
Systemic History		
Allergies	9	5.6
Cardiovascular disorders (MI, CAD, Afib, tachyarrhythmia, heart failure)	33	20.5
Cerebrovascular disorders	3	1.9
Diabetes	9	5.6
Hypercholesterolemia/Dyslipidemia	7	4.3
Hypertension	13	8.1
Hypothyroidism	11	6.8
Pulmonary disorders (COPD, embolism)	4	2.5
Renal disorders	5	3.1

The statistical evaluation revealed a significant association between the vaccine type and the glaucoma-onset duration following vaccination. The symptom onset duration in the patients who received the BNT162b2 (14.7 ± 27.58 days) and Ad26.COV2.S (5.5 ± 6.4 days) vaccines were significantly shorter compared with those who received mRNA-1273 (37.07 ± 66.11 days, p = 0.013) (Table 4). These findings were confirmed by a cumulative-incidence analysis, which showed a significant difference in the onset duration between BNT162b2 and mRNA-1273 (p = 0.05) (Figure 3). The analysis showed that there was no significant association between the onset interval and sex (p = 0.196), age (0.565), and history of COVID-19 (p = 0.08). Pearson's chi-square analysis showed that the frequency of glaucoma cases in patients who received the mRNA-1273 vaccine was significantly higher (p = 0.047) in the older age groups (sixth–seventh decade) (Table 5). A similar association was not observed in patients vaccinated with the BNT162b2 and Ad26.COV2.S vaccines. Additionally, we did not observe any significant association between the vaccine dose, sex, and onset interval.

Table 4. Analysis to assess factors associated with onset interval of glaucoma following SARS-CoV-2 vaccination.

	Percentage (n)	Mean Onset Interval (in Days)	Median Onset Interval (in Days)	p-Value
		Vaccine *		
BNT162b2	80.7% (130/161)	14.7 ± 2.42	5	0.013 *
mRNA-1273	16.7% (27/161)	37.07 ± 12.71	7	
Ad26.COV2.S	2.5% (4/161)	5.5 ± 3.2	3	
		Sex *		
Female	67.7% (109/161)	15.17 ± 2.98	4	0.196
Male	31.7% (51/161)	24.6 ± 6.65	9	
		Age *		
10–19	1.86% (3/161)	32 ± 31.03	1	0.565
20–29	5.6% (9/161)	21.88 ± 17.74	1	
30–39	6.8% (11/161)	29.81 ± 23.54	5	
40–49	8% (13/161)	12.46 ± 4.95	5	
50–59	32.3% (52/161)	14.90 ± 3.65	3.5	
60–69	13% (21/161)	27.04 ± 8.62	8	
70–79	21.7% (35/161)	15.57 ± 5.23	6	
80–89	8.7% (14/161)	20.71 ± 12.13	10	
90+	1.86% (3/161)	12 ± 10.51	2	
		Dosage *		
1	47.8% (77/161)	15.34 ± 4.26	4	0.268
2	36.6% (59/161)	23.64 ± 5.60	9	
3	8.07% (13/161)	17.61 ± 6.35	6	
Unknown	7.45% (12/161)			
		**History of COVID-19 ** **		
Yes	3.1% (5/161)	54.2 ± 32.5	33	0.08
No	96.27% (155/161)	17.18 ± 2.86	5	
Unknown	0.62% (1/161)			

* One-way ANOVA test; ** t-test.

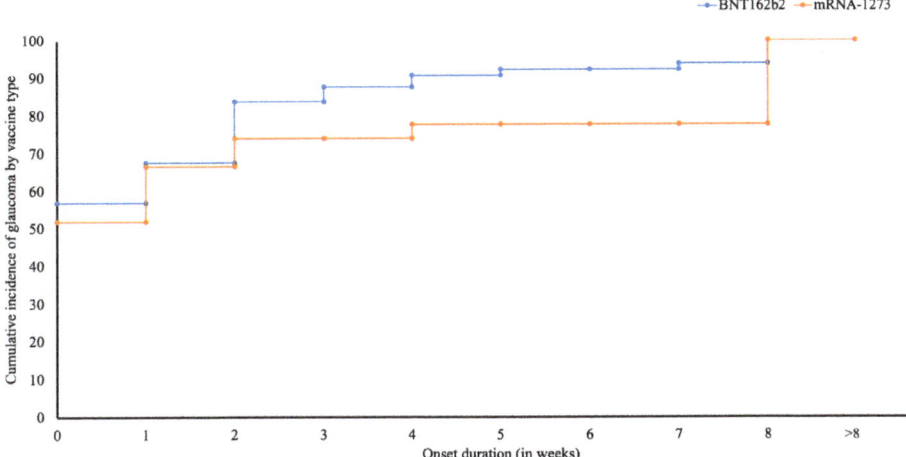

Figure 3. Cumulative-incidence analysis for glaucoma cases reported after administration of BNT162b2 and mRNA-1273 vaccines.

Table 5. Association analysis of age, sex, and onset interval with glaucoma following SARS-CoV-2 vaccination.

	BNT162b2 (Pfizer BioNTech)					mRNA-1273					Ad26.COV2.S			
	Unknown	1	2	3	χ^2	p-value	Unknown	1	2	χ^2	p-value	Unknown	1	χ^2	p-value
Age (in years)					19.17	0.742				26.2	0.047 *			1.333	0.995
10–19	0	0	2	0			0	0	0			0	1		
20–29	0	2	4	0			0	1	0			0	0		
30–39	2	6	2	0			1	1	0			0	0		
40–49	1	5	4	1			0	1	0			0	0		
50–59	4	16	16	4			0	0	1			0	2		
60–69	0	4	7	3			0	9	1			0	1		
70–79	1	14	13	4			0	5	2			0	0		
80–89	3	5	4	1			0	3	0			0	0		
90+	0	1	1	0			0	0	2			0	0		
Sex					0.555	0.906				0.905	0.636			1.333	0.248
Male	3	16	15	5			0	8	3			0	2		
Female	8	37	38	8			1	12	3			0	2		
Onset Interval (in days)					21.08	0.275				16.78	0.157			1.333	0.987
0	1	9	13	2			0	4	0			0	0		
1–7	3	25	16	5			1	9	0			0	3		
8–14	1	4	8	1			0	2	2			0	0		
15–21	4	10	6	1			0	2	0			0	1		
22–28	1	1	2	1			0	0	0			0	0		
29–35	1	1	2	0			0	0	1			0	0		
36–42	0	1	1	0			0	0	0			0	0		
43–49	0	0	0	0			0	0	0			0	0		
49–56	0	0	0	2			0	0	0			0	0		
56+	0	2	5	1			0	3	3			0	0		

* $p < 0.05$.

The patients were prescribed topical eye drops (*n* = 44), and surgical interventions (*n* = 29) were performed in the requisite cases. Laser iridotomy and shunt/valve placement surgeries were performed in 18 (11.2%) and 4 (2.5%) patients, respectively. None of the patients included in this study had a pre-existing iridotomy. Trabeculectomies were performed in two (1.2%) patients. The type of surgical intervention was not specified in seven (4.3%) patients. The patients were prescribed brimonidine (*n* = 5, 3.1%), dorzolamide (*n* = 6, 3.7%), timolol (*n* = 11, 6.8%), or Travoprost/Latanoprost (*n* = 2, 1.2%). The prescribed eye drops were not specified in 18 (11.2%) patients. The interventions were not known for more than half (*n* = 86, 53.4%) of the patients (Supplementary Table S3).

5. Discussion

Since initiation of the global vaccination in December 2020, several case reports have highlighted the ocular adverse events associated with the COVID-19 vaccines. The current study evaluates the temporal association between glaucoma and the SARS-CoV-2 vaccines, as there was a short interval between post-vaccination and the onset of the signs of glaucoma; however, further studies are required to evaluate the potential causal relationship [9]. Over the years, several studies have established the presence of the renin-angiotensin system in the human ciliary body and aqueous humor [10–12]. It has been speculated that binding of the spike proteins generated by SARS-CoV-2 vaccines (such as BNT162b2 and mRNA-1273) to angiotensin-converting enzyme 2 (ACE2) leads to angiotensin II overactivity, thereby increasing the aqueous-humor production and elevated intraocular pressure [13].

The ocular adverse events associated with the three vaccines approved in the United States include uveitis, Bell's and abducens nerve palsy, acute macular neuroretinopathy, central serous retinopathy, Grave's disease, Vogt–Koyanagi–Harada disease, retinal and ophthalmic vein thrombosis, and corneal-graft rejection [14–23]. Similar ocular disorders have also been observed in patients infected by the SARS-CoV-2 virus [24–26]. Recently, Choi and colleagues reported vision-threatening ocular adverse events in sixteen patients following SARS-CoV-2 vaccination [27]. Among these patients, the authors reported four cases of angle-closure glaucoma following the ChAdOx1 nCoV-19 vaccine and attributed it to the inflammation of the ciliary body due to vaccine-associated uveitis. Additionally, two cases of secondary angle-closure glaucoma post-vaccination have been reported in the literature. Behera and colleagues reported the case of a 60-year-old male with hemophilia who developed painful and sudden vision loss a day after receiving the ChAdOx1 nCoV-19 (Oxford AstraZeneca) vaccine due to acute angle-closure glaucoma secondary to a massive suprachoroidal hemorrhage [28]. In the other case, a 49-year-old male presented with progressive vision loss one day after the administration of the second dose of the BNT162b2 vaccine. The patient had a massive intraocular hemorrhage and was diagnosed with secondary angle-closure glaucoma, bullous retinal detachment, and massive intraocular hemorrhage [29]. The patient's presentation was attributed to the necrosis of a melanocytic lesion at the posterior edge of the ciliary body and choroid [29]. In another case report, Santovito and Pinna reported reduced vision, severe headache, and photophobia in a patient after vaccination with BNT162b2. The patient had no prior ocular history, and the authors could not establish a definitive diagnosis for the patient [16]. The pathogenesis of secondary glaucoma following vaccination can be explained by the underlying disorders, as observed in the abovementioned cases, or by trabecular dysfunction that is likely mediated by inflammatory responses and oxidative stress. Additionally, the fluctuations in the intraocular pressure also play a critical role in inducing metabolic stress [3].

The analysis of the VAERS data suggests an extremely low safety concern for glaucoma post-vaccination with BNT162b2, mRNA-1273, and Ad26.COV2.S. The estimated crude reporting rates in this study are comparable with the report by Wang and colleagues, who evaluated the data from the Australia Therapeutic Goods Administration Database of Adverse Event Notifications, the Canada Vigilance Adverse Reaction Database, the European Union Medicines Agency (EudraVigilance) System, and the United Kingdom

Medicines and Healthcare Products Regulatory Agency between December 2020 and August 2021 [30]. Although the glaucoma crude reporting rate is extremely low, it may be considered a "severe" adverse event because the fluctuations in the intraocular pressure can have a domino effect on the aqueous dynamics and optic nerve.

In this study, a substantial proportion of the patients were women and between 50 and 70 years old. The data analysis of this cohort shows that the patients typically presented with signs of glaucoma in the first 24–48 h post-vaccination (viz., elevated intraocular pressure), and the incidence was higher after the first dose. Most of the patients did not have a prior history of glaucoma; therefore, it is imperative that patients at risk of developing glaucoma remain vigilant post-vaccination. The onset interval of the disease was significantly shorter in the patients vaccinated with the BNT162b2 and Ad26.COV2.S vaccines compared with those vaccinated with the mRNA-1273 vaccine. The patients diagnosed with glaucoma after mRNA-1273 vaccination were between 60 and 80 years old. Although uveitis and other ocular inflammatory disorders are considered more common ocular adverse events associated with vaccination, only 4% of the patients were diagnosed with it. The pathogenesis of secondary glaucoma post-vaccination can be explained by the underlying disorders or trabecular dysfunction likely mediated by inflammatory responses and oxidative stress. In addition, increases or fluctuations in the intraocular pressure induce metabolic stress. However, there are no insights into the pathophysiologic mechanisms that can potentially cause open-angle glaucoma reported in many of the patients included in this study.

6. Limitations

This study, reporting glaucoma cases following SARS-CoV-2 vaccination, has several limitations. VAERS is a passive surveillance system which includes adverse event reports following administration of FDA approved vaccines, from pharmaceutical companies, physicians, drug regulators, and patients from all over the world. Despite the mandatory requirement to report vaccine-associated adverse events, underreporting and delayed reporting are common. In some cases, the submitted reports are incomplete and lack uniformity in the data reporting. Several reports have missing data points, such as ethnicity, that are considered important risk factors associated with glaucoma.

The absence of an unvaccinated control group impedes the relative-risk calculation. The pharmacovigilance associated with COVID-19 vaccines is limited to the European Union, the United States, Australia, Canada, and a few Asian countries. Hence, reports are not recorded from many developing countries, including India, where over one billion vaccine doses have been administered. Moreover, the data are absent for other approved vaccines, such as ChAdOx1 nCoV-19, ZyCoV-D, Sputnik, Covidecia, Sputnik, Sinopharm, Abdala, Zifivax, and Novavax.

The reports submitted by drug regulators, pharmaceutical companies, and physicians (~80%) can be relied on for the clinical diagnosis of glaucoma; however, cases in which patients self-reported are presumed to be glaucoma. The data in the literature suggest glaucoma underreporting; therefore, it can be assumed that the cases were grossly underreported. The lack of clinical (specifically vision and gonioscopy) data severely impedes the use of these data on the ability of the researchers to report the adverse effects in these reports convincingly. Additionally, there are no details of optic-nerve head cupping or visual-field defects on the perimetries; thus, what is labeled as glaucoma could also be secondary ocular hypertension, as access to detailed clinical history is not logistically possible and is limited by the Health Insurance Portability and Accountability Act (HIPPA) of 1996 [31].

In conclusion, the risk of glaucoma following vaccination with BNT162b2, mRNA-1273, and rAd26.COV2.S is extremely low. The majority of the patients in the cohort had primary open-angle glaucoma and had received the BNT162b2 vaccine. Most cases occurred after the first dose and within the first week following vaccination. Therefore, it is recommended that ophthalmologists and glaucoma specialists closely monitor the at-risk patients following vaccination.

Supplementary Materials: The following supporting information can be downloaded at: https://www.mdpi.com/article/10.3390/vaccines10101630/s1, Table S1: The country-wise distribution of glaucoma cases reported to the CDC VAERS; Table S2: State-wise crude reporting rates of glaucoma per million doses of SARS-CoV-2 vaccinations; Table S3: Therapeutic interventions reported in patients diagnosed with glaucoma following SARS-CoV-2 vaccination.

Author Contributions: Conceptualization, R.B.S. and P.I.; methodology, R.B.S. and P.I.; software, U.P.S.P.; validation, R.B.S., P.I. and U.P.S.P.; formal analysis, W.C., R.B.S., P.I. and U.P.S.P.; investigation, R.B.S.; resources, R.B.S. and P.I.; data curation, R.B.S., W.C. and U.P.S.P.; writing—original draft preparation, R.B.S. and W.C.; writing—review and editing, P.I.; visualization, R.B.S.; supervision, P.I.; project administration, R.B.S. and P.I. All authors have read and agreed to the published version of the manuscript.

Funding: This research received no external funding.

Institutional Review Board Statement: Because the study includes publicly available deidentified anonymous data, the University of Adelaide Human Research Ethics Committee exempted it from ethical review (Reference: 36024).

Informed Consent Statement: Patient consent was waived as this study includes publicly available, deidentified data.

Data Availability Statement: Publicly available datasets were analyzed in this study. These data can be found at https://wonder.cdc.gov/vaers.html (accessed on 30 April 2022).

Conflicts of Interest: Rohan Bir Singh (none), Uday Pratap Singh Parmar (none), Wonkyung Cho (none), Parul Ichhpujani (none).

References

1. Mathieu, E.; Ritchie, H.; Ortiz-Ospina, E.; Roser, M.; Hasell, J.; Appel, C.; Giattino, C.; Rodés-Guirao, L. A Global Database of COVID-19 Vaccinations. *Nat. Hum. Behav.* **2021**, *5*, 947–953. [CrossRef] [PubMed]
2. Centers for Disease Control the Vaccine Adverse Event Reporting System (VAERS) Request. Available online: https://wonder.cdc.gov/vaers.html (accessed on 18 May 2022).
3. Weinreb, R.N.; Aung, T.; Medeiros, F.A. The Pathophysiology and Treatment of Glaucoma: A Review. *JAMA* **2014**, *311*, 1901. [CrossRef] [PubMed]
4. Tham, Y.C.; Li, X.; Wong, T.Y.; Quigley, H.A.; Aung, T.; Cheng, C.Y. Global Prevalence of Glaucoma and Projections of Glaucoma Burden through 2040: A Systematic Review and Meta-Analysis. *Ophthalmology* **2014**, *121*, 2081–2090. [CrossRef] [PubMed]
5. Nickells, R.W.; Howell, G.R.; Soto, I.; John, S.W.M. Under Pressure: Cellular and Molecular Responses During Glaucoma, a Common Neurodegeneration with Axonopathy. *Annu. Rev. Neurosci.* **2012**, *35*, 153–179. [CrossRef] [PubMed]
6. Welcome to MedDRA | MedDRA. Available online: https://www.meddra.org/ (accessed on 18 May 2022).
7. Centers for Disease Control and Prevention (CDC) CDC WONDER FAQs. Available online: https://wonder.cdc.gov/wonder/help/faq.html#8 (accessed on 18 May 2022).
8. Centers for Disease Control and Prevention (CDC). The Vaccine Adverse Event Reporting System (VAERS) Data Request. Available online: https://wonder.cdc.gov/controller/datarequest/D8 (accessed on 7 June 2022).
9. Fedak, K.M.; Bernal, A.; Capshaw, Z.A.; Gross, S. Applying the Bradford Hill Criteria in the 21st Century: How Data Integration Has Changed Causal Inference in Molecular Epidemiology. *Emerg. Themes Epidemiol.* **2015**, *12*, 14. [CrossRef]
10. Savaskan, E.; Löffler, K.U.; Meier, F.; Müller-Spahn, F.; Flammer, J.; Meyer, P. Immunohistochemical Localization of Angiotensin-Converting Enzyme, Angiotensin II and AT1 Receptor in Human Ocular Tissues. *Ophthalmic Res.* **2004**, *36*, 312–320. [CrossRef]
11. Igic, R.; Robinson, C.J.G.; Milosevic, Z. Activity of Renin and Angiotensin I Converting Enzyme in Retina and Ciliary Body. *Lijec. Vjesn.* **1977**, *99*, 482–484.
12. Cullinane, A.B.; Leung, P.S.; Ortego, J.; Coca-Prados, M.; Harvey, B.J. Renin-Angiotensin System Expression and Secretory Function in Cultured Human Ciliary Body Non-Pigmented Epithelium. *Br. J. Ophthalmol.* **2002**, *86*, 676–683. [CrossRef]
13. Angeli, F.; Spanevello, A.; Reboldi, G.; Visca, D.; Verdecchia, P. SARS-CoV-2 Vaccines: Lights and Shadows. *Eur. J. Intern. Med.* **2021**, *88*, 1–8. [CrossRef]
14. Ozonoff, A.; Nanishi, E.; Levy, O. Bell's Palsy and SARS-CoV-2 Vaccines. *Lancet. Infect. Dis.* **2021**, *21*, 450–452. [CrossRef]
15. Fowler, N.; Mendez Martinez, N.R.; Pallares, B.V.; Maldonado, R.S. Acute-Onset Central Serous Retinopathy after Immunization with COVID-19 MRNA Vaccine. *Am. J. Ophthalmol. Case Rep.* **2021**, *23*, 101136. [CrossRef] [PubMed]

16. Santovito, L.S.; Pinna, G. Acute Reduction of Visual Acuity and Visual Field after Pfizer-BioNTech COVID-19 Vaccine 2nd Dose: A Case Report. *Inflamm. Res.* **2021**, *70*, 931–933. [CrossRef] [PubMed]
17. Wasser, L.M.; Roditi, E.; Zadok, D.; Berkowitz, L.; Weill, Y. Keratoplasty Rejection After the BNT162b2 Messenger RNA Vaccine. *Cornea* **2021**, *40*, 1070–1072. [CrossRef]
18. Phylactou, M.; Li, J.P.O.; Larkin, D.F.P. Characteristics of Endothelial Corneal Transplant Rejection Following Immunisation with SARS-CoV-2 Messenger RNA Vaccine. *Br. J. Ophthalmol.* **2021**, *105*, 893–896. [CrossRef] [PubMed]
19. Rallis, K.I.; Ting, D.S.J.; Said, D.G.; Dua, H.S. Corneal Graft Rejection Following COVID-19 Vaccine. *Eye* **2022**, *36*, 1319–1320. [CrossRef]
20. Ivanov, K.; Garanina, E.; Rizvanov, A.; Khaiboullina, S. Inflammasomes as Targets for Adjuvants. *Pathogens* **2020**, *9*, 252. [CrossRef] [PubMed]
21. Bayas, A.; Menacher, M.; Christ, M.; Behrens, L.; Rank, A.; Naumann, M. Bilateral Superior Ophthalmic Vein Thrombosis, Ischaemic Stroke, and Immune Thrombocytopenia after ChAdOx1 NCoV-19 Vaccination. *Lancet* **2021**, *397*, e11. [CrossRef]
22. Papasavvas, I.; Herbort, C.P. Reactivation of Vogt-Koyanagi-Harada Disease under Control for More than 6 Years, Following Anti-SARS-CoV-2 Vaccination. *J. Ophthalmic Inflamm. Infect.* **2021**, *11*, 21. [CrossRef]
23. Singh, R.B.; Parmar, U.P.S.; Kahale, F.; Agarwal, A.; Tsui, E. Vaccine-Associated Uveitis Following SARS-CoV-2 Vaccination: A CDC-VAERS Database Analysis. *Ophthalmology* **2022**, *8*, 27. [CrossRef]
24. Wu, P.; Duan, F.; Luo, C.; Liu, Q.; Qu, X.; Liang, L.; Wu, K. Characteristics of Ocular Findings of Patients with Coronavirus Disease 2019 (COVID-19) in Hubei Province, China. *JAMA Ophthalmol.* **2020**, *138*, 1291. [CrossRef]
25. Gupta, A.; Madhavan, M.V.; Sehgal, K.; Nair, N.; Mahajan, S.; Sehrawat, T.S.; Bikdeli, B.; Ahluwalia, N.; Ausiello, J.C.; Wan, E.Y.; et al. Extrapulmonary Manifestations of COVID-19. *Nat. Med.* **2020**, *26*, 1017–1032. [CrossRef] [PubMed]
26. Li, J.P.O.; Lam, D.S.C.; Chen, Y.; Ting, D.S.W. Novel Coronavirus Disease 2019 (COVID-19): The Importance of Recognising Possible Early Ocular Manifestation and Using Protective Eyewear. *Br. J. Ophthalmol.* **2020**, *104*, 297–298. [CrossRef] [PubMed]
27. Choi, M.; Seo, M.H.; Choi, K.E.; Lee, S.; Choi, B.; Yun, C.; Kim, S.W.; Kim, Y.Y. Vision-Threatening Ocular Adverse Events after Vaccination against Coronavirus Disease 2019. *J. Clin. Med.* **2022**, *11*, 3318. [CrossRef] [PubMed]
28. Behera, G.; Jossy, A.; Deb, A.K.; Neelakandan, S.; Basavarajegowda, A. Spontaneous Suprachoroidal Haemorrhage in Haemophilia Coincident with ChAdOx1 NCoV-19 Vaccine. *Eur. J. Ophthalmol.* **2022**, 112067212210982. [CrossRef]
29. Wagle, A.; Wu, B.; Gopal, L.; Sundar, G. Necrosis of Uveal Melanoma Post-COVID-19 Vaccination. *Indian J. Ophthalmol.* **2022**, *70*, 1837. [CrossRef]
30. Wang, M.T.M.; Niederer, R.L.; McGhee, C.N.J.; Danesh-Meyer, H.V. COVID-19 Vaccination and the Eye. *Am. J. Ophthalmol.* **2022**, *240*, 79–98. [CrossRef]
31. Health Insurance Portability and Accountability Act of 1996 (HIPAA) | CDC. Available online: https://www.cdc.gov/phlp/publications/topic/hipaa.html (accessed on 19 May 2022).

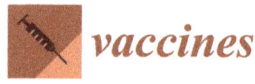

Case Report

A Case of Atypical Unilateral Optic Neuritis Following BNT162b2 mRNA COVID-19 Vaccination

Shuntaro Motegi, Takayuki Kanda and Masaru Takeuchi *

Department of Ophthalmology, National Defense Medical College, 3-2 Namiki, Tokorozawa 359-8513, Japan
* Correspondence: masatake@ndmc.ac.jp; Tel.: +81-42-995-1211; Fax: +81-42-995-5332

Abstract: Background: We report a case of atypical unilateral optic neuritis after receiving the BNT162b2 mRNA-based COVID-19 vaccine. Case Presentation: An 86-year-old man complained of blurred vision and decreased visual acuity in his right eye 8 days after receiving the second BNT162b2 mRNA-based COVID-19 vaccine and was referred to our hospital. He also had pain with eye movement. Best corrected visual acuity (BCVA) in the right eye was 20/200 and critical flicker frequency dropped to 16 Hz. Relative afferent pupillary defect was positive and central scotomas were observed on visual field analysis. Fundus examination and SD-OCT revealed optic disc swelling and apparent thickening of the retinal nerve fiber layer around the optic disc in the right eye. Although either an increase in CRP or ESR on laboratory tests, demyelinating lesion on MRI, or positive of anti-MOG antibodies or anti-AQP4 antibodies were not observed, fluorescein angiography presented only hyperfluorescence of the optic disc in the right eye, but there were no findings such as papillary deficiency and choroidal delay that would suggest ischemic optic neuropathy. We diagnosed atypical optic neuritis developed after the SARS-CoV-2 mRNA-based vaccination and initiated oral corticosteroid therapy. One month later, the optic disc swelling disappeared and BCVA improved to 20/100; however, the central scotoma remained and no further improvement in visual function OD was obtained. Conclusions: An atypical acute idiopathic optic neuritis can occur after receiving the second vaccination with BNT162b2, which may present a limited response to corticosteroid therapy.

Keywords: COVID-19; optic neuritis; mRNA vaccine; vaccination

Citation: Motegi, S.; Kanda, T.; Takeuchi, M. A Case of Atypical Unilateral Optic Neuritis Following BNT162b2 mRNA COVID-19 Vaccination. *Vaccines* **2022**, *10*, 1574. https://doi.org/10.3390/vaccines10101574

Academic Editor: Vincenzo Baldo

Received: 18 August 2022
Accepted: 16 September 2022
Published: 20 September 2022

Publisher's Note: MDPI stays neutral with regard to jurisdictional claims in published maps and institutional affiliations.

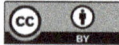

Copyright: © 2022 by the authors. Licensee MDPI, Basel, Switzerland. This article is an open access article distributed under the terms and conditions of the Creative Commons Attribution (CC BY) license (https:// creativecommons.org/licenses/by/ 4.0/).

1. Background

Coronavirus disease 2019 (COVID-19) remains rampant worldwide, with the development of vaccines against the causative virus severe acute respiratory syndrome coronavirus 2 (SARS-CoV-2) progressing rapidly with an urgent demand. Several vaccines have been approved for emergency use for the prevention of COVID-19, though critical adverse events of the vaccines have not been fully investigated.

Multiple sclerosis (MS) or neuromyelitis optica spectrum disorders (NMOSD) after COVID-19 vaccination have been reported [1–6], while a complication of optic neuritis (ON) is also known [7–10]. Although idiopathic ON after COVID-19 vaccination is also reported [11–15], those visual prognoses are generally favorable. We report a case of atypical unilateral ON after receiving the BNT162b2 mRNA-based COVID-19 vaccine, in which the recovery of visual functions was restricted despite corticosteroid therapy.

2. Case Presentation

An 86-year-old man who complained of blurred vision and decreased visual acuity in the right eye visited a local eye clinic. This patient had received the second dose of the BNT162b2 mRNA-based COVID-19 vaccine 8 days before the onset of his ocular symptoms. Since the patient was also aware of pain with eye movement, he was referred to our hospital on suspicion of optic neuritis. He had a history of arrhythmia, but had no abnormalities such as flu-like symptoms before vaccination. At presentation, the best-corrected visual acuity (BCVA) was 20/200 in the right eye (OD) and 20/20 in the left eye (OS), with intraocular pressure (IOP) 14 mmHg OD and 15 mmHg OS. Critical flicker frequency (CFF) was 16 Hz OD and 47 Hz OS. Relative afferent pupillary defect (RAPD) OD was observed and fundus examination revealed optic disc swelling OD (Figure 1A,B). Fluorescein angiography (FA) OD showed only hyperfluorescence of the optic disc (Figure 1C,D), with no findings such as papillary filling deficiency and choroidal delay that would suggest ischemic optic neuropathy. Humphrey's visual field analysis (HFA) and spectral domain optical coherence tomography (SD-OCT) OD revealed central scotomas (Figure 1E,F) and apparent thickening of the retinal nerve fiber layer (RNFL) around the optic disc (Figure 2). Alternatively, laboratory tests including erythrocyte sedimentation rate (ESR) and C-reactive protein (CRP) indicated no abnormal values. Anti-myelin oligodendrocyte glycoprotein (MOG) antibodies or anti-aquaporin 4 (AQP4) antibodies were also examined by commercial-based cell-based assays (CBAs) using live transfected cells, but were negative. Intracranial magnetic resonance imaging (MRI) indicated neither a contrast-enhanced effect of gadolinium on the optic nerve nor abnormalities such as demyelinating lesions. Non-arteritic anterior ischemic optic neuropathy (NA-AION) was suspected based on the patient's age and his medical history of arrhythmia; however, FA findings and HFA results were consistent with acute idiopathic optic neuritis OD, contrary to NA-AION. Since the patient had received the second BNT162b2 mRNA-based COVID-19 vaccine 8 days before the onset of ocular symptoms OD, a side effect of the COVID-19 vaccine was suspected to be the possible cause. Considering the patient's advanced age, methylprednisolone pulse administration was avoided and oral corticosteroid therapy was initiated from 0.6 mg/kg. One month later, although the optic disc swelling OD had gradually resolved (Figure 3A,B) and BCVA OD had improved to 20/100, the central scotoma remained (Figure 3C,D) and no further improvement in visual function OD was obtained. There was no inflammation in the left eye during these events.

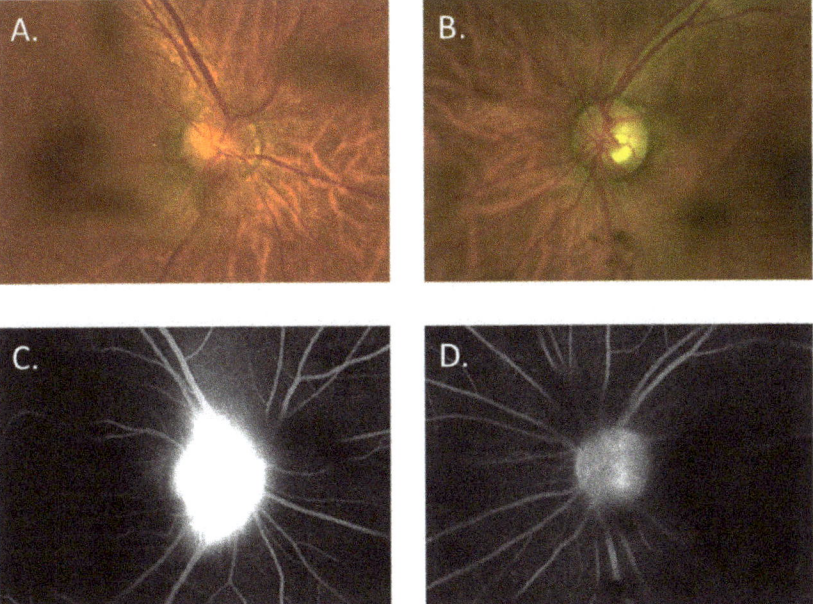

Figure 1. *Cont.*

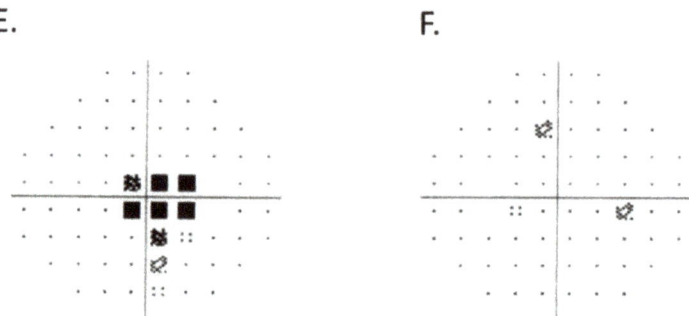

Figure 1. (**A**,**B**) color fundus photographs of the right eye (**A**) and left eye (**B**) 8 days after receiving the second COVID-19 vaccination. (**C**,**D**) fluorescein angiography findings in the right eye (**C**) and left eye (**D**) at the late stage. (**E**,**F**) Humphrey's visual field analysis of the right eye (**E**) and left eye (**F**).

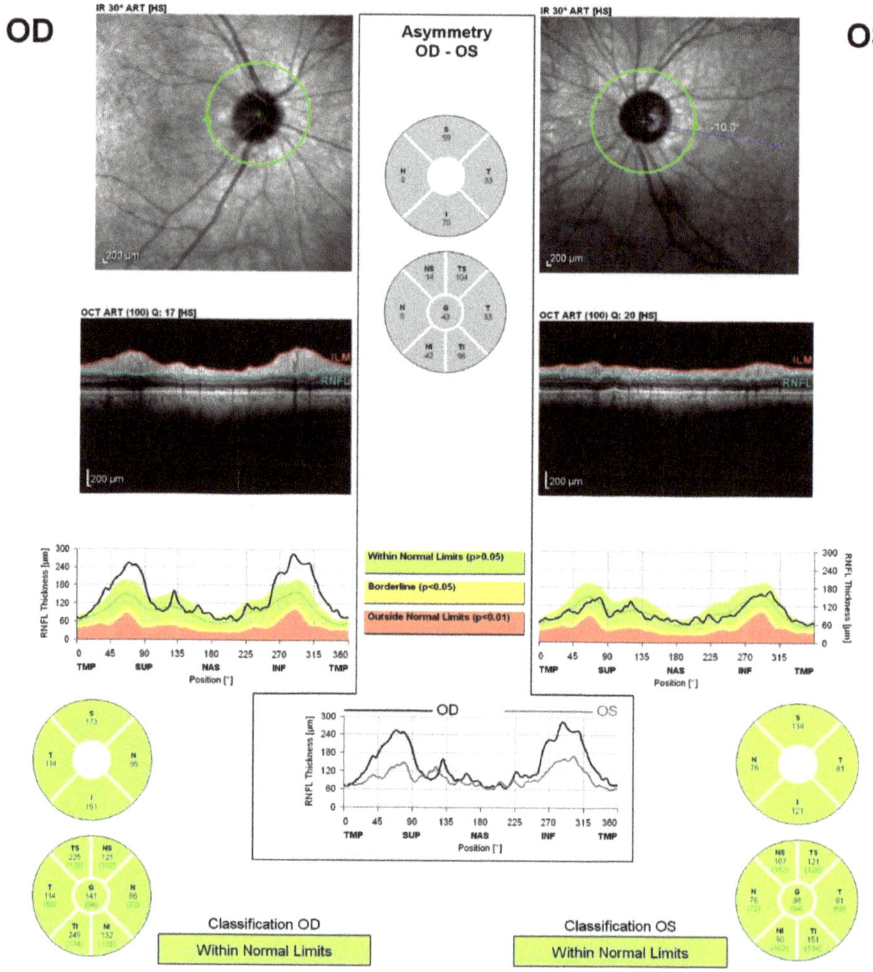

Figure 2. Retinal nerve fiber layer thickness around the optic nerve head of the right eye (**OD**) and left eye (**OS**) measured by spectral domain optical coherence tomography.

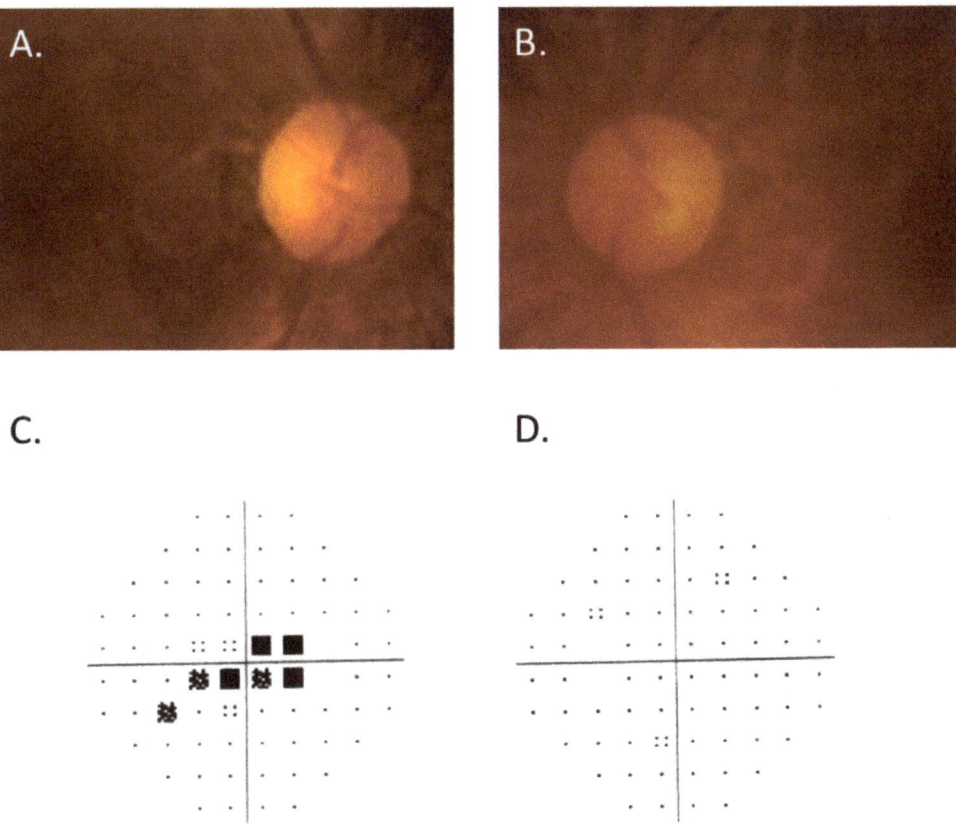

Figure 3. (**A**,**B**) color fundus photographs of the right eye (**A**) and left eye (**B**) 1 month after receiving the second COVID-19 vaccination. (**C**,**D**) Humphrey's visual field analysis of the right eye (**C**) and left eye (**D**).

3. Discussion

Optic neuropathy is suspected as one of adverse events of the COVID-19 vaccine, which includes ON associated with or without demyelinating CNS diseases [7–16], NA-AION [17–24], and NMOSD [8,9]. Lotan et al. reviewed 14 case reports and 2 case series by electronic searches of the published literature regarding neuro-ophthalmological complications of COVID-19 vaccines and reported that optic neuritis was the most common, occurring in 61 of 76 cases (80.3%) [25]. We reviewed the previous reports of newly onset optic neuropathy after receiving COVID-19 vaccines and compared clinical manifestations, management, and outcomes in Table 1. The onset after receiving COVID-19 vaccines ranged from 1 day to 3 weeks, in which 7 of all 26 cases (26.9%) were associated with relapsing-remitting multiple sclerosis (RRMS) or NMOSD, with 10 cases (38.5%) idiopathic ON. High-dose pulse steroid therapy was useful in most cases and their visual prognosis was favorable. Although visual acuity was not fully recovered in 3 cases [13], those were not as high as in this case. NA-AION was also reported in 8 cases (30.8%), with ON suspected in some cases.

Table 1. Published cases reports of optic neuropathy after receiving COVID-19 vaccines.

	Author (Year)	Age (Sex)	Medical History	Clinical Presentation	Diagnosis	Vaccine	Time between Vaccination and Symptoms	Treatment	Final Visual Acuity
1	Ayman G Elnahry (2021) [11]	69 (female)	None	Bilateral vision loss	Bilateral optic neuritis	mRNA (Pfizer-BioNTech) 2nd dose	16 days	1000 mg/day intravenous methylprednisolone (IVMP) for 5 days,	Stable
		32 (female)	None	Blurred vision OS	Optic neuritis OS	Viral vector (Oxford–AstraZeneca) 1st dose	5 days	1000 mg/day IVMP for 3 days	20/20
2	Henrique M. Leber (2021) [16]	32 (female)	None	Vision loss and pain OS	Bilateral optic neuritis and thyroiditis	Inactivated (Sinovac) 2nd dose	12 h	1000 mg/day IVMP for 5 days	20/20 OD 20/25 OS
3	Rika Tsukii (2021) [17]	55 (female)	None	Visual field disturbance OD	Non-arteritic anterior ischemic optic neuropathy (NA-AION) OD	mRNA (Pfizer-BioNTech) 1st dose	7 days	No treatment	20/20
4	Valentina Arnao (2022) [14]	Middle-age (female)	None	Bilateral blurred vision and pain	Bilateral optic neuritis	Viral vector (Oxford–AstraZeneca) 1st dose	14 days	1000 mg/day IVMP for 5 days	Recovered
5	Jiajun Wang (2022) [12]	21 (female)	None	Blurred vision OD with ocular rotation pain	Optic neuritis OD	Inactivated (Sinopharm) 2nd dose	3 weeks	800 mg/day IVMP for 3 days	20/20
		38 (female)	None	Blurred vision OD	Optic neuritis OD	Inactivated (Sinopharm) 1st dose	3 weeks	1000 mg/day IVMP for 3 days	20/20
6	Madhurima Roy (2022) [13]	27 (female)	None	Progressive blurring of vision OS	Optic neuritis OS	Viral vector (Covishield) 1st dose	9 days	1000 mg/day IVMP for 3 days	20/40
		48 (female)	None	Painless gradual diminution of vision OS	Optic neuritis OS	Viral vector (Covishield) 2nd dose	5 days	1000 mg/day IVMP for 3 days	20/30
		40 (male)	None	Blurring vision in both eyes	Bilateral optic neuritis	Viral vector (Covishield) 1st dose	12 days	Steroid therapy	20/30 OD 20/40 OS
7	Mahsa Khayat-Khoei (2022) [7]	26 (female)	None	Blurred vision and pain OD	New onset relapsing-remitting multiple sclerosis (RRMS)	mRNA (Moderna) 2nd dose	14 days	1000 mg/day IVMP for 5 days	-
		64 (male)	RRMS	Vision changes and pain OD	Multiple sclerosis (MS) exacerbation	mRNA (Pfizer-BioNTech) 2nd dose	1 day	1000 mg/day IVMP for 3 days	-
		33 (male)	none	Blurred vision OS	New onset RRMS	mRNA (Pfizer-BioNTech) 2nd dose	1 day	1000 mg/day IVMP for 3 days	-
		48 (female)	clinically isolated demyelinating syndrome (CIS)	Pain OD, Lhermitte's, balance/gait	Conversion from CIS to RRMS	mRNA (Pfizer-BioNTech) 1st dose	15 days	1000 mg/day IVMP for 3 days	-
8	Christian García-Estrada (2022) [15]	19 (female)	None	Vision loss and pain OS	Optic neuritis OS	Viral vector (Janssen) 1st dose	1 week	1000 mg/day IVMP for 5 days	20/20

Table 1. Cont.

	Author (Year)	Age (Sex)	Medical History	Clinical Presentation	Diagnosis	Vaccine	Time between Vaccination and Symptoms	Treatment	Final Visual Acuity
9	Yelda Yıldız Tascı (2022) [8]	32 (male)	Graves' disease	Ocular pain and blurred vision OD	Neuromyelitis optica spectrum disorders (NMOSD) OD	Inactivated (Sinovac) 1st dose	14 days	1000 mg/day IVMP for 5 days	20/20
10	Sai A Nagaratnam (2022) [10]	36 (female)	None	Bilateral vision loss and subjective color desaturation, painful eye movements and fatigue	Bilateral optic neuritis	Viral vector (Oxford–AstraZeneca ChAdOx1) 1st dose	14 days	1000 mg/day IVMP for 3 days	20/16 OD 20/20 OS
11	Bader Shirah (2022) [9]	31 (female)	Systemic lupus erythematosus (SLE)	Painful eye movements and blurred vision OS	NMOSD OS	mRNA (Pfizer-BioNTech) 2nd dose	14 days	1000 mg/day IVMP for 2 days	-
12	Wen-Yun Lin (2022) [18]	61 (female)	Hypertension and hyperlipidemia	Blurred vision OS	NA-AION OS	Viral vector (Oxford–AstraZeneca ChAdOx1) 2nd dose	7 days	Oral prednisolone 60 mg/day	20/80
13	Abdelrahman M Elhusseiny (2022) [19]	51 (male)	None	Vision loss OS	NA-AION OS	mRNA (Pfizer-BioNTech) 2nd dose	1 day	Oral prednisone over 1 month	20/400
14	Sonia Valsero Franco (2022) [20]	53 (male)	None	Bilateral vision loss	Suspected bilateral NA-AION	mRNA (Pfizer-BioNTech) 1st dose OD mRNA (Pfizer-BioNTech) 2nd dose OS	7 days 10 days	Acetazolamide 750 mg/day	20/20 OD 20/40 OS
		65 (male)	Arterial hypertension	Blurred vision OD	Suspected NA-AION OD	mRNA (Pfizer-BioNTech) 1st dose	12 days	No treatment	20/200
15	Snezhana Murgova (2022) [21]	45 (male)	Arterial hypertension	Visual disturbance OD	NA-AION OD	mRNA (Pfizer-BioNTech) 2nd dose	10 days	Vasodilators and anti-platelet therapy	20/20
16	Seung Ah Chung (2022) [22]	65 (female)	None	Sudden inferior visual field loss OD	NA-AION OD	Viral vector (Oxford–AstraZeneca ChAdOx1) 2nd dose	15 days	1000 mg/day IVMP for 3 days	20/200
17	Ilay Caliskan (2022) [23]	43 (female)	None	Blurred vision and movement-associated pain OD	NMOSD OD	mRNA (Pfizer-BioNTech) 2nd dose	1 day	IVMP and plasma exchange	-
18	Srinivasan Sanjay (2022) [24]	50s (Female)	Non-arteritic anterior ischaemic optic neuropathy (NA-AION) OD	Vision loss OS	NA-AION OS	Viral vector (Covishield) 1st dose	4 days	Oral aspirin 75 mg for 1 month	20/20

Clinically, it is often challenging to differentiate ON from NA-AION, with the diagnosis usually based on the patient's background, clinical findings, and multimodal images. In this case, NA-AION OD was primarily suspected based on the medical history of arrhythmia, the patient's age, negative result for anti-MOG or anti-AQP4 antibodies, no elevation of ESR or CRP, and no associated neurological signs or abnormalities on an intracranial MRI. However, FA presented only hyperfluorescence of the optic disc, without papillary filling deficiency or choroidal delay suggesting AION was negative. In addition, visual field test results provide the critical clue of the diagnosis. It is well known that central scotomas are highly characteristic of ON, while an inferior altitudinal defect along the horizontal meridian, particularly in the nasal periphery, is characteristic of AION [26]. Although a worse visual outcome in this case is also differentiating features of NA-AION, eye movement pain, FA findings, and central scotomas without the horizontal meridian led us to diagnose acute ON rather than NA-AION.

Hypotheses indicating a causal relationship between COVID-19 vaccination and ON are yet to be proved, but the close temporal association between symptom onset and vaccination strongly supports that possibility. BNT162b2 is a nucleoside-modified mRNA vaccine, which is translated into the SARS-CoV-2 spike protein by the host's ribosomes, followed by antigen processing and presentation to local immune cells for subsequent neutralizing antibody production and T-cell-mediated immune response [27]. Since there have also been several reports regarding optic neuritis developed after SARS-CoV-2 infection, we speculate that adverse events after receiving the COVID-19 vaccine are probably attributed to the adaptive immune response evoked by the vaccination, and/or the spike protein itself.

The autoimmune mechanism evoked by molecular mimicry of viral proteins and the immunological involvement of adjuvants have been suggested to underlie the development of ON following COVID-19 vaccination [7,28]. Visual prognosis of ON associated with RRMS or idiopathic ON with autoimmune nature is generally favorable by high-dose pulse steroid therapy. The reasons for the inadequate recovery of visual function in this case are speculated to be the avoidance of methylprednisolone pulse administration due to the patient's advanced age and the impairment of tissue repair associated with aging.

In conclusion, we encountered a case of unilateral atypical ON occurring after the second BNT162b2 mRNA-based COVID-19 vaccination. Warnings should be given to ophthalmologists and physicians about the risk of atypical optic neuritis after COVID-19 vaccination.

Author Contributions: Conception, T.K. and M.T.; Design, M.T.; Acquisition, S.M. and T.K.; Analysis, S.M. and T.K.; Data interpretation, S.M., T.K., and M.T.; Writing—original draft preparation, S.M. and M.T.; Writing—review and editing, S.M. and M.T. All authors have read and agreed to the published version of the manuscript. All authors have agreed to be both personally accountable for their own contributions and ensure that questions related to the accuracy or integrity of any part of the manuscript are answered.

Funding: The authors received no specific funding for this work.

Institutional Review Board Statement: Ethics approval was not applicable. The authors declare that they adhered to the CARE guidelines/methodology.

Informed Consent Statement: Written informed consent was obtained from the patient for publication of this case report and any accompanying images. A copy of the written consent is available for review by the editor of this journal.

Data Availability Statement: Not applicable.

Acknowledgments: The authors thank Eiko Machida, Kiyoko Yamada, Tomomi Nakamura, and Saeko Kanno for their contribution to the present report.

Conflicts of Interest: The authors declare no conflict of interest.

References

1. Chen, S.; Fan, X.R.; He, S.; Zhang, J.W.; Li, S.J. Watch out for neuromyelitis optica spectrum disorder after inactivated virus vaccination for COVID-19. *Neurol. Sci* **2021**, *42*, 3537–3539. [CrossRef] [PubMed]
2. Ozgen Kenangil, G.; Ari, B.C.; Guler, C.; Demir, M.K. Acute disseminated encephalomyelitis-like presentation after an inactivated coronavirus vaccine. *Acta Neurol. Belg.* **2021**, *121*, 1089–1091. [CrossRef] [PubMed]
3. Román, G.C.; Gracia, F.; Torres, A.; Palacios, A.; Gracia, K.; Harris, D. Acute Transverse Myelitis (ATM):Clinical Review of 43 Patients With COVID-19-Associated ATM and 3 Post-Vaccination ATM Serious Adverse Events With the ChAdOx1 nCoV-19 Vaccine (AZD1222). *Front. Immunol.* **2021**, *12*, 653786. [CrossRef] [PubMed]
4. Pagenkopf, C.; Südmeyer, M. A case of longitudinally extensive transverse myelitis following vaccination against Covid-19. *J. Neuroimmunol.* **2021**, *358*, 577606. [CrossRef]
5. Ismail, I.I.; Salama, S. A systematic review of cases of CNS demyelination following COVID-19 vaccination. *J. Neuroimmunol.* **2022**, *362*, 577765. [CrossRef]
6. Badrawi, N.; Kumar, N.; Albastaki, U. Post COVID-19 vaccination neuromyelitis optica spectrum disorder: Case report & MRI findings. *Radiol. Case Rep.* **2021**, *16*, 3864–3867. [CrossRef]
7. Khayat-Khoei, M.; Bhattacharyya, S.; Katz, J.; Harrison, D.; Tauhid, S.; Bruso, P.; Houtchens, M.K.; Edwards, K.R.; Bakshi, R. COVID-19 mRNA vaccination leading to CNS inflammation: A case series. *J. Neurol.* **2022**, *269*, 1093–1106. [CrossRef]
8. Yildiz Tasci, Y.; Nalcacoglu, P.; Gumusyayla, S.; Vural, G.; Toklu, Y.; Yesilirmak, N. Aquaporin-4 protein antibody-associated optic neuritis related to neuroendocrine tumor after receiving an inactive COVID-19 vaccine. *Indian J. Ophthalmol.* **2022**, *70*, 1828–1831. [CrossRef]
9. Shirah, B.; Mulla, I.; Aladdin, Y. Optic Neuritis Following the BNT162b2 mRNA COVID-19 Vaccine in a Patient with Systemic Lupus Erythematosus Uncovering the Diagnosis of Neuromyelitis Optica Spectrum Disorders. *Ocul. Immunol. Inflamm.* **2022**, *18*, 1–3. [CrossRef]
10. Nagaratnam, S.A.; Ferdi, A.C.; Leaney, J.; Lee, R.L.K.; Hwang, Y.T.; Heard, R. Acute disseminated encephalomyelitis with bilateral optic neuritis following ChAdOx1 COVID-19 vaccination. *BMC Neurol.* **2022**, *22*, 54. [CrossRef]
11. Elnahry, A.G.; Asal, Z.B.; Shaikh, N.; Dennett, K.; Abd Elmohsen, M.N.; Elnahry, G.A.; Shehab, A.; Vytopil, M.; Ghaffari, L.; Athappilly, G.K.; et al. Optic neuropathy after COVID-19 vaccination: A report of two cases. *Int. J. Neurosci.* **2021**, 1–7. [CrossRef] [PubMed]
12. Wang, J.; Huang, S.; Yu, Z.; Zhang, S.; Hou, G.; Xu, S. Unilateral optic neuritis after vaccination against the coronavirus disease: Two case reports. *Doc. Ophthalmol.* **2022**, *145*, 65–70. [CrossRef] [PubMed]
13. Roy, M.; Chandra, A.; Roy, S.; Shrotriya, C. Optic neuritis following COVID-19 vaccination: Coincidence or side-effect?—A case series. *Indian J. Ophthalmol.* **2022**, *70*, 679–683. [CrossRef] [PubMed]
14. Arnao, V.; Maimone, M.B.; Perini, V.; Giudice, G.L.; Cottone, S. Bilateral optic neuritis after COVID vaccination. *Neurol. Sci.* **2022**, *43*, 2965–2966. [CrossRef]
15. Garcia-Estrada, C.; Gomez-Figueroa, E.; Alban, L.; Arias-Cardenas, A. Optic neuritis after COVID-19 vaccine application. *Clin. Exp. Neuroimmunol.* **2022**, *13*, 72–74. [CrossRef]
16. Leber, H.M.; Sant'Ana, L.; Konichi da Silva, N.R.; Raio, M.C.; Mazzeo, T.; Endo, C.M.; Nascimento, H.; de Souza, C.E. Acute Thyroiditis and Bilateral Optic Neuritis following SARS-CoV-2 Vaccination with CoronaVac: A Case Report. *Ocul. Immunol. Inflamm.* **2021**, *29*, 1200–1206. [CrossRef]
17. Tsukii, R.; Kasuya, Y.; Makino, S. Nonarteritic Anterior Ischemic Optic Neuropathy following COVID-19 Vaccination: Consequence or Coincidence. *Case Rep. Ophthalmol. Med.* **2021**, *2021*, 5126254. [CrossRef]
18. Lin, W.Y.; Wang, J.J.; Lai, C.H. Non-Arteritic Anterior Ischemic Optic Neuropathy Following COVID-19 Vaccination. *Vaccines (Basel)* **2022**, *10*, 931. [CrossRef]
19. Elhusseiny, A.M.; Sanders, R.N.; Siddiqui, M.Z.; Sallam, A.B. Non-arteritic Anterior Ischemic Optic Neuropathy with Macular Star following COVID-19 Vaccination. *Ocul. Immunol. Inflamm.* **2022**, 1–4. [CrossRef] [PubMed]
20. Valsero Franco, S.; Fonollosa, A. Ischemic Optic Neuropathy After Administration of a SARS-CoV-2 Vaccine: A Report of 2 Cases. *Am. J. Case Rep.* **2022**, *23*, e935095. [CrossRef]
21. Murgova, S.; Balchev, G. Ophthalmic manifestation after SARS-CoV-2 vaccination: A case series. *J. Ophthalmic Inflamm. Infect* **2022**, *12*, 20. [CrossRef] [PubMed]
22. Chung, S.A.; Yeo, S.; Sohn, S.Y. Nonarteritic Anterior Ischemic Optic Neuropathy Following COVID-19 Vaccination: A Case Report. *Korean J. Ophthalmol.* **2022**, *36*, 168–170. [CrossRef]
23. Caliskan, I.; Bulus, E.; Afsar, N.; Altintas, A. A Case With New-Onset Neuromyelitis Optica Spectrum Disorder Following COVID-19 mRNA BNT162b2 Vaccination. *Neurologist* **2022**, *27*, 147–150. [CrossRef] [PubMed]
24. Sanjay, S.; Acharya, I.; Rawoof, A.; Shetty, R. Non-arteritic anterior ischaemic optic neuropathy (NA-AION) and COVID-19 vaccination. *BMJ Case Rep. CP* **2022**, *15*, e248415. [CrossRef] [PubMed]
25. Lotan, I.; Lydston, M.; Levy, M. Neuro-Ophthalmological Complications of the COVID-19 Vaccines: A Systematic Review. *J. Neuroophthalmol.* **2022**, *42*, 154–162. [CrossRef]
26. Gerling, J.; Meyer, J.H.; Kommerell, G. Visual field defects in optic neuritis and anterior ischemic optic neuropathy: Distinctive features. *Graefes Arch. Clin. Exp. Ophthalmol.* **1998**, *236*, 188–192. [CrossRef]

27. Polack, F.P.; Thomas, S.J.; Kitchin, N.; Absalon, J.; Gurtman, A.; Lockhart, S.; Perez, J.L.; Perez Marc, G.; Moreira, E.D.; Zerbini, C.; et al. Safety and Efficacy of the BNT162b2 mRNA Covid-19 Vaccine. *N. Engl. J. Med.* **2020**, *383*, 2603–2615. [CrossRef]
28. Karussis, D.; Petrou, P. The spectrum of post-vaccination inflammatory CNS demyelinating syndromes. *Autoimmun. Rev.* **2014**, *13*, 215–224. [CrossRef]

MDPI
St. Alban-Anlage 66
4052 Basel
Switzerland
www.mdpi.com

Vaccines Editorial Office
E-mail: vaccines@mdpi.com
www.mdpi.com/journal/vaccines

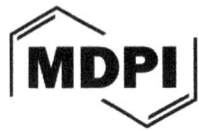

Disclaimer/Publisher's Note: The statements, opinions and data contained in all publications are solely those of the individual author(s) and contributor(s) and not of MDPI and/or the editor(s). MDPI and/or the editor(s) disclaim responsibility for any injury to people or property resulting from any ideas, methods, instructions or products referred to in the content.

www.ingramcontent.com/pod-product-compliance
Lightning Source LLC
LaVergne TN
LVHW070632100526
838202LV00012B/789